AF687140

A Clinician's Guide to Mood Disorders

A Clinician's Guide to Mood Disorders

Edited by Peter Garner

hayle
medical

New York

Hayle Medical,
750 Third Avenue, 9th Floor,
New York, NY 10017, USA

Visit us on the World Wide Web at:
www.haylemedical.com

© Hayle Medical, 2017

This book contains information obtained from authentic and highly regarded sources. Copyright for all individual chapters remain with the respective authors as indicated. All chapters are published with permission under the Creative Commons Attribution License or equivalent. A wide variety of references are listed. Permission and sources are indicated; for detailed attributions, please refer to the permissions page and list of contributors. Reasonable efforts have been made to publish reliable data and information, but the authors, editors and publisher cannot assume any responsibility for the validity of all materials or the consequences of their use.

ISBN: 978-1-63241-458-8

The publisher's policy is to use permanent paper from mills that operate a sustainable forestry policy. Furthermore, the publisher ensures that the text paper and cover boards used have met acceptable environmental accreditation standards.

Trademark Notice: Registered trademark of products or corporate names are used only for explanation and identification without intent to infringe.

Printed in the United States of America.

Cataloging-in-Publication Data

A clinician's guide to mood disorders / edited by Peter Garner.
p. cm.
Includes bibliographical references and index.
ISBN 978-1-63241-458-8
1. Affective disorders. 2. Psychology, Pathological. 3. Depression, Mental. I. Garner, Peter.
RC537 .C55 2017
616.852 7--dc23

Table of Contents

Preface

The main aim of this book is to educate learners and enhance their research focus by presenting diverse topics covering this vast field. This is an advanced book which compiles significant studies by distinguished experts. This book addresses successive solutions to the challenges arising in the area of application, along with it; the book provides scope for future developments.

Mood disorders encompass a wide array of mood issues, such as major depressive disorder, dysthymic disorder, bipolar disorder, etc. This book is a valuable compilation of topics, ranging from the basic to the most complex advancements in the field of mood disorders. This text will prove helpful for researchers and psychiatrists working in this field as it presents the varied dimensions of this disorder. This book sheds light on the various causes and treatments of mood disorder through the extensive use of examples and case studies. It is an invaluable source of knowledge for those interested in this field of study. The readers would gain knowledge that would broaden their perspective about mood disorders.

It was a great honour to edit this book, though there were challenges, as it involved a lot of communication and networking between me and the editorial team. However, the end result was this all-inclusive book covering diverse themes in the field.

Finally, it is important to acknowledge the efforts of the contributors for their excellent chapters, through which a wide variety of issues have been addressed. I would also like to thank my colleagues for their valuable feedback during the making of this book.

Editor

1

Caveats of chronic exogenous corticosterone treatments in adolescent rats and effects on anxiety-like and depressive behavior and hypothalamic-pituitary-adrenal (HPA) axis function

Patti Waters and Cheryl M McCormick*

Abstract

Background: Administration of exogenous corticosterone is an effective preclinical model of depression, but its use has involved primarily adult rodents. Using two different procedures of administration drawn from the literature, we explored the possibility of exogenous corticosterone models in adolescence, a time of heightened risk for mood disorders in humans.

Methods: In experiment 1, rats were injected with 40 mg/kg corticosterone or vehicle from postnatal days 30 to 45 and compared with no injection controls on behavior in the elevated plus maze (EPM) and the forced swim test (FST). Experiment 2 consisted of three treatments administered to rats from postnatal days 30 to 45 or as adults (days 70 to 85): either corticosterone (400 μg/ml) administered in the drinking water along with 2.5% ethanol, 2.5% ethanol or water only. In addition to testing on EPM, blood samples after the FST were obtained to measure plasma corticosterone. Analysis of variance (ANOVA) and alpha level of $P < 0.05$ were used to determine statistical significance.

Results: In experiment 1, corticosterone treatment of adolescent rats increased anxiety in the EPM and decreased immobility in the FST compared to no injection control rats. However, vehicle injected rats were similar to corticosterone injected rats, suggesting that adolescent rats may be highly vulnerable to stress of injection. In experiment 2, the intake of treated water, and thus doses delivered, differed for adolescents and adults, but there were no effects of treatment on behavior in the EPM or FST. Rats that had ingested corticosterone had reduced corticosterone release after the FST. Ethanol vehicle also affected corticosterone release compared to those ingesting water only, but differently for adolescents than for adults.

Conclusions: The results indicate that several challenges must be overcome before the exogenous corticosterone model can be used effectively in adolescents.

Background

The World Health Organization has found mood disorders such as anxiety and depression to be a major contributor to disability and loss of years of health in women and in men [1]. Stressful experiences are implicated in the pathogenesis of mood disorders, and dysregulation of the hypothalamic-pituitary-adrenal (HPA) axis is a key feature of depression in particular (reviewed in [2-6]). Clinical research indicates that adolescence is a time of increased risk for mood disorders (reviewed in [7,8]). Changes in the reactivity of the stress systems during times of biological transitions, such as those occurring in the nervous system and gonadal systems during adolescence, are proposed to underlie the increased vulnerability [9].

The use of animal models, though not without limitations, is recognized as an important approach to understanding mood disorders [10,11]. Animal models of depression based on environmental stress (repeated

* Correspondence: cmccormick@brocku.ca
Department of Psychology and Centre for Neuroscience, Brock University, St Catharines, Ontario, Canada

stress exposures administered by the experimenter) have high face and construct validity [12]. Until recently, however, the focus has been on stressors in perinatal life or in adulthood rather than in adolescence [13]. Limitations of many animal models of environmental stress include the lack of control over individual differences and variation in procedures from laboratory to laboratory, which lead to inconsistencies in the literature (reviewed in [14,15]). These limitations may be especially relevant in investigations of adolescent rats, given the sensitivity of gonadal maturation to environmental factors, the ongoing development of the HPA axis, and the relatively short time frame in which adolescent development occurs [13]. One classification system for adolescence (a transitional period with no clear 'onset' or 'offset') involves three stages, a prepubescence/early adolescence period from postnatal days 21 (when rats are typically weaned in the laboratory) to 34, a mid-adolescence period from postnatal days 34 to 46 (time in which most rats first exhibit the physical markers of puberty, such as vaginal opening and balanopreputial separation), and a late adolescence period from postnatal days 46 to 59 [16-18].

The effects of chronic or repeated stress in humans and in animal models are mediated primarily by the prolonged elevations of glucocorticoids (cortisol in humans, corticosterone in rodents) that are the endpoint of activation of the HPA axis [19,20]. Thus, repeated administration of exogenous corticosterone has been proposed as an effective means of circumventing some of the limitations of animal models of chronic stress exposures (reviewed in [14]). Although there is much evidence to indicate that repeated treatment with corticosterone produces reliable changes in a variety of depressive-like behaviors (reviewed in [14]), this approach has yet to be explored in adolescence. One exception is a study of a low dose of corticosterone (20 mg/ml) administered in the drinking water for 2 months (early adolescence into adulthood), which was found to decrease depression-like behavior in male mice [21]. Thus, more studies are required to assess the use of exogenous corticosterone as an animal model using higher doses and within a timeframe limited to adolescence.

Our laboratory has used a social instability stress model in rats to investigate the consequences of exposure to stressors in mid-adolescence (daily 1 h isolation and change of cage partner from postnatal days 30 to 45) (reviewed in [22]). Although social instability stress in adolescence produces lasting changes in neurogenesis and decrements in performance of hippocampal-dependent tasks (for example, [23,24]), effects on anxiety-like and depressive behavior have been modest [25,26], perhaps because of habituation of corticosterone release to the repeated stress procedures in male rats [27]. Thus, in the present experiments, we investigated the effects of repeated administration of exogenous corticosterone over the same timeframe as our adolescent social instability procedure on anxiety-like and depressive behavior. In experiment 1, we used a 40 mg/kg injection of corticosterone and in experiment 2 we used a 400 mg/ml dose administered in the drinking water; both doses and administration procedures have been used extensively with adult rats (for example, injection [28-30] and in water [31-33]). Vehicle and no treatment controls were included in both experiments, and an adult treatment comparison group was included in experiment 2. In both experiments, 24 h after the last treatment day, anxiety-like behavior was evaluated using the elevated plus maze and after another 24 h, depressive behavior was evaluated using the forced swim test, both well validated measures (reviewed in [34,35]). In experiment 2, blood samples were obtained at timepoints after the end of the forced swim test to evaluate treatment effects on stress-induced corticosterone release. The aim of the experiments was to assess the potential of exogenous corticosterone as a model for adolescent mood disorders. The main hypothesis of both experiments was that chronic treatment with exogenous corticosterone in adolescence would increase anxiety-like and depressive behavior in rats.

Methods

Experiment 1

Animals

Male Long-Evans rats (n = 24) were obtained from Charles River (St Constant, Quebec, Canada) at 22 days of age. Rats were housed in pairs in polycarbonate cages and were provided with a plastic tube in each cage for enrichment throughout the experiment. Rats were identified by tail coloring with a felt tip marker. The rats were kept on a 12 h light, 12 h dark light cycle, and were given unlimited access to rat chow and water. All experimental procedures were consistent with National Institutes of Health Guide for Care and Use of Laboratory Animals (Publication No. 85-23, revised 1985), and Canadian Council on Animal Care guidelines and were approved by the Brock University Institutional Animal Care and Use Committee.

Treatment

Starting on postnatal day 30, rats were randomly assigned to one of three treatment conditions. The CORT group (n = 8) was given a daily injection subcutaneously for 16 days of 40 mg/kg/ml corticosterone (Steraloids, Newport, RI, USA) (procedure as in [36,37]) suspended in isotonic saline and 2% Tween 80 (Sigma-Aldrich, St Louis, MO, USA). The VEHIC group (n = 8) was injected daily with vehicle for 16 days. After injection, the rat was returned to the home cage, and each pair of rats that shared a cage was administered the same treatment. Previous research has found this dose of corticosterone injection to produce plasma corticosterone levels of approximately 2,100 ng/ml 1-4 h after the injection [37]. The rats were weighed once every 3 days, and the injection volume was adjusted accordingly. The NO-INJ (no injection, n = 8) control group was not disturbed except for cage maintenance and was weighed only on postnatal days 30 and 45 (first and last injection days). Rats were tested in the elevated plus maze on postnatal day 46 and in the forced swim test on postnatal day 47.

Elevated plus maze

The elevated plus maze (EPM), first described by Pellow and colleagues [38], is a well validated measure of anxiety in rodents [34]. The EPM relies on conflict between the propensity of rodents to explore novel territory and their fear of open and elevated areas. The EPM consisted of four arms 50 cm in length, and walls enclosing two arms (closed arms) 42 cm in height constructed out of grey painted plywood. The sides of the open arms had 1.3 cm high ledges. The maze was raised 79 cm off the ground and was kept in a separate room from the colony. During testing, the maze was illuminated with dim white light and white noise (approximately 60 dB) was played. Each rat was placed in the closed arm at the end farthest from the center and was allowed to explore the maze for 5 min. All sessions were videotaped, and tapes were later scored while blind to treatment condition. Tapes were scored for time spent in the open arm (with more time on the open arm, higher percent time on open arm, and higher percentage of open arm entries all indicative of less anxiety) and center hub as well as the total number of entries into closed arms (used as an index of locomotor activity), rears (when the rat stands on its hind legs) and head dips (when the rat reaches its head over the edge of the open arm). Rears and dips are considered measures of exploratory behavior that are exhibited more when less anxious.

Forced swim test

The forced swim test (FST) is a measure of behavioral despair (for example, [39]) and consisted of a clear cylinder 20.3 cm in diameter filled 24.1 cm high with water such that a rat was unable to touch the bottom or climb over the side. The water was warmed to 26°C, and it was changed for each rat. Rats were placed in the water and left in the tank for 15 min in experiment 1 and 20 min in experiment 2 (longer time in experiment 2 was used for maximal corticosterone release). All sessions were videotaped, and tapes were later scored while blind to treatment condition. Behavioral measures for analysis were derived from the literature (for example, [40,41]) and included the following four behaviors: swimming (quick movements of forelimbs and/or hindlimbs, including swimming in circles and pedaling), climbing (in a vertical position, pawing at the side of the cylinder with front paws and leveraging the body slightly out of the water), diving (head under water, swimming to the bottom of cylinder, including circling at the bottom) and immobility (reduced movement including floating and slow circling or pedaling). Diving occurred with very low frequency, and was thus not included in statistical analyses. Climbing reflects the most vigorous attempt at escape whereas immobility is the measure considered to represent depressive-like behavior.

Classically the FST is administered in two sessions that are 24 h apart, with latency to immobility and time spent immobile measured in the second session and the first session considered the means to induce a depressive state (for example, [39]). However, stressors or chronic manipulations are found to produce depression-like states and thus differences among groups can be found in the first session (for example, [28,36,42]). Further, the effects of chronic corticosterone treatment for 21 days in adults were the same whether tested with a 1 day version of the test or a 2 day version [29]. Therefore, the experiments described here used a one-session test.

Experiment 2

Animals, treatment, and procedure

Male Long-Evans rats were obtained from Charles River at 22 days of age (n = 20) or at 64 days of age (n = 20) and were housed in age-matched pairs as in experiment 1. Starting on postnatal day 30 or 70, the drinking water was replaced for the CORT-ETOH rats (n = 8 per age group) with a solution of 400 μg/ml corticosterone (Steraloids) dissolved in 2.5% ethanol. To ensure that any effects observed were the result of corticosterone treatment and not ethanol exposure, a second group was given 2.5% ethanol to drink (ETOH rats, n = 6 per group). The WATER rats (n = 6 per group) continued to receive tap water. Each solution was colored with a different food coloring to be easily distinguished from one another. After 16 days, on postnatal day 46 or 86, treatment was removed and tap water was provided to all. During treatment, the mass of water consumed was measured every 2 days. Rats were weighed before and after the 16 days of treatment, but were not handled during the course of treatment, except for cage cleaning thrice weekly. Using weight at the start and end of treatment, the dose of ethanol and of corticosterone consumed by the pair of rats in a cage over a 2 day period was calculated. To calculate the doses of ethanol and corticosterone, the density of each solution was determined by weighing 1 ml of each solution, because consumption was measured in mass. Using the beginning and ending weights, the approximate weight on day 8 of treatment was extrapolated, and the ethanol and corticosterone doses for days 7 and 8 were calculated based on this weight. All rats in this experiment were tested on the EPM on either postnatal day 46 or 47 and on the FST on postnatal day 47 or 87 using the methods described for experiment 1.

Collection and measurement of plasma corticosterone

To determine the amount of corticosterone released after the FST, blood was collected by tail nick from each rat immediately, 45 min and 90 min after removal from the test. No baseline was obtained before the FST in order that behavior in the FST would not be affected by the blood sampling. Blood samples were centrifuged at 3,000 rpm and 4°C for 20 min. Plasma was collected and stored at -20°C until corticosterone was measured using enzyme-linked immunosorbent assay kits (Neogen, Lansing, MI, USA). Corticosterone was extracted from the samples using ethyl ether and the samples were reconstituted in a buffer provided in the kit. The assay was run entirely as specified in the instructions for the kit, except that the reconstituted samples were diluted twofold compared to the kit instructions in order for the stress levels of corticosterone to be readable within the standard curve. The minimum detection level for the assay is 1 μg per tube. The antiserum crossreacts with deoxycorticosterone (38%), and only slightly with cortisol (1.1%), testosterone (0.12%), and estradiol (<0.01%). The intra-assay and interassay reliabilities were both less than 10%.

Results and discussion

Experiment 1

Weight

There were no group differences in weight on postnatal day 30 ($F_{1,21}$ = 0.02, P = 0.93), but by postnatal day 45, corticosterone injected (CORT) rats weighed less than vehicle injected (VEHIC) and no injection (NO-INJ) rats ($F_{1,21}$ = 10.78, P = 0.001, see Figure 1). The finding of reduced weight gain of CORT rats is consistent with the evidence of reduced weight gain or weight loss after exogenous corticosterone treatment in adult rats (for example, [28,36]) and after chronic stressors in adolescent and in adult rats (for example, [43-45]).

EPM

Although vehicle injection had no effect on weight gain, both VEHIC and CORT treated rats had increased anxiety-like behavior compared to NO-INJ rats. NO-INJ rats spent more time on the open arm ($F_{1,21}$ = 7.96, P = 0.003, see Figure 2) than did VEHIC (P = 0.002) and CORT (P = 0.002) rats, which did not differ (P = 0.78). The same pattern of significant differences as time in the open arm were obtained for the percentage of time in the open arm using time in open and closed arms

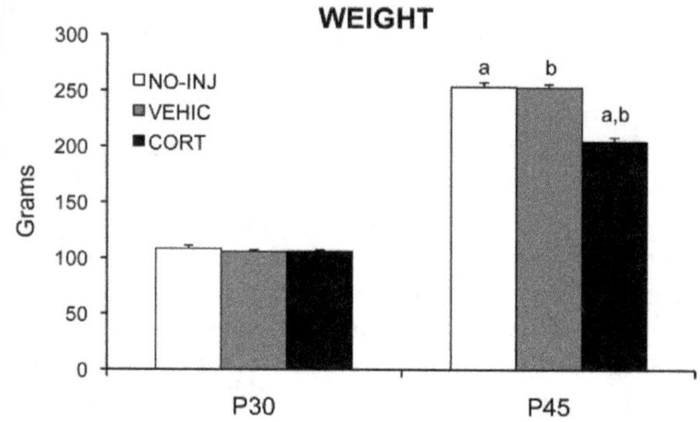

Figure 1 Mean (SEM) weight at postnatal day 30 (P30) and P45, the first and last day of treatment for the corticosterone injected (CORT), vehicle injected (VEHIC) and no injection (NO-INJ) groups. Matched letters indicate significant (P < 0.05) differences between groups.

without time in the hub as a denominator ($F_{1,21}$ = 7.96, P = 0.003, (mean, ± SEM) = VEHIC rats (6.4%, ± 2.6), CORT rats (7.6%, ± 1.6), and NO-INJ rats (23.7%, ± 5.0)). Differences were less marked using percentage of open arm entries relative to total arm entries as the index of anxiety ($F_{1,21}$ = 3.65, P = 0.045, with only VEHIC rats having a lower percentage of open arm entries (20.8%, ± 6.8) than NO-INJ rats (37.7%, ± 2.75), and neither group different from CORT rats (29.8%, ± 1.9)). NO-INJ rats reared and head dipped more than did VEHIC and CORT rats, which did not differ ($F_{1,21}$ = 32.45, P < 0.0001, $F_{1,21}$ = 10.41, P < 0.0001, $F_{1,21}$ = 4.76, P = 0.02, see Figure 2). The differences among the groups in time spent in the hub of the EPM and the number of closed arm entries were not significant ($F_{1,21}$ = 2.72, P = 0.09 and $F_{1,21}$ = 3.11, P = 0.07).

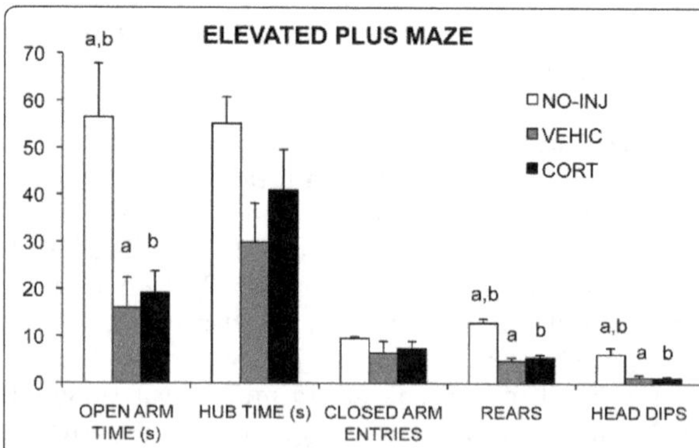

Figure 2 Mean (SEM) of the behavioral measures for the elevated plus maze (EPM) for corticosterone injected (CORT), vehicle injected (VEHIC) and no injection (NO-INJ) groups. Matched letters indicate significant (P < 0.05) differences between groups within each behavioral measure.

These results suggest that stress of injection is sufficient in adolescence to increase anxiety-like behavior. Although acute injections are known to be a mild stressor (for example, [46]), adult rodents readily habituate to repeated injections (for example, [47,48]). Further, in studies of adults, even when a higher number of injections were used than the 16 used here, differences are observed between vehicle-treated and corticosterone-treated groups [28,29,36,49]. Thus, adolescents may be more sensitive to injection stress than are adults.

FST

There was no main effect or interaction of group and time on climbing or immobility (all $P > 0.19$) (see Figure 3). The interaction of group and time on swimming approached significance ($F_{4,42} = 2.48$, $P = 0.06$). The three groups did not differ in latency to immobility ($P = 0.72$, data not shown). To explore the possibility that group differences were masked by low power by inclusion of several timepoints in the analysis (shorter times than 15 min have been used for analysis by others, for example [29]), a multivariate analysis of variance (MANOVA) was computed for climbing, immobility, and swimming, using only the first 5 min in the FST. The multivariate test of group was significant (Pillai's trace $F_{6,40} = 2.73$, $P = 0.025$), with significant between subject effects for immobility ($F_{2,21} = 4.32$, $P = 0.027$) and for swimming ($F_{2,21} = 6.78$, $P = 0.005$). Post hoc analyses indicated that CORT rats spent less time immobile and more time swimming than did NO-INJ rats and more time swimming than VEHIC rats (all $P < 0.05$) (see Figure 3).

Thus, the effects of treatment were limited to the first 5 min of the test and were in the opposite direction than predicted. The measure of depressive behavior in the FST is immobility, and thus CORT rats showed less depressive behavior than did NO-INJ rats. The VEHIC rats' behavior fell between that of the CORT and NO-INJ rats. An alternative explanation is that the increased swimming and decreased immobility of CORT rats is a reflection of their increased anxiety evident in the EPM. Anxiety symptoms are as common as depressed mood is among people meeting the criteria for major depressive disorder [50], and there is evidence that anxiety may be a precursor for the development of depression [51]. Nevertheless, there is increasing evidence of both shared and distinct neural mechanisms underlying anxiety and depressive behaviors (for example, [52]).

Others also have reported the apparent contradiction of increased anxiety and decreased depressive behaviors in animal models. For example, knockout (KO) mice for the 5-hydroxytryptamine $(5HT)_{1A}$ receptor also exhibited increased anxiety in an open field test and increased swimming and decreased immobility in the FST [53]. The authors interpreted the behavior in the FST as

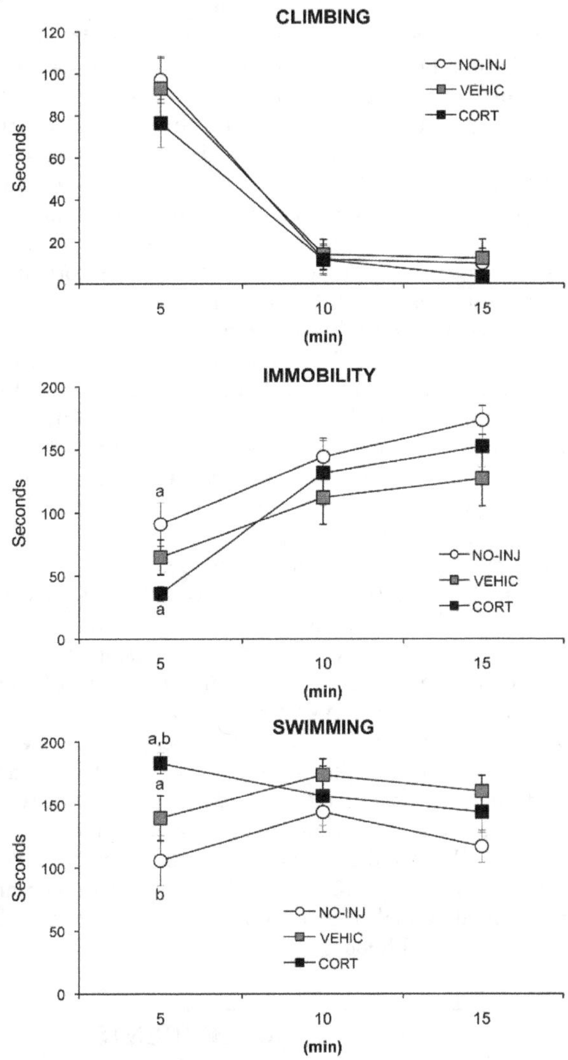

Figure 3 Mean (SEM) of the behavioral measures for the forced swim test (FST) for corticosterone injected (CORT), vehicle injected (VEHIC) and no injection (NO-INJ) groups. Matched letters indicate significant ($P < 0.05$) differences between groups within each behavioral measure.

further evidence of increased anxiety and emotional reactivity rather than to decreased depression, and they suggested the differences in KO mice might involve increased serotonergic turnover. More recently, KO mice of the $5HT_{1A}$ autoreceptor had increased anxiety and did not differ from controls in the FST, whereas KO mice of the $5HT_{1A}$ heteroreceptor had increased immobility in the FST and did not differ in anxiety from controls [52]. In adults, chronic injection of corticosterone decreases neural responsiveness to serotonin (for example, [54]) and increases depressive behavior in the

FST (for example, [28,29,36]). One possibility for the difference in the results of the previous studies in adults whereby injection of corticosterone increased depressive behavior compared to our finding of reduced depressive behavior (or increased anxiety) for adolescents is that our study involved fewer injections than those in studies of adults (16 versus 21 injections). A stronger possibility is that the differences between the studies of adults and ours with adolescents are because of developmental differences in susceptibility to the effects of stress/corticosterone. Studies of adults have found more robust differences between vehicle injected and corticosterone injected groups, thus adults may be less susceptible to injection stress than are adolescents. The ongoing maturation of neural circuitry underlying emotional behavior, which is evident, for example, in the different responses of adolescent and adult rats to selective serotonin reuptake inhibitors (for example, [55]), may render the circuitry more vulnerable.

In experiment 2, we eliminated the possibility of stress of injection by administering corticosterone in the drinking water. The method, which involves dissolving corticosterone in ethanol, was based on established procedures that have effectively mimicked many of the effects of chronic stress in adult rats (for example, [31-33]). Because the comparable studies available were conducted only in adults, we were concerned that ethanol alone may have an effect in adolescents. Thus, two control groups were used, one group was given 2.5% ethanol to drink and the other was given water only. To better assess the specificity of effects to developmental stage, an additional three experimental groups received treatment in adulthood.

Experiment 2

Weight

There were no group differences in weight on postnatal day 30 ($F_{1,17} = 0.54$, $P = 0.93$), but by the 16th day of treatment on postnatal day 45, CORT-ETOH rats had gained less weight than ETOH and WATER rats, which did not differ ($F_{1,17} = 4.37$, $P = 0.029$, see Figure 4). There were no weight differences for the adult groups on the first day of treatment ($F_{1,17} = 2.84$, $P = 0.09$), but by the 16th day of treatment, CORT-ETOH rats had gained less weight than ETOH and WATER rats, which did not differ ($F_{1,17} = 13.85$, $P < 0.0001$, see Figure 4). Thus, the effects of corticosterone treatment in the drinking water were similar to the results in other studies (for example, [31,56]) and to the effect of corticosterone injection in experiment 1, and the effects were comparable for adolescents and adults. No effect of 2.5% ethanol was observed on weight.

Intake

Treatment altered the intake of the three groups differently for adolescents than for adults. For adolescents, there was an interaction of treatment day and group ($F_{2,14} = 3.25$, $P = 0.04$): The intake of CORT-ETOH rats was less than that of ETOH rats ($P = 0.01$) and less than that of WATER rats on day 16 of treatment ($P < 0.0001$) (see Figure 5a). For adults, although the intake of CORT-ETOH rats was less than that of the other groups, only the effect of treatment day was significant ($F_{2,14} = 6.42$, $P = 0.01$), whereby intake increased over days (see Figure 5b). Thus for adults, there seemed to be an immediate aversion to corticosterone that reduced intake throughout, whereas in adolescents, corticosterone did not reduce drinking initially. The reduced

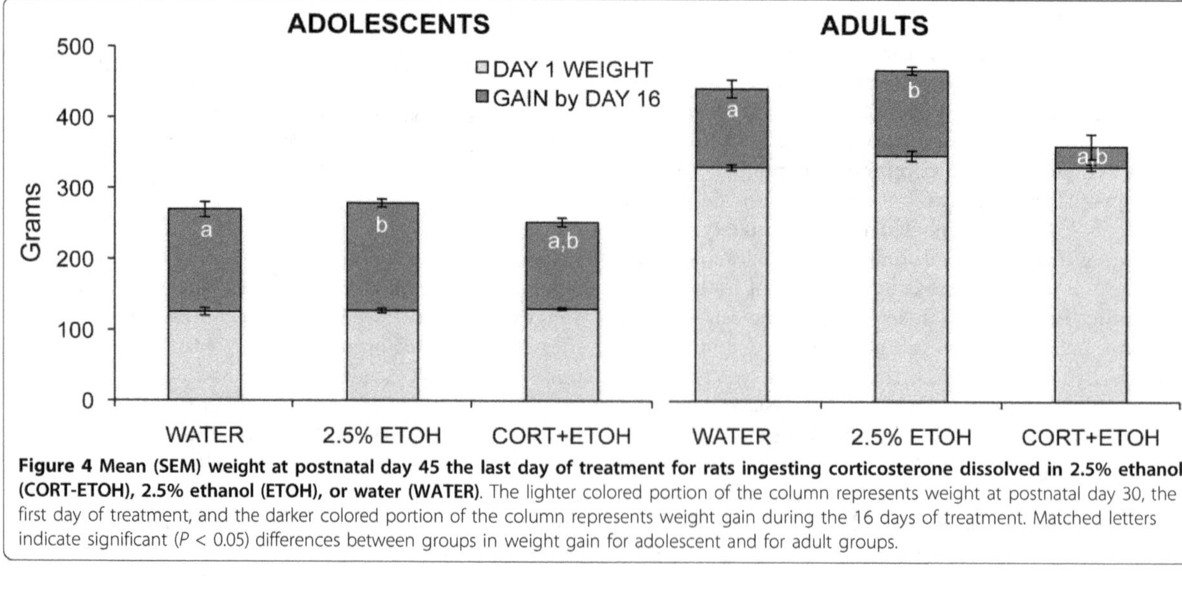

Figure 4 Mean (SEM) weight at postnatal day 45 the last day of treatment for rats ingesting corticosterone dissolved in 2.5% ethanol (CORT-ETOH), 2.5% ethanol (ETOH), or water (WATER). The lighter colored portion of the column represents weight at postnatal day 30, the first day of treatment, and the darker colored portion of the column represents weight gain during the 16 days of treatment. Matched letters indicate significant ($P < 0.05$) differences between groups in weight gain for adolescent and for adult groups.

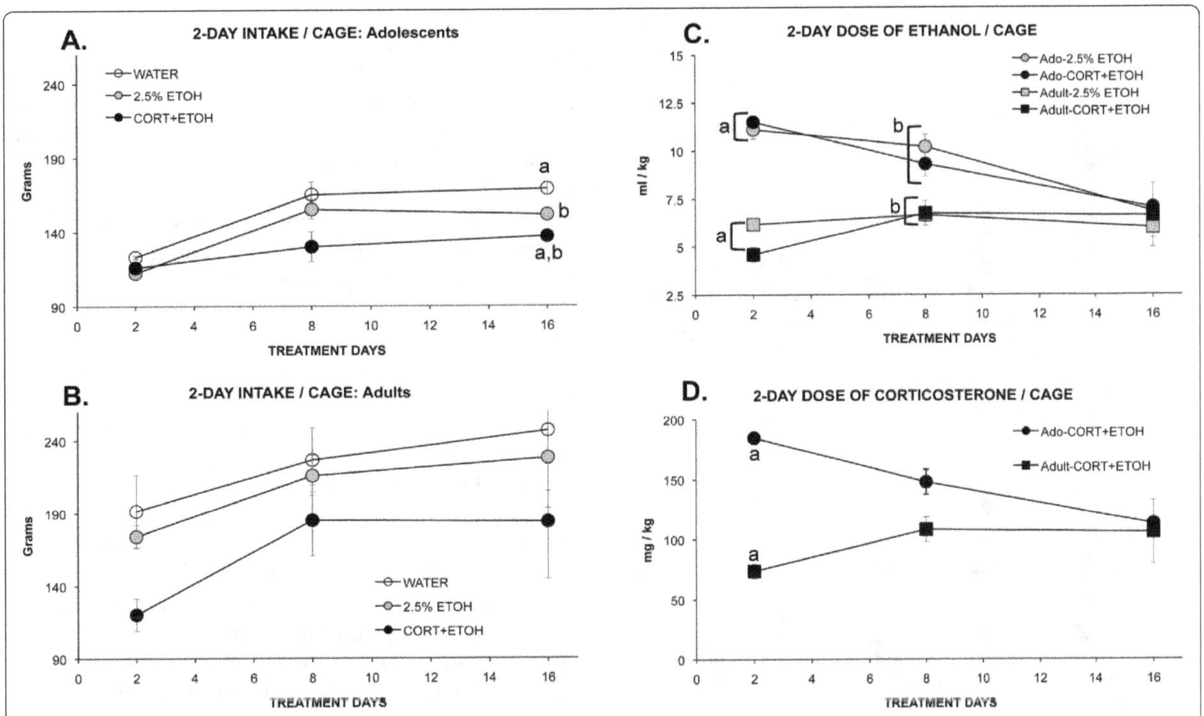

Figure 5 Mean (SEM) intake of fluid in grams in 2 days per pair of rats during 16 days of treatment for rats ingesting corticosterone dissolved in 2.5% ethanol (CORT-ETOH), 2.5% ethanol (ETOH), or water (WATER) as adolescents (a) or as adults (b). (c) Shows the dose of ethanol consumed by body weight and **(d)** provides the dose of corticosterone consumed by body weight. Matched letters indicate significant ($P < 0.05$) differences between groups on a treatment day. The main effect of treatment day was significant in (b), in (c) for adolescents only, and in (d) for both adolescents and adults, although in opposite directions (all $P < 0.05$).

drinking by day 16 of CORT-ETOH adolescent rats may be related to their reduced body weight or to an aversion that was slower to develop. For neither age group was the intake of rats drinking 2.5% ethanol different from those rats drinking water only.

The interaction of treatment day and age was significant for the dose of ethanol consumed (ml/kg) ($F_{2,14}$ = 15.99, $P < 0.0001$): For adolescents, the dose of ethanol consumed (ml/kg) decreased over treatment days ($F_{2,10}$ = 84.95, $P < 0.0001$) similarly for the CORT-ETOH and ETOH rats (see Figure 5c). For adults, there was no effect of, or interaction of, treatment day and group. The higher dose of ethanol ingested by adolescents than by adults was significant only at treatment day 2 and 8 (both $P < 0.0001$). The interaction of age × treatment day was significant for the dose of corticosterone (mg/kg) consumed by the CORT-ETOH groups ($F_{2,14}$ = 6.42, $P = 0.01$): For adolescents, the dose of corticosterone (mg/kg) consumed by the CORT-ETOH rats declined over time ($F_{2,6}$ = 309.3, $P < 0.0001$), and for adults ($F_{2,6}$ = 91.5, $P < 0.0001$), the dose of corticosterone (mg/kg) consumed increased over time (see Figure 5d). The higher dose of corticosterone ingested by adolescents than by adults was significant only at treatment day 2 ($P = 0.02$). These results highlight the difficulty in administering comparable dosages in drinking water to rats of different stages of development.

EPM and FST

There were no differences among the groups for any of the EPM measures for either adolescents (all $P > 0.32$) or adults (all $P > 0.13$). Adolescents spent less time in the center hub than did adults, but no other age difference was significant ($F_{1,34}$ = 4.26, $P = 0.047$) (see Figure 6). Although there was effect of time for the FST measures, with climbing and swimming decreasing and immobility increasing with time for both age groups (see Figure 7), the only effect of group was a group × time interaction ($F_{6,51}$ = 2.63, $P = 0.027$) for time spent climbing by adults. No group comparison, however, was significant at any timepoint.

There are several possibilities for the lack of an effect of corticosterone treatment on anxiety-like and depressive behavior when administered in the drinking water compared to when injected. One possibility is that we would have uncovered behavioral differences among the groups using a broader range of tests of anxiety-like and

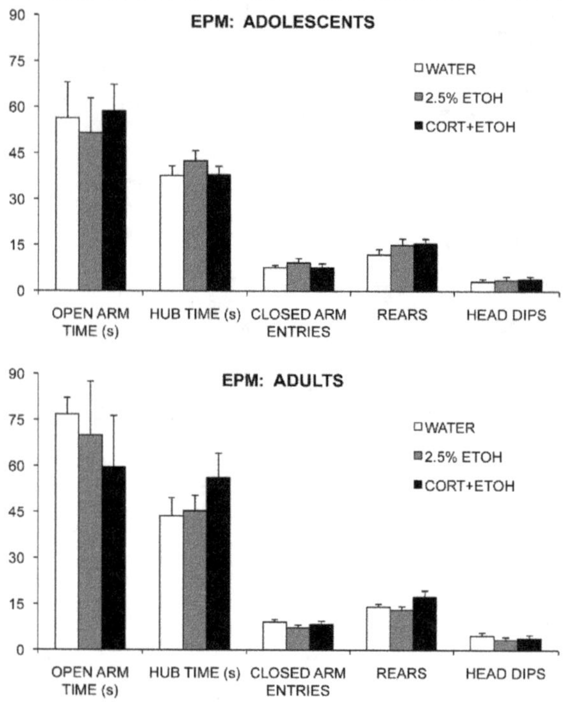

Figure 6 Mean (SEM) of the behavioral measures for the elevated plus maze (EPM) for rats ingesting corticosterone dissolved in 2.5% ethanol (CORT-ETOH), 2.5% ethanol (ETOH), or water (WATER) as adolescents (upper panel) or as adults (lower panel). Matched letters indicate significant ($P < 0.05$) differences between treatment groups for each behavioral measure within each age group.

depressive behavior. Another possibility is that, at least in adolescence, corticosterone is not as effective at altering emotional behavior in the absence of actual stressful experiences, such as injection. Of note, in experiment 1, the effect of injection of corticosterone on behavior was only marginally greater than that of injection of vehicle. Exogenous corticosterone and chronic stress do not always have the same effects when directly compared. Although both 21 days of 400 μg/ml corticosterone in drinking water and 21 days of chronic stress (restraint 6 h/day) caused retraction of hippocampal dendrites, only chronic stress impaired spatial memory [57], and the two manipulations differed in their effects on fear conditioning [33] and had the opposite effects on proteins involved in synaptic plasticity in the piriform cortex [58]. Whereas 21 days of injection of corticosterone decreased the number of cells expressing reelin in the hippocampus, 21 days of daily restraint did not [59]. Nevertheless, the differential effects of chronic stress versus exogenous administration of corticosterone do not explain the absence of an effect of corticosterone observed in experiment 2.

Another possibility is that 16 days is insufficient to have an effect with 400 μg/ml in the drinking water, especially when the pharmacokinetics of this method of delivery differs from a bolus injection, which is more similar to that produced by a bout of restraint. Consistent with the possibility that dose may be a factor is that injections of 10 mg/kg corticosterone in adult rats are sufficient to cause dendritic retraction in the hippocampus (for example, [60,61]) but higher doses are required to increase depressive behavior in the FST [28]. Lastly, the evidence for an effect of corticosterone delivered in the drinking water on anxiety and depressive behavior is not as substantial as it is for corticosterone delivered by injection. The available studies used mice rather than rats and lower doses (<50 μg/ml) and found reduced depressive behavior when provided for 1 to 4 days [62], increased depressive behavior when provided for 14 days and tested 2 weeks later [63], but did not affect depressive behavior in the FST when provided for 4 weeks [64]. Thus, given the advantages of administering corticosterone in the drinking water (for example, no handling or injection of the animals is involved), it would be worthwhile to test the effects of the 400 μg/ml dose provided over a longer time frame on behavior.

Plasma corticosterone

Baseline samples were not collected before the FST to prevent interference with subsequent behavior. Plasma concentrations of corticosterone obtained at timepoints after the FST indicated that both corticosterone treatment and the 2.5% ethanol vehicle altered HPA function. For adolescents, the interaction of sampling time and group was significant ($F_{4,34} = 5.73$, $P = 0.001$) (see Figure 8). At removal from the FST and 45 min later, CORT-ETOH rats had lower corticosterone concentrations than had WATER rats (both $P < 0.0001$). ETOH rats had lower corticosterone concentrations than had WATER rats only immediately after removal from the FST ($P = 0.001$). Group differences were not significant 90 min after the FST.

For adults, the interaction of sampling time and group was significant ($F_{4,34} = 16.55$, $P < 0.0001$) (see Figure 8). On removal from the FST and 45 min later, CORT-ETOH rats had lower corticosterone concentrations than had ETOH (both $P < 0.0001$) and WATER rats (both $P < 0.01$), and ETOH rats had higher corticosterone concentrations than had WATER rats (both $P < 0.05$). The groups did not differ 90 min after the FST.

Reduced adrenal function after lengthy exogenous treatment with high doses of corticosterone is a typical finding, because of the reduction in size of the adrenal gland caused by exogenous corticosterone, which is in contrast to the increase in size of the adrenal produced by chronic stress (for example, [28,31]). Thus, the lack of effect of treatment on behavior cannot be attributed

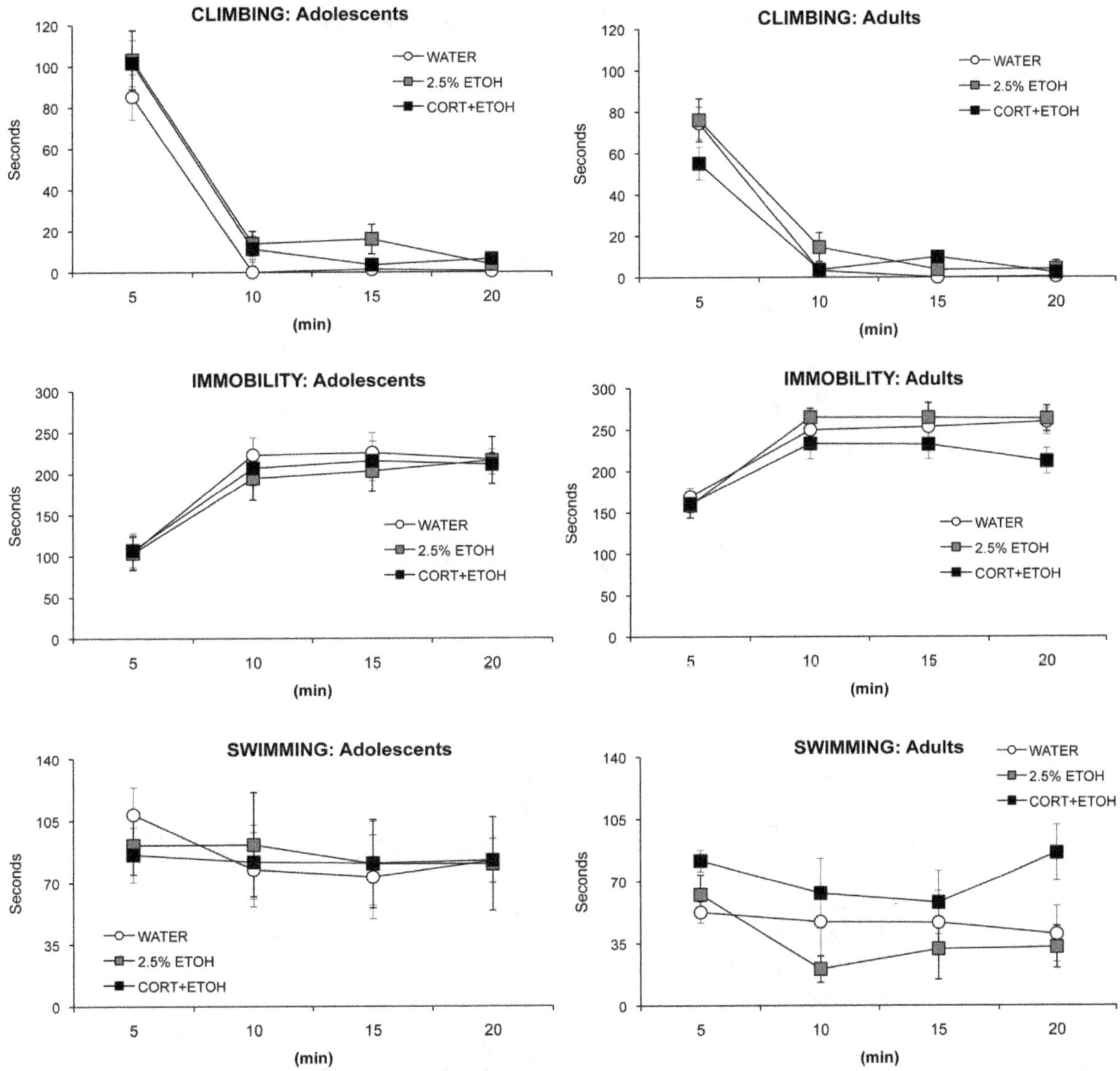

Figure 7 Mean (SEM) of the behavioral measures for the behavioral measures for the forced swim test (FST) for rats ingesting corticosterone dissolved in 2.5% ethanol (CORT-ETOH), 2.5% ethanol (ETOH), or water (WATER) as adolescents (left panels) or as adults (right panels).

to a lack of delivery of the treatment. The effect of 2.5% ethanol vehicle on corticosterone release was unexpected, as most studies of corticosterone in the drinking water have not included a 'no 2.5% ethanol' control group (for example, [33,56,58,65]). In adolescents, the low dose of ethanol in the drinking water reduced corticosterone release after the FST, but not to the same extent that corticosterone and ethanol combined did. In adults, ethanol prolonged corticosterone release after the FST. Whether the effect of ethanol involved effects on the adrenal gland or at a higher level of control of the HPA axis in either adolescents or adults is unknown. After acute or chronic ethanol exposure to adult rodents, usually heightened HPA function is reported, with changes evident at all levels of the HPA axis (such as increased adrenal weight/corticosterone content, higher expression of pituitary pro-opiomelanocortin (POMC) mRNA, of hypothalamic corticotropin-releasing hormone (CRH) mRNA) that are consistent with higher stress-induced corticosterone release (for

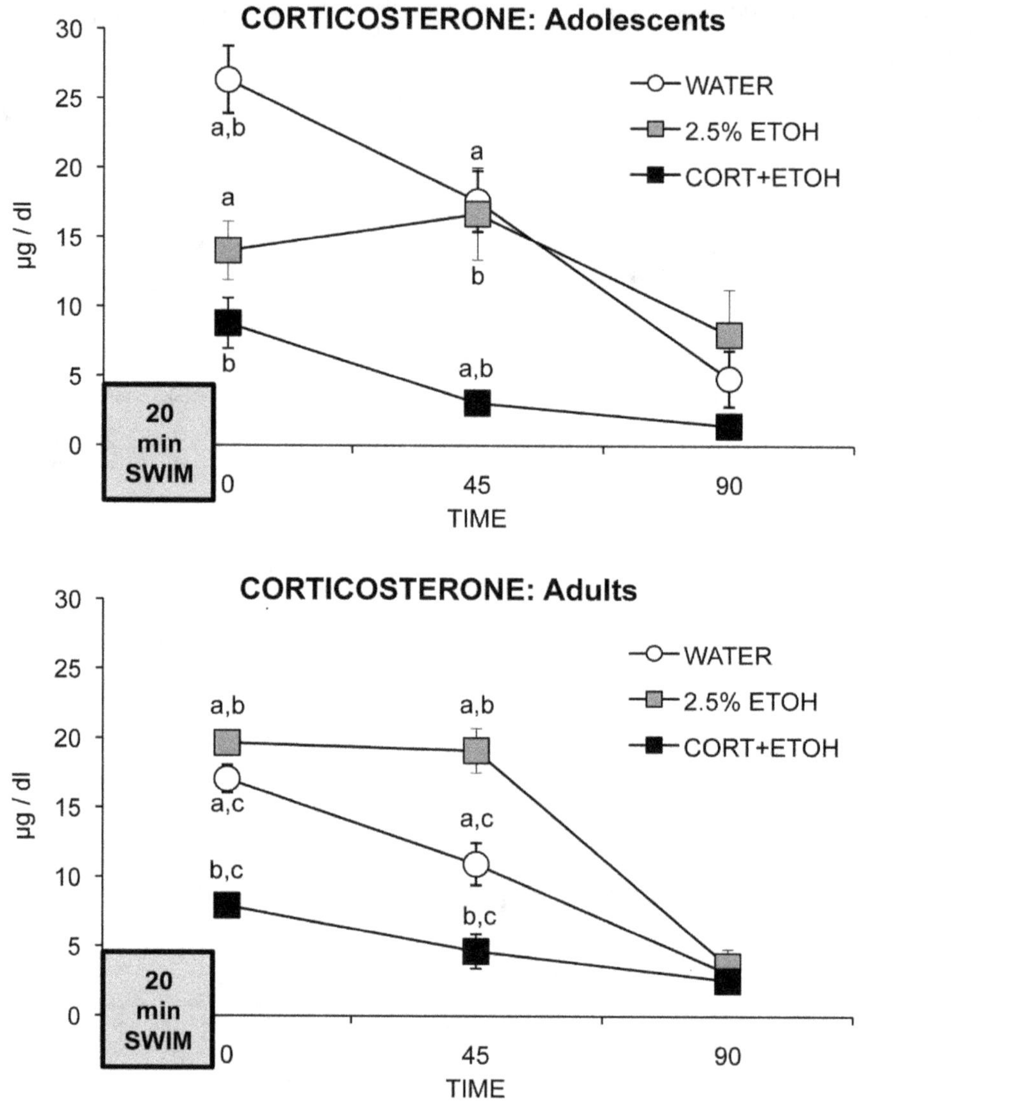

Figure 8 Mean (SEM) concentrations of corticosterone at timepoints after removal from the forced swim test (FST) for rats ingesting corticosterone dissolved in 2.5% ethanol (CORT-ETOH), 2.5% ethanol (ETOH), or water (WATER) as adolescents (upper panel) or as adults (lower panel). Matched letters indicate significant ($P < 0.05$) differences between treatment groups at a timepoint within each age group.

example, [66-70] although for evidence of dampened HPA function after alcohol exposure, see [71]).

The differences in the effects of ethanol in the two age groups may reflect differences in their developmental stage (for example, [72]) or that the dose of ethanol consumed was higher for adolescents than for adults. In adults, although activation of the HPA axis was found to a first dose of alcohol, self-administration or experimenter administration of alcohol was found to dampen HPA responses to subsequent stressors up to 24 days after removal of the alcohol (reviewed in [71]). One study of adolescent exposure to ethanol (alcohol vapors) found evidence of reduced HPA function when tested in adults [73]. In contrast, binge drinking (3 g/kg/day) beginning at postnatal day 37 increased the expression of secretagogues of ACTH in the paraventricular nucleus of the hypothalamus in adolescence [74]. Such studies, however, involved much higher doses than used here (for example, a bolus injection of 4.5 mg/kg to a rat is far more than the 200 mg/kg highest dose consumed by a pair of rats over a 48 h period in the present study). Nevertheless, the present results suggest that a no vehicle control group should be used in future studies using ethanol as a vehicle for corticosterone.

Conclusions

Administration of exogenous corticosterone has proven to be an effective preclinical model of depression in adult rodents to study the relationships among stress, glucocorticoids, and depression (reviewed in [14]). The findings of the present experiments suggest there are challenges to overcome in the use of exogenous corticosterone to investigate the heightened vulnerability of adolescents to stressors. First, the stress of injection masks potential effects of exogenous corticosterone in adolescents, whereas robust differences between vehicle-injected and corticosterone-injected subjects are found routinely in adults [14]. Second, corticosterone delivered in the drinking water does not allow for sufficient control of dosing for comparable treatment in adolescents and adults. Administration procedures that do not involve ethanol, such as the use of corticosterone hemisuccinate rather than corticosterone, are recommended, because even the low dose of ethanol used here affected corticosterone release in both adolescents and adults. Further, although the dose of corticosterone used (400 μg/ml) represents the high end of doses administered in such a way, 16 days of treatment did not produce effects on behavior in the EPM and the FST, although many studies have found chronic stress in adolescence to affect behavior in the EPM and the FST within shorter timeframes (reviewed in [13]). Thus, although this route of administration overcomes the problem of stress of injection, the more sustained pattern of corticosterone exposure through such oral administration may not allow for marked effects on mood-related behavior to be observed in rats. In sum, the present results highlight challenges to overcome in the use of exogenous corticosterone treatments in animal models to study sensitivity to stress and mood disorders in adolescence.

Clinicians have long recognized there are unique features to mood disorders in adolescence compared to in adulthood, irrespective of whether or not a mood disorder is the same fundamental disease at each age (for example, [75]). In humans, anxiety is primarily a disorder of childhood and adolescence, with anxiety in adults stemming from adolescence, and stress is a risk factor for anxiety in adolescence [76,77]. Immaturity of the relevant regulatory mechanisms in adolescence is thought to underlie the difference in performance on behavioral tests of anxiety of adolescent and adult rats [78,79]. In experiment 1, injected and corticosterone-treated adolescents had increased anxiety-like behavior compared to control rats, with little difference observed in depressive behavior. Similar treatments in adult rats found greater increases in depressive behavior than in anxiety [14]. These results suggest there are age differences in the behavioral expression of exposure to corticosterone that may parallel the developmental stage-specific manifestations of mood disorders in humans. In humans, the age of onset for depression is later than for anxiety, which also suggests that the maturation of relevant neural circuitries may determine which mood disorder or symptom is evident at each age. These points underscore the relevance of animal models for understanding the pathogenesis of mood disorders and the importance of investigating the range of developmental stages in both preclinical and clinical studies.

Acknowledgements

The research was completed in partial fulfillment of the requirements for the Master of Arts degree (PW). The research was supported by grants from the Natural Sciences and Engineering Research Council, the Canadian Foundation for Innovation, and the Ontario Innovation Trust (CMM). We thank Feather Nixon for assistance in data collection.

Authors' contributions

PW and CMM contributed equally to the design, analysis, and writing of the manuscript. PW implemented the research and collected the data. Both authors read and approved the final manuscript.

Authors' information

Patti Waters, MA, Department of Psychology, Brock University, 500 Glenridge Avenue, St Catharines, Ontario, L2S 3A1, Canada. Cheryl M McCormick, PhD, Canada Research Chair in Behavioural Neuroscience, Professor, Centre for Neuroscience and Department of Psychology, Brock University 500 Glenridge Avenue, St Catharines, Ontario, L2S 3A1, Canada.

Competing interests

The authors declare that they have no competing interests.

References

1. Mathers C, Fat G, Boema JT: *The Global Burden of Disease: 2004 Update* Geneva, Switzerland: World Health Organization; 2008.
2. Bao AM, Meynen G, Swaab DF: **The stress system in depression and neurodegeneration: focus on the human hypothalamus.** *Brain Res Rev* 2008, **57**:531-553.
3. Risch N, Herrell R, Lehner T, Liang KY, Eaves L, Hoh J, Griem A, Kovacs M, Ott J, Merikangas KR: **Interaction between the serotonin transporter gene (5-HTTLPR), stressful life events, and risk of depression: a meta-analysis.** *JAMA* 2009, **301**:2462-2471.
4. Wang J: **Work stress as a risk factor for major depressive episodes.** *Psychol Med* 2005, **35**:865-871.
5. Pariante CM, Lightman SL: **The HPA axis in major depression: classical theories and new developments.** *Trends Neurosci* 2008, **31**:464-468.
6. Kessler RC, McLaughlin KA, Green JG, Gruber MJ, Sampson NA, Zaslavsky AM, Aguilar-Gaxiola S, Alhamzawi AO, Alonso J, Angermeyer M, Benjet C, Bromet E, Chatterji S, de Girolamo G, Demyttenaere K, Fayyad J, Florescu S, Gal G, Gureje O, Haro JM, Hu CY, Karam EG, Kawakami N, Lee S, Lépine JP, Ormel J, Posada-Villa J, Sagar R, Tsang A, Ustün TB, Vassilev S, Viana MC, Williams DR: **Childhood adversities and adult psychopathology in the WHO World Mental Health Surveys.** *Br J Psychiatry* 2010, **197**:378-385.
7. Reardon LE, Leen-Feldner EW, Hayward C: **A critical review of the empirical literature on the relation between anxiety and puberty.** *Clin Psychol Rev* 2009, **29**:1-23.

8. Grant KE, Compas BE, Stuhlmacher AF, Thurm AE, McMahon SD, Halpert JA: **Stressors and child and adolescent psychopathology: moving from markers to mechanisms of risk.** *Psychol Bull* 2003, **129**:447-466.
9. Dorn LD, Chrousos GP: **The neurobiology of stress: understanding regulation of affect during female biological transitions.** *Sem Reprod Endocrinol* 1997, **15**:19-35.
10. Anisman H, Matheson K: **Stress, depression, and anhedonia: caveats concerning animal models.** *Neurosci Biobehav Rev* 2005, **29**:525-546.
11. Cryan JF, Slattery DA: **Animal models of mood disorders: recent developments.** *Curr Opin Psychiatr* 2007, **20**:1-7.
12. McArthur R, Borsini F: **Animal models of depression in drug discovery: A historical perspective.** *Pharmacol Biochem Behav* 2006, **84**:436-452.
13. McCormick CM, Mathews IZ, Thomas C, Waters P: **Investigations of HPA function and the enduring consequences of stressors in adolescence in animal models.** *Brain Cog* 2010, **72**:73-85.
14. Sterner EY, Kalynchuk LE: **Behavioral and neurobiological consequences of prolonged glucocorticoid exposure in rats: relevance to depression.** *Prog Neuropsychopharm Biol Psychiatry* 2010, **34**:777-790.
15. Willner P: **Chronic mild stress (CMS) revisited: consistency and behavioural-neurobiological concordance in the effects of CMS.** *Neuropsychobiology* 2005, **52**:90-110.
16. Tirelli E, Laviola G, Adriani W: **Ontogenesis of behavioral sensitization and conditioned place preference induced by psychostimulants in laboratory rodents.** *Neurosci Biobehav Rev* 2003, **27**:163-178.
17. Spear LP: **The adolescent brain and age-related behavioral manifestations.** *Neurosci Biobehav Rev* 2000, **24**:417-463.
18. McCormick CM, Mathews IZ: **Adolescent development, hypothalamic-pituitary-adrenal function, and programming of adult learning and memory.** *Prog Neuropsychopharm Biol Psychiatry* 2010, **34**:756-765.
19. Brown E: **Effects of glucocorticoids on mood, memory, and the hippocampus. Treatment and preventive therapy.** *Ann NY Acad Sci* 2009, **1179**:41-55.
20. Tata DA, Anderson BJ: **The effects of chronic glucocorticoid exposure on dendritic length, synapse numbers and glial volume in animal models: implications for hippocampal volume reductions in depression.** *Physiol Behav* 2010, **99**:186-193.
21. Xu Z, Zhang Y, Hou B, Gao Y, Wu Y, Zhang C: **Chronic corticosterone administration from adolescence through early adulthood attenuates depression-like behaviors in mice.** *J Affect Disord* 2011, **131**:128-135.
22. McCormick CM: **An animal model of social instability stress in adolescence and risk for drugs of abuse.** *Physiol Behav* 2010, **99**:194-203.
23. Morrissey MD, Mathews IZ, McCormick CM: **Enduring deficits in contextual and auditory fear conditioning after adolescent, not adult, social instability stress in male rats.** *Neurobiol Learn Mem* 2011, **95**:46-56.
24. McCormick CM, Nixon F, Thomas C, Lowie B, Dyck J: **Hippocampal cell proliferation and spatial memory performance after social instability stress in adolescence in female rats.** *Behav Brain Res* 2010, **208**:23-29.
25. Mathews IZ, Wilton A, Styles A, McCormick CM: **Heightened neuroendocrine function in males to a heterotypic stressor and increased depressive behaviour in females after adolescent social stress in rats.** *Behav Brain Res* 2008, **190**:33-40.
26. McCormick CM, Smith C, Mathews IZ: **Effects of chronic social stress in adolescence on anxiety and neuroendocrine response to mild stress in male and female rats.** *Behav Brain Res* 2008, **187**:228-238.
27. McCormick CM, Merrick A, Secen J, Helmreich DL: **Social instability in adolescence alters the central and peripheral hypothalamic-pituitary-adrenal responses to a repeated homotypic stressor in male and female rats.** *J Neuroendocrinol* 2007, **19**:116-126.
28. Johnson SA, Fournier NM, Kalynchuk LE: **Effect of different doses of corticosterone on depression-like behavior and HPA axis responses to a novel stressor.** *Behav Brain Res* 2006, **168**:280-288.
29. Marks W, Fournier NM, Kalynchuk LE: **Repeated exposure to corticosterone increases depression-like behavior in two different versions of the forced swim test without altering nonspecific locomotor activity or muscle strength.** *Physiol Behav* 2009, **98**:67-72.
30. Barr AM, Brotto LA, Phillips AG: **Chronic corticosterone enhances the rewarding effect of hypothalamic self-stimulation in rats.** *Brain Res* 2000, **875**:196-201.
31. Magarinos AM, Orchinik M, McEwen BS: **Morphological changes in the hippocampal CA3 region induced by non-invasive glucocorticoid administration: a paradox.** *Brain Res* 1998, **809**:314-318.
32. Pekary AE, Sattin A, Blood J, Furst S: **TRH and TRH-like peptide expression in rat following episodic or continuous corticosterone.** *Psychoneuroendocrinology* 2008, **33**:1183-1197.
33. Conrad CD, MacMillan DD, Tsekhanov S, Wright RL, Baran SE, Fuchs RA: **Influence of chronic corticosterone and glucocorticoid receptor antagonism in the amygdala on fear conditioning.** *Neurobiol Learn Mem* 2004, **81**:185-199.
34. Wall PM, Messier C: **Methodological and conceptual issues in the use of the elevated plus-maze as a psychological measurement instrument of animal anxiety-like behavior.** *Neurosci Biobehav Rev* 2001, **25**:275-286.
35. Castagne V, Moser P, Roux S, Porsolt RD: **Rodent models of depression: forced swim and tail suspension behavioral despair tests in rats and mice.** *Curr Protoc Neurosci* 2011, **55**:8.10A.11-18.10A.14.
36. Kalynchuk LE, Gregus A, Boudreau D, Perrot-Sinal TS: **Corticosterone increases depression-like behavior, with some effects on predator odor-induced defensive behavior, in male and female rats.** *Behav Neurosci* 2004, **118**:1365-1377.
37. Sousa N, Madeira MD, Paula-Barbosa MM: **Effects of corticosterone treatment and rehabilitation on the hippocampal formation of neonatal and adult rats. An unbiased stereological study.** *Brain Res* 1998, **794**:199-210.
38. Pellow S, Chopin P, File S, Briley M: **Validation of open:closed arm entries in an elevated plus maze as measure of anxiety the rat.** *J Neurosci Meth* 1985, **14**:149-167.
39. Porsolt RD, Anton G, Blavet N, Jalfre M: **Behavioral despair in rats: a new model sensitive to antidepressant treatments.** *Eur J Pharmacol* 1978, **47**:379-391.
40. Perrot-Sinal TS, Gregus S, Boudreau D, Kalynchuk LE: **Sex and repeated restraint interact to affect cat dor-induced defensive behavior in adult rats.** *Brain Res Bull* 2004, **1027**:161-172.
41. Cryan JF, Valentino RJ, Lucki I: **Assessing substrates underlying the behavioral effects of antidepressants using the modified rat forced swimming test.** *Neurosci Biobehav Rev* 2005, **29**:547-569.
42. Overstreet DH, Griebel G: **Antidepressant-like effects of CRF1 receptor antagonist SSR125543 in an animal model of depression.** *Eur J Pharmacol* 2004, **497**:49-53.
43. McCormick CM, Robarts D, Gleason E, Kelsey JE: **Stress during adolescence enhances locomotor sensitization to nicotine in adulthood in female, but not male, rats.** *Horm Behav* 2004, **46**:458-466.
44. Haller J, Fuchs E, Halasz J, Makara GB: **Defeat is a major stressor in males while social instability is stressful mainly in females: towards the development of a social stress model in female rats.** *Brain Res Bull* 1999, **50**:33-39.
45. Stone EA, Quartermain D: **Greater behavioral effects of stress in immature as compared to mature male mice.** *Physiol Behav* 1997, **63**:143-145.
46. Cameron HA, Gould E: **Adult neurogenesis is regulated by adrenal steroids in the dentate gyrus.** *Neuroscience* 1994, **61**:203-209.
47. Ryabinin AE, Wang YM, Finn DA: **Different levels of Fos immunoreactivity after repeated handling and injection stress in two inbred strains of mice.** *Pharmacol Biochem Behav* 1999, **63**:143-151.
48. Izumi J, Washizuka M, HayashiKuwabara Y, Yoshinaga K, Tanaka Y, Ikeda Y, Kiuchi Y, Oguchi K: **Evidence for a depressive-like state induced by repeated saline injections in Fischer 344 rats.** *Pharmacol Biochem Behav* 1997, **57**:883-888.
49. Lee B, Shim I, Lee HJ, Yang Y, Hahm DH: **Effects of acupuncture on chronic corticosterone-induced depression-like behavior and expression of neuropeptide Y in the rats.** *Neurosci Lett* 2009, **453**:151-156.
50. Drevets WC: **Prefrontal cortical-amygdalar metabolism in major depression.** *Ann N Y Acad Sci* 1999, **877**:614-637.
51. Paul SM: **Anxiety and depression: a common neurobiological substrate?** *J Clin Psychiatry* 1988, **49**:13-16.
52. Richardson-Jones JW, Craige CP, Nguyen TH, Kung HF, Gardier AM, Dranovsky A, David DJ, Guiard BP, Beck SG, Hen R, Leonardo ED: **Serotonin-1A autoreceptors are necessary and sufficient for the normal formation of circuits underlying innate anxiety.** *J Neurosci* 2011, **31**:6008-6018.
53. Parks CL, Robinson PS, Sibille E, Shenk T, Toth M: **Increased anxiety of mice lacking the serotonin(1A) receptor.** *Proc Natl Acad Sci USA* 1998, **95**:10734-10739.
54. Karten YJG, Nair SM, van Essen L, Sibug R, Joels M: **Long-term exposure to high corticosterone levels attenuates serotonin responses in rat hippocampal CA1 neurons.** *Proc Natl Acad Sci USA* 1999, **96**:13456-13461.

55. Karanges E, Li KM, Motbey C, Callaghan PD, Katsifis A, McGregor IS: **Differential behavioural and neurochemical outcomes from chronic paroxetine treatment in adolescent and adult rats: a model of adverse antidepressant effects in human adolescents?** *Int J Neuropsychopharmacol* 2011, **14**:491-504.
56. Pung T, Zimmerman K, Klein B, Ehrich M: **Corticosterone in drinking water: altered kinetics of a single oral dose of corticosterone and concentrations of plasma sodium, albumin, globulin, and total protein.** *Tox Indust Health* 2003, **19**:171-182.
57. Conrad CD, McLaughlin KJ, Harman JS, Foltz C, Wieczorek L, Lightner E, Wright RL: **Chronic glucocorticoids increase hippocampal vulnerability to neurotoxicity under conditions that produce CA3 dendritic retraction but fail to impair spatial recognition memory.** *J Neurosci* 2007, **27**:8278-8285.
58. Nacher J, Pham K, Gil-Fernandez V, McEwen BS: **Chronic restraint stress and chronic corticosterone treatment modulate differentially the expression of molecules related to structural plasticity in the adult rat piriform cortex.** *Neuroscience* 2004, **126**:503-509.
59. Lussier AL, Caruncho HJ, Kalynchuk LE: **Repeated exposure to corticosterone, but not restraint, decreases the number of reelin-positive cells in the adult rat hippocampus.** *Neurosci Lett* 2009, **460**:170-174.
60. Woolley C, Gould E, McEwen BS: **Exposure to excess glucocorticoids alters dendritic morphology of adult hippocampal pyramidal neurons.** *Brain Res* 1990, **531**:225-231.
61. Watanabe Y, Gould E, Cameron HA, Daniels DC, McEwen BS: **Phenytoin prevents stress-induced and corticosterone-induced atrophy of CA3 pyramidal neurons.** *Hippocampus* 1992, **2**:431-435.
62. Stone EA, Lin Y: **An anti-immobility effect of exogenous corticosterone in mice.** *Eur J Pharmacol* 2008, **580**:135-142.
63. Gourley SL, Kiraly DD, Howell JL, Olausson P, Taylor JR: **Acute hippocampal brain-derived neurotrophic factor restores motivational and forced swim performance after corticosterone.** *Biol Psychiatry* 2008, **64**:884-890.
64. David DJ, Samuels BA, Rainer Q, Wang JW, Marsteller D, Mendez I, Drew M, Craig DA, Guiard BP, Guilloux JP, Artymyshyn RP, Gardier AM, Gerald C, Antonijevic IA, Leonardo ED, Hen R: **Neurogenesis-dependent and -independent effects of fluoxetine in an animal model of anxiety/depression.** *Neuron* 2009, **62**:479-493.
65. Enkel T, Koch M: **Chronic corticosterone treatment impairs trace conditioning in rats with a neonatal medial prefrontal cortex lesion.** *Behav Brain Res* 2009, **203**:173-179.
66. Ellis FW: **Effect of ethanol on plasma corticosterone levels.** *J Pharmacol Exper Therapeut* 1966, **153**:121-127.
67. Buck HM, Hueston CM, Bishop C, Deak T: **Enhancement of the hypothalamic-pituitary-adrenal axis but not cytokine responses to stress challenges imposed during withdrawal from acute alcohol exposure in Sprague-Dawley rats.** *Psychopharmacology* .
68. Rasmussen DD, Boldt BM, Bryant CA, Mitton DR, Larsen SA, Wilkinson CW: **Chronic daily ethanol and withdrawal: 1. Long-term changes in the hypothalamo-pituitary-adrenal axis.** *Alcohol Clin Exp Res* 2000, **24**:1836-1849.
69. Ogilvie KM, Rivier C: **Gender difference in hypothalamic-pituitary-adrenal axis response to alcohol in the rat: activational role of gonadal steroids.** *Brain Res* 1997, **766**:19-28.
70. Silveri MM, Spear LP: **Characterizing the ontogeny of ethanol-associated increases in corticosterone.** *Alcohol* 2004, **32**:145-155.
71. Allen CD, Lee SY, Koob GF, Rivier CL: **Immediate and prolonged effects of alcohol exposure on the activity of the hypothalamic-pituitary-adrenal axis in adult and adolescent rats.** *Brain Behav Immun* 2011, **25**:550-560.
72. Spear LP, Varlinskaya EI: **Sensitivity to ethanol and other hedonic stimuli in an animal model of adolescence: implications for prevention science?** *Dev Psychobiol* 2010, **52**:236-243.
73. Allen CD, Rivier CL, Lee SY: **Adolescent alcohol exposure alters the central brain circuits known to regulate the stress response.** *Neuroscience* 2011, **182**:162-168.
74. Przybycien-Szymanska MM, Rao YS, Pak TR: **Binge-pattern alcohol exposure during puberty induces sexually dimorphic changes in genes regulating the HPA axis.** *Am J Physiol Endocrinol Metab* 2009, **298**:E320-328.
75. Cantwell DP, Baker L: **Manifestations of depressive affect in adolescence.** *J Youth Adolesc* 1991, **20**:121-133.
76. Rockhill C, Kodish I, DiBattisto C, Macias M, Varley C, Ryan S: **Anxiety disorders in children and adolescents.** *Curr Probl Pediatr Adolesc Health Care* 2010, **40**:66-99.
77. Beesdo K, Knappe S, Pine DS: **Anxiety and anxiety disorders in children and adolescents: developmental issues and implications for DSM-V.** *Psychiatr Clin North Am* 2009, **32**:483-524.
78. Doremus TL, Varlinskaya EI, Spear LP: **Age-related differences in elevated plus maze behavior between adolescent and adult rats.** *Ann N Y Acad Sci* 2004, **1021**:427-430.
79. Genn RF, Tucci SA, Thomas A, Edwards JE, File SE: **Age-associated sex differences in response to food deprivation in two animal tests of anxiety.** *Neurosci Biobehav Rev* 2003, **27**:155-161.

2

Early handling attenuates enhancement of glucocorticoid receptors in the prefrontal cortex in an animal model of post-traumatic stress disorder

Sophie A George[1*], Stephanie A Stout[1], Melissa Tan[1], Dayan Knox[1,3] and Israel Liberzon[1,2]

Abstract

Background: Changes in glucocorticoid receptors (GRs) have been implicated in the pathogenesis of stress related psychiatric disorders such as depression and post-traumatic stress disorder (PTSD). Abnormal adaptation of the stress-response system following traumatic stress can lead to an altered hypothalamic-pituitary-adrenal axis that may contribute to PTSD development. Indeed, elevated GR expression in the hippocampus and prefrontal cortex linked to PTSD-like characteristics have been reported in the validated animal model of PTSD, single-prolonged stress. These findings implicate increased levels of GRs in the development of post-traumatic psychopathology and suggest that exploration of GR-targeted interventions may have potential for PTSD prevention. Early handling during the neonatal phase alters GR expression and is proposed to confer resilience to stress. We therefore examined the effects of combined early handling and single prolonged stress treatments on GR expression.

Methods: Timed pregnant dams gave birth to pups that were subjected to early handling (n = 11) or control (n = 13) procedures during the neonatal phase. At postnatal day 45 animals underwent single prolonged stress or a control procedure. Rats were euthanized one day later and GR levels were assayed using western blot electrophoresis.

Results: Single prolonged stress exposure enhanced GR expression in the hippocampus and prefrontal cortex. Early handling treatment protected against single prolonged stress-induced enhancement of GR expression in the prefrontal cortex, but not in the hippocampus.

Conclusions: These data are a first step in highlighting the importance of targeting GR systems in prevention/resilience and may suggest that preventive strategies targeting GR upregulation might be particularly effective when prefrontal rather than hippocampal GRs are the target.

Keywords: Hippocampus, HPA axis, Maternal care, Single prolonged stress, Stress

Background

Stress initiates a cascade of neuroendocrine events in the hypothalamic-pituitary-adrenal (HPA) axis, which ultimately leads to increased secretion of the glucocorticoid hormone cortisol from the adrenal glands. Activity of the HPA axis is tightly controlled through complex regulatory mechanisms of glucocorticoid negative feedback. Glucocorticoids regulate the secretion of corticotropin-releasing factor and adrenocorticotropic hormone, from the hypothalamus and pituitary, respectively [1-4]. In addition, receptor sites within the hippocampus and prefrontal cortex play an important role in the regulation of HPA axis activity [2,5]. Following chronic or traumatic stress, inappropriate adaptation of the HPA axis can lead to pathological states; specifically, changes in glucocorticoid receptors (GRs) have been implicated in the pathogenesis of stress related psychiatric disorders such as post-traumatic stress disorder (PTSD) [6] and symptoms

* Correspondence: alicegeo@med.umich.edu
[1]Department of Psychiatry, University of Michigan, 4250 Plymouth Road, Ann Arbor, MI 48109, USA
Full list of author information is available at the end of the article

of PTSD are believed to reflect trauma-induced changes that lead to long-term dysfunctional stress regulation [7-9].

PTSD is characterized by increased cortisol suppression to dexamethasone, believed to result from an increased number or sensitivity of GRs [10]. Recently, in a prospective study, van Zuiden et al. reported higher levels of GR as a risk factor for subsequent development of PTSD in a sample of soldiers [11,12]. Findings from animal models further support changes in GR as the potential mechanism for the development of PTSD symptoms. In addition to reproducing cardinal symptoms of PTSD, such as hyperarousal and elevated fast feedback of the HPA axis [13-16], increased GR levels have been found in the single prolonged stress (SPS) [16-18] and predator exposure models in the hippocampus and prefrontal cortex [19]. In concert, pretreatment with GR antagonists prevents PTSD-like phenotypes in both SPS and predator exposure models [14,20]. Furthermore, in a recent "dismantling" study in which full SPS (involving restraint, forced swim, and ether exposure) was compared to the effect of different components of SPS (i.e., two of three stressors), only those animals that were exposed to the full SPS procedure and demonstrated the greatest degree of upregulation of GR in the hippocampus and prefrontal cortex, exhibited deficits in retention of extinction memories – a mechanism that is proposed to contribute to an inability to retain new safe memories and prevent recovery from trauma [19,21,22]. Together, these findings implicate altered GRs in the development of some aspects of post-traumatic psychopathology, and suggest that exploration of GR-targeted interventions may have potential for PTSD resilience/prevention.

Levine [23-25], and subsequently others (e.g., [26]), demonstrated that glucocorticoid responses to stress were modulated by early life environmental events and could result in stable changes to HPA axis reactivity, most notably via alterations in GR gene expression in the hippocampus and frontal cortex [27]. Early handling (EH), which involves brief daily separation from the mother during the neonatal phase is one such manipulation that has a documented effect on GR expression. EH increases the frequency of maternal behaviors [28,29] and thus increases GR expression and confers resilience to later stress [30,31]. Meany et al. demonstrated that EH enhances the availability of GRs [32], which in turn attenuates stress-induced HPA axis responsivity, as evidenced by attenuated glucocorticoid release in response to stress and reduced anxiety-like behaviors in adulthood [23,27,30,32].

While a number of previous studies have demonstrated that EH can attenuate the effects of chronic stress on inducing HPA axis reactivity [33-35], the effects of EH in animal models of PTSD have not been examined. Given the documented role of GR upregulation in the etiology of PTSD and the demonstration that "traumatic" stress as described in the SPS model increases GR expression, we hypothesized that EH would protect against the GR enhancement that develops following SPS. The goal of this study was to examine the combined effects of EH and single prolonged stress on GR expression. We chose to examine GR changes in the hippocampus and prefrontal cortex because of their documented role in the protective effect of EH [27], as well in the development of SPS-induced changes following traumatic stress [16,19].

Methods

Animals

Timed-pregnant dams (Charles River, Portage, MI, USA) were delivered to the Veterans Affairs Veterinary Medical Unit at approximately gestation day 16. Dams were singly housed in a temperature and humidity controlled environment, on a 12 hour light–dark cycle, and had *ad lib* access to standard laboratory chow and water. All experimental procedures were approved by the Veteran Affairs Institutional Animal Care Usage Committee and were in accordance with the National Institute of Health Guide for the Care and Use of Laboratory Animals. The day of birth of the litter was marked as postnatal day (PND) 0. Litter sizes varied naturally between 6 and 12, and on PND 2, animals were culled to ensure that equivalent numbers of males and females were present in each litter. The animals in this experiment were drawn from eight litters, and the number of animals in each litter from which data was sampled ranged from 4–12. Pups were subjected to EH or animal facility reared (AFR) treatments [36]. Briefly, EH litters received 15 minutes of daily maternal separation for 21 days. AFR rats were left undisturbed, except for bi-weekly cage maintenance. On PND 23, pups were weaned and housed in same sex sibling pairs.

SPS and brain homogenate preparation

On PND 45, 24 male Sprague–Dawley rats were assigned to the SPS (AFR = 7, EH = 5) or control (AFR = 6, EH = 6) groups. SPS rats were exposed to two hours of restraint, followed by 20 minutes of forced swimming in a 55 L container. After 15 minutes recuperation rats were exposed to 70 mL of ether in a desiccator until general anesthesia was induced (typically less than five minutes). Rats were then returned to their home cages for a seven day quiescent period. The SPS procedure refers to the application of the three stressors plus the seven day quiescent period. The quiescent period has been demonstrated to be critical for the development of PTSD-like physiological and behavioral abnormalities following SPS [15,37]. Animals assigned to the control group were left undisturbed in their home cages for the duration of SPS.

Following SPS (i.e., 8 days after the application of acute stressors), rats were euthanized by rapid decapitation, their brains were removed, flash frozen in chilled isopentane and stored in a −80°C freezer for later processing. Brains were then thawed to −20°C in a cryostat and the prefrontal cortex was dissected, approximately 1.00 mm anterior to Bregma [38]. The cerebrum was separated from the brain stem, thawed on ice, and the hippocampus was removed. The prefrontal cortex and hippocampus were sonicated separately in homogenization buffer (50 mM Trizma base, 1 mM ethylenediaminetetra-acetic acid, 10% sucrose, 4% sodium dodecyl sulfate, 2X protease inhibitor cocktail (Roche USA), pH 7.0 to 7.4), centrifuged at 105,000 *xg* for 45 minutes, homogenates decanted, and protein content determined using a Pierce BCA kit (Sigma-Aldrich, St. Louis, MO, USA). Approximately 40 μg of protein was diluted into a 1X Lamelli sample buffer and stored in a −80°C freezer until the western blot assay was performed.

Western blot electrophoresis

Western blot for total GR (cytoplasm and nucleus) was adapted from Spencer et al. [39] and conducted as previously described [19]. Briefly, samples heated at 70°C for 7 minutes were electrophoresed on 7.5% Tris HCl gels (Bio-Rad Laboratories, Inc., Hercules, CA, USA) along with a molecular weight ladder (Li-COR, Lincoln, NE, USA). Proteins in gels were transferred onto nitrocellulose membranes and blocked in blocking buffer (BB) (5% non-fat milk and 0.05% Tween-20 in tris-buffered saline (TBS)). Nitrocellulose membranes were then probed for GR by incubating membranes with a rabbit polyclonal GR antibody (Santa Cruz Biotechnology Inc., Santa Cruz, CA, USA; M-20, diluted 1:500 in BB) for 2 hours. After several washes in 0.05% Tween-20 in TBS, nitrocellulose membranes were incubated with an IRDye 800 conjugated anti-rabbit IgG secondary antibody (Li-COR, diluted 1:2,000 in BB) for 1 hour. Nitrocellulose membranes were then rinsed with TBS and scanned using a Li-COR Odyssey Scanner for visualization of GR bands.

After probing nitrocellulose membranes for GR, the same membranes were probed for actin related protein (Arp) which was used as the reference protein as previously described [40]. Nitrocellulose membranes were incubated with a rabbit polyclonal Arp antibody (Santa Cruz Antibodies, Arp-2, diluted 1:2,000 in BB), washed in 0.05% Tween-20 in TBS, and then incubated with the secondary antibody (Li-COR, 1:8,000 in BB). Nitrocellulose membranes were rinsed with TBS and scanned in a Li-COR Odyssey scanner in order to visualize Arp bands.

Images of scanned nitrocellulose membranes were analyzed using Odyssey software (Li-COR). The integrated intensity of the GR and Arp bands were expressed as a ratio (GR/Arp) and used as a relative measure of GR levels. Each gel contained representative samples from each of the treatment groups (Additional file 1). Samples were initially run in duplicate, but after a small coefficient of variance was established, single samples were run subsequently. GR levels were subjected to two factor analysis with the factors neonatal treatment (EH vs. AFR) and stress treatment (SPS vs. control). GR in the hippocampus and prefrontal cortex were analyzed separately. Main and simple effects were analyzed using analysis of variance (ANOVA), while main and simple comparisons were analyzed using *t*-test with a Bonferroni correction where necessary. Criterion of significance for all tests was set at $P < 0.05$.

Results

Prominent bands were observed between the 100 kDa and 75 kDa molecular weight markers for GR, and 50 kDa and 37 kDa for Arp in both hippocampus and prefrontal cortex (Figure 1). These bands correspond closely to previously determined locations for GR and Arp using the primary antibodies described in the Methods section.

An ANOVA of GR expression in the prefrontal cortex revealed a significant SPS × EH interaction ($F_{(1,20)} = 7.077$, $P = 0.015$). Post hoc comparisons revealed higher GR signal in SPS animals in comparison to controls in AFR treated groups ($t_{(11)} = 2.856$, $P = 0.016$), but this effect was not present in the EH exposed groups ($t_{(9)} = 0.626$, $P = 0.547$), suggesting that SPS-induced enhancement of

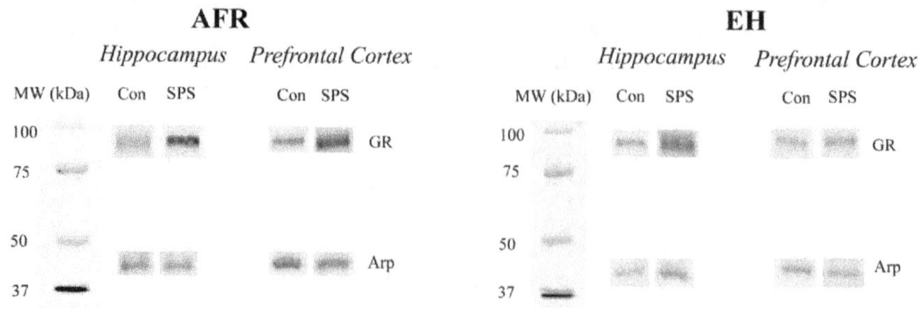

Figure 1 Representative protein bands from all treatment groups in this study. MW: Molecular weight markers; AFR: Animal facility reared; EH: Early handling; SPS: Single prolonged stress; Con: Control; GR: Glucocorticoid receptor; Arp: Actin related protein.

GR expression in prefrontal cortex was effectively prevented by EH. An ANOVA of hippocampal GR revealed a significant main effect of SPS ($F_{(1,17)} = 4.929$, $P = 0.04$) with higher GR signal in SPS-exposed animals; however, there was no SPS × EH interaction ($F_{(1,17)} = 1.487$, $P = 0.239$) or main effect of EH ($F_{(1,17)} = 0.851$, $P = 0.369$), suggesting that EH did not attenuate SPS-induced increases in GR expression in the hippocampus. These data are illustrated in Figure 2.

Discussion

In the present experiments SPS enhanced GR expression in the hippocampus and prefrontal cortex, replicating findings previously reported by ourselves and others [16,18,19]. EH, on the other hand, attenuated SPS-induced enhancement of GR in the prefrontal cortex, suggesting that EH may be protective against some of the SPS-induced changes implicated in PTSD pathophysiology. Interestingly, while affecting GR in prefrontal cortex, EH did not attenuate SPS-induced enhancement of GR in the hippocampus suggesting that there are regional differences in GR expression following combined effects of early life environment and stressors experienced in adulthood. It has long been suggested that early life experiences may lead to developmental changes that result in stable alterations to HPA axis and potentially confer resilience to later stress. To our knowledge, this is the first report of the combined effects of early life experiences and later "traumatic" stress on GR expression. Given the established role of GR in HPA axis regulation and stress reactivity [30,31] as well as in the pathophysiology of the SPS model of PTSD [16], these findings may have some implications for understanding mechanisms of resilience to traumatic stress, and of the regional differences that may be critical in moderating the protective effect of early life experiences to later life stressors. While intriguing, the functional implications of these GR expression changes will need to be examined in order to further establish the significance of

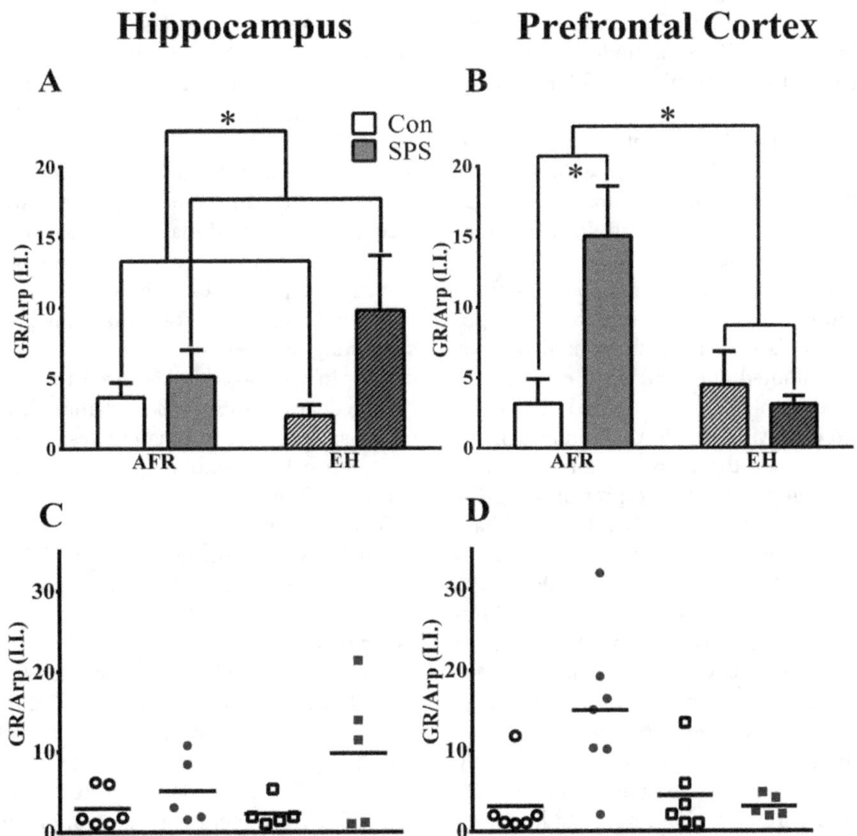

Figure 2 The effects of early handling (EH) and single prolonged stress on mean relative glucocorticoid levels in the (A) hippocampus and (B) prefrontal cortex. (C,D) Scatter plots showing individual data points from animals included in this experiment. *$P < 0.05$. AFR: Animal facility reared; EH: Early handling; SPS: Single prolonged stress; Con: Control; GR: Glucocorticoid receptor; Arp: Actin related protein; I.I.: Integrated intensity.

this finding. In addition, given the heterogeneity of the prefrontal cortex, in particular with respect to regulation of stress reactivity conferred by environmental influences [41], it would be interesting to further examine whether different subregions of the prefrontal cortex contribute differentially to the effect reported herein.

Differential changes in GR expression between frontal cortex and hippocampus following stress manipulations have been previously reported by our laboratory [19] as well as by others. Indeed, in Meaney's seminal paper in which the effect of EH on GR in the frontal cortex and hippocampus is first described, GR in the hippocampus was increased in EH animals compared to non-handled controls irrespective of post-weaning housing conditions [32]. However, this was not the case in the frontal cortex in which post-weaning housing condition moderated GR expression. These data suggest that hippocampal changes in GR may be more stable and enduring than those in the frontal cortex, resonating with our own finding, in which hippocampal GRs were found to be less sensitive to environmental effects than GRs in the prefrontal cortex.

The precise functional role of hippocampal and prefrontal cortex GRs are not known, although a wealth of data suggests that receptor sites within the hippocampus and prefrontal cortex play an important role in the regulation of HPA axis activity [2,5]. Recent data from our own laboratory, in which full SPS (comprised of all three stressors) was compared to partial SPS procedures (e.g., restraint + ether or forced swim + restraint), demonstrated that exposure to ether alone was sufficient to alter prefrontal GR levels, while multiple combined stressors were required to alter GR levels in the hippocampus. Moreover, the behavioral data from this study indicated that the combined effect of serial exposure to all three stressors (restraint, forced swim and ether) was required in order to observe extinction retention deficits. These results suggest that the mere enhancements in GR expression in the hippocampus and prefrontal cortex might be insufficient to lead to PTSD-relevant behavioral deficits, but "threshold" change in these regions is required for SPS-induced extinction retention deficits to manifest. Together with the present data, these findings suggest that the ability of EH to attenuate SPS-induced enhancement in prefrontal GR levels should be interpreted with caution as they may not necessarily translate to resilience in PTSD-relevant behavioral outcomes. Addressing this question directly, for instance by examining the effect of EH on extinction retention deficits in SPS animals, will be an important goal of future studies.

Interestingly, in these experiments we did not detect effects of EH alone on total GR expression. This is in contrast to the findings reported by Meaney et al., in which EH was found to increase baseline levels of unbound cytoplasmic GR. There are several possibilities that may explain this apparent discrepancy; EH effects are known to be mediated by FKBP5 protein modulating GR sensitivity to ligands [42]. Thus, when FKBP5 is bound to GR, binding of glucocorticoids to GRs is reduced. It is therefore possible that EH could increase GR sensitivity by attenuating FKBP5-GR binding. Because radioimmunoassays are typically used to assay unbound cytoplasmic GR, these assays rely on protein-ligand binding and therefore a treatment that increases GR sensitivity could be interpreted as an increase in unbound cytoplasmic GR. Thus, the differing approaches to measuring GR levels may explain these apparently contradictory findings. Alternatively, there were a number of other methodological differences that may underlie the difference in baseline EH findings between the two studies. For example, different strains of rat were used and the age at which GR was measured was different, as were post-weaning housing conditions, all of which have been suggested to impact GR expression [32].

Interestingly, in Meaney's model [32], increases in GR expression are interpreted as functionally beneficial, with EH increasing GR expression and conferring later resilience to stress. Accordingly, prolonged maternal separation, which reduces GR expression, is proposed to have adverse consequences, resulting in vulnerability to later stress. Conversely, our data suggest that GR increases following SPS relate to greater functional impairment [19]. The differences in the developmental stages at which GR changes are initiated may be critical to the behavioral impact of GR changes, explaining the seemingly conflicting results. The present data shows that EH prevents trauma-induced increases in GR in adult fully-grown animals, thus suggesting that early life EH protects against later increases in GR, possibly because of a more efficient negative feedback system which clamps down the HPA axis response following traumatic stress. Critically, both studies confirm EH results in changes in GR expression that likely result in resilience but further research is clearly needed to examine the precise mechanisms by which EH modulates GR expression following different stressors and in different brain regions.

Conclusions

While a number of previous studies have demonstrated that EH can attenuate the effects of chronic stress on inducing HPA axis reactivity, to our knowledge, this is the first study to examine the effects of EH in an animal model of PTSD. The data reported here suggest that the early life environment may have an important role in later responses to traumatic stress, and suggest that regional differentiation in GR expression may be important characteristic of the effects. These data, while limited to a measure of protein expression, underscore the importance of targeting GR systems in prevention/resilience and suggest that preventive strategies targeting GR upregulation may be more effective when prefrontal rather than hippocampal GRs are the target.

Additional file

Additional file 1: Representative example of a western blot assay. The data presented in this manuscript were obtained from a larger research project that examined the effects of a number of neonatal treatments and single prolonged stress on GR expression in the hippocampus and prefrontal cortex. This additional data file shows a representative example of a western blot assay.

Abbreviations

AFR: Animal facility reared; Arp: Actin related protein; BB: Blocking buffer; EH: Early handling; GR: Glucocorticoid receptor; HPA: Hypothalamic-pituitary-adrenal axis; PND: Postnatal day; PTSD: Post-traumatic stress disorder; SPS: Single prolonged stress; TBS: Tris-buffered saline.

Competing interests

The authors declare that they have no competing interests.

Author contributions

SG was the primary writer of the manuscript. She also contributed to data collection, statistical analyses and interpretation of the data. DK contributed to the conception and design of the experiment, statistical analyses and interpretation of the data. He supervised the data acquisition and substantially contributed to the drafting and revision of the manuscript. SS and MT were primarily responsible for acquisition of data. They conducted all early handling protocols and stress procedures and carried out initial statistical analyses. IL bore overall responsibility for conception and design of the study, and interpretation of the data. He made critical revisions to the manuscript. All authors read and approved the final manuscript.

Acknowledgements

The research in this manuscript was supported by a VA Merit award and Department of Defense grant W81XWH-08-1-0661 awarded to Israel Liberzon. We would like to thank Dr. Sarah Clinton for her valuable contribution.

Author details

[1]Department of Psychiatry, University of Michigan, 4250 Plymouth Road, Ann Arbor, MI 48109, USA. [2]Ann Arbor Veterans Affairs Hospital, 2215 Fuller Road, Ann Arbor, MI 49105, USA. [3]Present address: Department of Psychology, University of Delaware, 108 Wolf Hall, Newark, DE 19716, USA.

References

1. Dallman MF, Akana SF, Jacobson L, Levin N, Cascio CS, Shinsako J: **Characterization of corticosterone feedback regulation of ACTH secretion.** *Ann N Y Acad Sci* 1987, **512**:402–414.
2. de Kloet ER: **Brain corticosteroid receptor balance and homeostatic control.** *Front Neuroendocrinol* 1991, **12**:95–164.
3. Jacobson L, Sapolsky R: **The role of the hippocampus in feedback regulation of the hypothalamic-pituitary-adrenocortical axis.** *Endocr Rev* 1991, **12**:118–134.
4. Feldman S, Weidenfeld J: **Neural mechanisms involved in the corticosteroid feedback effects on the hypothalamo-pituitary-adrenocortical axis.** *Prog Neurobiol* 1995, **45**:129–141.
5. Diorio D, Viau V, Meaney MJ: **The role of the medial prefrontal cortex (cingulate gyrus) in the regulation of hypothalamic-pituitary-adrenal responses to stress.** *J Neurosci* 1993, **13**:3839–3847.
6. Yehuda R: **Biology of posttraumatic stress disorder.** *J Clin Psychiatry* 2001, **62**(Suppl 17):41–46.
7. Heim C, Nemeroff CB: **Neurobiology of posttraumatic stress disorder.** *CNS Spectr* 2009, **14**:13–24.
8. Yehuda R: **Clinical relevance of biologic findings in PTSD.** *Psychiatr Q* 2002, **73**:123–133.
9. de Kloet CS, Vermetten E, Geuze E, Kavelaars A, Heijnen CJ, Westenberg HG: **Assessment of HPA-axis function in posttraumatic stress disorder: pharmacological and non-pharmacological challenge tests, a review.** *J Psychiatr Res* 2006, **40**:550–567.
10. Yehuda R, Boisoneau D, Lowy MT, Giller EL Jr: **Dose–response changes in plasma cortisol and lymphocyte glucocorticoid receptors following dexamethasone administration in combat veterans with and without posttraumatic stress disorder.** *Arch Gen Psychiatry* 1995, **52**:583–593.
11. van Zuiden M, Geuze E, Willemen HL, Vermetten E, Maas M, Heijnen CJ, Kavelaars A: **Pre-existing high glucocorticoid receptor number predicting development of posttraumatic stress symptoms after military deployment.** *Am J Psychiatry* 2011, **168**:89–96.
12. van Zuiden M, Kavelaars A, Geuze E, Olff M, Heijnen CJ: **Predicting PTSD: Pre-existing vulnerabilities in glucocorticoid-signaling and implications for preventive interventions.** *Brain Behav Immun* 2013, **30**:12–21.
13. Khan S, Liberzon I: **Topiramate attenuates exaggerated acoustic startle in an animal model of PTSD.** *Psychopharmacology (Berl)* 2004, **172**:225–229.
14. Kohda K, Harada K, Kato K, Hoshino A, Motohashi J, Yamaji T, Morinobu S, Matsuoka N, Kato N: **Glucocorticoid receptor activation is involved in producing abnormal phenotypes of single-prolonged stress rats: a putative post-traumatic stress disorder model.** *Neuroscience* 2007, **148**:22–33.
15. Liberzon I, Krstov M, Young EA: **Stress-restress: effects on ACTH and fast feedback.** *Psychoneuroendocrinology* 1997, **22**:443–453.
16. Liberzon I, Lopez JF, Flagel SB, Vazquez DM, Young EA: **Differential regulation of hippocampal glucocorticoid receptors mRNA and fast feedback: relevance to post-traumatic stress disorder.** *J Neuroendocrinol* 1999, **11**:11–17.
17. Kozlovsky N, Matar MA, Kaplan Z, Zohar J, Cohen H: **A distinct pattern of intracellular glucocorticoid-related responses is associated with extreme behavioral response to stress in an animal model of post-traumatic stress disorder.** *Eur Neuropsychopharmacol* 2009, **19**:759–771.
18. Wang HT, Han F, Shi YX: **Activity of the 5-HT1A receptor is involved in the alteration of glucocorticoid receptor in hippocampus and corticotropin-releasing factor in hypothalamus in SPS rats.** *Int J Mol Med* 2009, **24**:227–231.
19. Knox D, Nault T, Henderson C, Liberzon I: **Glucocorticoid receptors and extinction retention deficits in the single prolonged stress model.** *Neuroscience* 2012, **223**:163–173.
20. Adamec R, Muir C, Grimes M, Pearcey K: **Involvement of noradrenergic and corticoid receptors in the consolidation of the lasting anxiogenic effects of predator stress.** *Behav Brain Res* 2007, **179**:192–207.
21. Liberzon I, Garfinkel SN: **Functional neuroimaging in post-traumatic stress disorder.** In *Post-Traumatic Stress Disorder.* Edited by LeDoux JE, Keane T, Shiromani P. New York: Humana Press; 2009:297–317.
22. Pitman RK, Rasmusson AM, Koenen KC, Shin LM, Orr SP, Gilbertson MW, Milad MR, Liberzon I: **Biological studies of post-traumatic stress disorder.** *Nat Rev Neurosci* 2012, **13**:769–787.
23. Levine S: **Infantile experience and resistance to physiological stress.** *Science* 1957, **126**:405.
24. Levine S, Alpert M, Lewis GW: **Infantile experience and the maturation of the pituitary adrenal axis.** *Science* 1957, **126**:1347.
25. Levine S: **Maternal and environmental influences on the adrenocortical response to stress in weanling rats.** *Science* 1967, **156**:258–260.
26. Zarrow MX, Campbell PS, Denenberg VH: **Handling in infancy: increased levels of the hypothalamic corticotropin releasing factor (CRF) following exposure to a novel situation.** *Proc Soc Exp Biol Med* 1972, **141**:356–358.
27. Meaney MJ, Diorio J, Francis D, Widdowson J, LaPlante P, Caldji C, Sharma S, Seckl JR, Plotsky PM: **Early environmental regulation of forebrain glucocorticoid receptor gene expression: implications for adrenocortical responses to stress.** *Dev Neurosci* 1996, **18**:49–72.
28. Barnett SA, Burn J: **Early stimulation and maternal behaviour.** *Nature* 1967, **213**:150–152.
29. Lehmann J, Feldon J: **Long-term biobehavioral effects of maternal separation in the rat: consistent or confusing?** *Rev Neurosci* 2000, **11**:383–408.
30. Francis DD, Meaney MJ: **Maternal care and the development of stress responses.** *Curr Opin Neurobiol* 1999, **9**:128–134.
31. Lee MHS, Williams DI: **Changes in licking behaviour of rat mother following handling of young.** *Anim Behav* 1974, **22**:679–681.

32. Meaney MJ, Aitken DH, Bodnoff SR, Iny LJ, Tatarewicz JE, Sapolsky RM: **Early postnatal handling alters glucocorticoid receptor concentrations in selected brain regions.** *Behav Neurosci* 1985, **99**:765–770.
33. Papaioannou A, Gerozissis K, Prokopiou A, Bolaris S, Stylianopoulou F: **Sex differences in the effects of neonatal handling on the animal's response to stress and the vulnerability for depressive behaviour.** *Behav Brain Res* 2002, **129**:131–139.
34. Panagiotaropoulos T, Papaioannou A, Pondiki S, Prokopiou A, Stylianopoulou F, Gerozissis K: **Effect of neonatal handling and sex on basal and chronic stress-induced corticosterone and leptin secretion.** *Neuroendocrinology* 2004, **79**:109–118.
35. Oines E, Murison R, Mrdalj J, Gronli J, Milde AM: **Neonatal maternal separation in male rats increases intestinal permeability and affects behavior after chronic social stress.** *Physiol Behav* 2012, **105**:1058–1066.
36. Meaney MJ, Aitken DH, Viau V, Sharma S, Sarrieau A: **Neonatal handling alters adrenocortical negative feedback sensitivity and hippocampal type II glucocorticoid receptor binding in the rat.** *Neuroendocrinology* 1989, **50**:597–604.
37. Knox D, George SA, Fitzpatrick CJ, Rabinak CA, Maren S, Liberzon I: **Single prolonged stress disrupts retention of extinguished fear in rats.** *Learn Mem* 2012, **19**:43–49.
38. Paxinos G, Watson C: *The Rat Brain in Stereotaxic Coordinates.* 2nd edition. San Diego: Academic Press; 1986.
39. Spencer RL, Kalman BA, Cotter CS, Deak T: **Discrimination between changes in glucocorticoid receptor expression and activation in rat brain using western blot analysis.** *Brain Res* 2000, **868**:275–286.
40. Knox D, Nault T, Henderson C, Liberzon I: **Glucocorticoid receptors and extinction retention deficits in the single prolonged stress model.** *Neuroscience* 2012, **223**:163–173.
41. Lehmann ML, Herkenham M: **Environmental enrichment confers stress resiliency to social defeat through an infralimbic cortex-dependent neuroanatomical pathway.** *J Neurosci* 2011, **31**:6159–6173.
42. Binder EB: **The role of FKBP5, a co-chaperone of the glucocorticoid receptor in the pathogenesis and therapy of affective and anxiety disorders.** *Psychoneuroendocrinology* 2009, **34**(Suppl 1):S186–S195.

3

Predicting post-trauma stress symptoms from pre-trauma psychophysiologic reactivity, personality traits and measures of psychopathology

Scott P Orr[1,2*], Natasha B Lasko[1,2], Michael L Macklin[1,2], Suzanne L Pineles[3,4], Yuchiao Chang[5] and Roger K Pitman[1]

Abstract

Background: Most individuals exposed to a traumatic event do not develop post-traumatic stress disorder (PTSD), although many individuals may experience sub-clinical levels of post-traumatic stress symptoms (PTSS). There are notable individual differences in the presence and severity of PTSS among individuals who report seemingly comparable traumatic events. Individual differences in PTSS following exposure to traumatic events could be influenced by pre-trauma vulnerabilities for developing PTSS/PTSD.

Methods: Pre-trauma psychological, psychophysiological and personality variables were prospectively assessed for their predictive relationships with post-traumatic stress symptoms (PTSS). Police and firefighter trainees were tested at the start of their professional training (i.e., pre-trauma; n = 211) and again several months after exposure to a potentially traumatic event (i.e., post-trauma, n = 99). Pre-trauma assessments included diagnostic interviews, psychological and personality measures and two psychophysiological assessment procedures. The psychophysiological assessments measured psychophysiologic reactivity to loud tones and the acquisition and extinction of a conditioned fear response. Post-trauma assessment included a measure of psychophysiologic reactivity during recollection of the traumatic event using a script-driven imagery task.

Results: Logistic stepwise regression identified the combination of lower IQ, higher depression score and poorer extinction of forehead (corrugator) electromyogram responses as pre-trauma predictors of higher PTSS. The combination of lower IQ and increased skin conductance (SC) reactivity to loud tones were identified as pre-trauma predictors of higher post-trauma psychophysiologic reactivity during recollection of the traumatic event. A univariate relationship was also observed between pre-trauma heart rate (HR) reactivity to fear cues during conditioning and post-trauma psychophysiologic reactivity.

Conclusion: The current study contributes to a very limited literature reporting results from truly *prospective* examinations of pre-trauma physiologic, psychologic, and demographic predictors of PTSS. Findings that combinations of lower estimated IQ, greater depression symptoms, a larger differential corrugator EMG response during extinction and larger SC responses to loud tones significantly predicted higher PTSS suggests that the process(es) underlying these traits contribute to the pathogenesis of subjective and physiological PTSS. Due to the low levels of PTSS severity and relatively restricted ranges of outcome scores due to the healthy nature of the participants, results may underestimate actual predictive relationships.

Keywords: Stress disorders, Post-traumatic, Conditioning, Startle, Imagery, Psychophysiology, Risk factors

* Correspondence: Scott_Orr@hms.harvard.edu
[1]Department of Psychiatry, Massachusetts General Hospital and Harvard Medical School, Charlestown, MA, USA
[2]Department of Veterans Affairs Medical Center, Manchester, NH, USA
Full list of author information is available at the end of the article

Background

Most individuals exposed to a traumatic event do not develop post-traumatic stress disorder (PTSD); however, many individuals may experience varying amounts of sub-clinical levels of post-traumatic stress symptoms (PTSS). Notable differences in the presence and severity of PTSS have been found among individuals reporting traumatic events that would appear to be comparably stressful [1–3]. This raises the possibility that some individuals may have pre-trauma vulnerabilities for developing PTSS or diagnosable PTSD.

Increased vulnerability to PTSS has been found to be associated with individual difference factors such as: personal history of depressive disorders [4,5], anxiety disorders [4] as well as introversion [6] and neuroticism [4,6,7]. Underlying these various vulnerabilities may be a common factor termed, "negative affectivity." Clark, Watson and Mineka [8] have described negative affectivity as a "...stable, heritable, and highly general trait dimension with a multiplicity of aspects ranging from mood to behavior" that is "...broadly related to psychopathology, including indices of both anxiety and depression..." (p. 104). Thus, negative affectivity would encompass a range of characteristics demonstrated to be highly correlated with each other and potentially with PTSS, including: anxiety, introversion, neuroticism, electrodermal lability, slowed habituation rate and increased conditionability [6,7,9].

Numerous studies have demonstrated concurrent associations between psychologic and psychophysiologic factors and PTSD symptoms. This research has primarily used cross-sectional study designs, i.e., comparisons are made between individuals with and without PTSD. From such studies it is difficult, if not impossible, to determine whether the observed differences are a consequence of developing PTSD or might represent pre-existing differences that are associated with risk for developing PTSD. We examined the PTSD literature to identify well-standardized psychologic and psychophysiologic measures that have been found to discriminate between individuals with and without PTSD in at least one or more published studies and that might serve as risk markers for the development of PTSD. The candidate variables we selected from this review as potential risk markers, in addition to age, education, gender and race, are listed in Table 1.

Briefly, studies of psychologic measures have found individuals with, compared to without, PTSD to have greater: general psychiatric symptoms e.g., [10–13], depression symptoms e.g., [11,12,14–16], state and/or trait anxiety e.g., [11–15,17–19] and neuroticism e.g., [16,20–23]. Whereas, greater: IQ [16,24–27], extraversion [22,28], openness [29] and agreeableness [22,23] have been observed in individuals without, compared to with, PTSD.

Table 1 Pre-trauma Predictor Variable Means and SDs for Individuals Exposed to a Traumatic Event (N = 99)

Variable	M	SD
Psychometric Measures		
SCL-90-R GSI	0.3	0.4
BDI	2.5	3.2
WAIS-R EST-IQ	101.8	10.0
STAI-T	31.2	8.2
NEO-PI-R Domain		
Neuroticism	46.7	8.0
Extroversion	54.7	8.2
Openness	48.0	11.3
Agreeableness	48.0	9.4
Loud-tone Psychophysiologic Measures		
Heart rate		
Pre-tone level (bpm)	71.6	11.6
Mean response (√bpm)	0.6	0.9
Response slope	0.1	1.0
Skin conductance		
Pre tone level (μS)	7.2	5.6
Mean response (√μS)	0.6	0.3
Response slope	-0.4	0.2
Trials to criterion	9.7	4.2
Electromyogram		
Mean response (√μV)	2.3	1.7
Fear-conditioning Psychophysiologic Measures		
SC Orienting Response	0.6	0.7
Differential Response		
Acquisition Phase		
SC (μS)	0.2	0.5
EMG (μv)	0.2	2.9
HR (bpm)	1.0	5.7
Extinction Phase		
SC (μS)	-0.1	0.5
EMG (μV)	-0.7	4.4
Response to CS + trials		
Acquisition Phase		
SC (μS)	0.6	0.6
EMG (μv)	2.5	3.0
HR (bpm)	5.8	4.8
Extinction Phase		
SC (μS)	0.2	0.4
EMG (μV)	3.1	4.2

Note: SCL-90-R GSI = Symptom Checklist 90-Revised, Global Severity Score; BDI = Beck Depression Inventory; WAIS-R EST-IQ = Estimated WAIS-R Full Scale IQ from Shipley Institute of Living Scale; STAI-S = State/Trait Anxiety Inventory-State score; bpm = beats per minute; S = Siemens; V = volts; SC = skin conductance; HR = heart rate; Orienting Response = mean response to first presentation of the CS + and the CS- during the habituation phase; Acquisition and extinction response to CS + trials = mean response to CS + trials during the acquisition and extinction phases, respectively; habituation, acquisition, and extinction differential responses = the mean CS interval response to CS + trials minus the mean CS interval response to CS- trials for the habituation, acquisition, and extinction phases, respectively; CS = conditioned stimulus.

Of particular note, research cited above suggests that lower IQ and the personality traits of increased neuroticism, lower extraversion and lower agreeableness are pre-trauma predictors of increased risk for PTSD and/or PTSS.

Studies of psychophysiologic reactivity to startling stimuli and fear conditioning have reported several reliable differences between individuals with and without PTSD. The startle response represents a form of unconditioned reactivity to sudden, unexpected stimuli such as a loud noise that is mediated by brainstem neural circuitry [30] but is influenced by higher psychological processes such as emotional state. Magnitude of the eyeblink response is commonly used as the prototypical measure of startle in humans. However, startling acoustic stimuli can also produce increased skin conductance (SC) and heart rate (HR) responses, indicating that there are autonomic, as well as muscular, features of startle. The magnitude of reactivity to startling stimuli and rate of decline in response magnitude over repeated presentations of a startle stimulus, i.e., habituation, have been extensively used as measures of anxiety and/or emotional state. There is a substantial literature demonstrating larger magnitude: eyeblink e.g., [17,31,32], skin conductance e.g., [19,32,33] and heart rate e.g., [10,17, 19,31,33–36] responses to loud noise or tone stimuli in individuals with, compared to without, PTSD. Of particular note, findings from a recent prospective study of firefighter trainees suggests that eyeblink and SC response magnitudes to loud tones predict the development of greater PTSS following exposure to a traumatic event [37]. In contrast, there is now compelling evidence that larger HR response magnitude to loud tones is an acquired feature of PTSD [36,38]. Slower habituation of SC responses e.g., [10,17,33,35,36], HR responses [34] and eyeblink responses [38] have also been observed in individuals with PTSD. There is some evidence that slower habituation of SC and eyeblink responses, as measured by the number of trials to no-response, may be acquired features of PTSD [38].

Psychophysiologic studies of acquisition and extinction of conditioned fear responses have also demonstrated differences between individuals with and without PTSD. Fear conditioning provides a measure of an individual's propensity to associate a neutral cue with an aversive outcome. This propensity can be assessed from the strength of the conditioned response that is established during acquisition, as well as from its resistance to extinction. Measures of SC activity have been commonly used to assess human fear conditioning; measures of HR and facial EMG activity have been less frequently used. Over the past three decades, differential fear conditioning, a procedure that pairs one of two neutral stimuli with a mildly aversive unconditioned stimulus (UCS), has been widely used to study conditioned fear in humans. This conditioning procedure allows for the calculation of differential response scores, calculated as the average response to the conditioned stimulus (CS+) paired with the UCS minus the average response to the stimulus (CS-) not paired with the UCS. These scores reflect the amount of conditioned responding to the fear cue (CS+) during acquisition and extinction. Individuals with PTSD have been found to show larger differential SC [11,14], corrugator EMG [11] and HR [11,18] responses during acquisition and larger SC [11,14,39] responses during extinction. Of particular relevance to the present work is the recent finding from a study of firefighter trainees that the magnitude of the differential corrugator EMG response during acquisition and extinction was significantly correlated with PTSS following exposure to a traumatic event [40].

To date, only a very few studies have addressed whether the aforementioned psychologic and psychophysiologic measures represent pre-trauma vulnerability markers or are consequences of developing PTSD/PTSS. From a practical standpoint, the identification of vulnerability markers for PTSD could have important practical implications related to screening and targeting early intervention for at-risk individuals working in high-risk occupations. From a theoretical standpoint, addressing whether or not psychologic and psychophysiologic features associated with PTSS represent pre-trauma or acquired traits has substantial implications for understanding the pathogenesis of PTSS and PTSD.

The work reported here assessed pre-trauma psychologic and psychophysiologic measures in order to evaluate their ability to predict the development of PTSD/PTSS severity following exposure to an intervening traumatic event. In order to increase the likelihood of finding participants who would be exposed to a traumatic event at some proximate point following pre-trauma assessment, we recruited firefighter and police trainees at the time of their initial training. The pre-trauma assessment included structured diagnostic interviews, standard psychometrics, and psychophysiologic reactivity to loud-tones and differential fear conditioning. Participants were closely followed for the occurrence of a traumatic event that met the DSM-IV PTSD Category A1 criterion during the course of their new professional duties. After such a traumatic event, the participant was invited to return for psychodiagnostic, psychometric and psychophysiologic assessments. As part of the post-trauma assessment, psychophysiologic reactivity to individually-tailored imagery scripts was measured as a non-subjective measure of emotional reactivity to the traumatic event.

The primary goal of the work reported here was to prospectively identify the best combination of psychologic and psychophysiologic variables that predicted PTSD/PTSS following exposure to a potentially traumatic event.

Based upon the sparse but most relevant literature mentioned above, we hypothesized that individuals with higher PTSD/PTSS following exposure to a traumatic event would show the following pre-trauma traits: 1) greater conditionability (i.e., stronger acquisition and slower extinction of an aversively conditioned differential corrugator EMG response); 2) larger magnitude eyeblink EMG and SC responses to loud tones; 3) a higher mean SC level; 4) lower IQ; and 5) lower extraversion, higher neuroticism, and lower agreeableness scores on the Revised NEO Personality Inventory [41].

Methods

Participants

Three hundred eight firefighter/EMT and police trainees initially provided written informed consent to participate, which was obtained from all participants in accordance with the requirements of the Human Research Committee at the Massachusetts General Hospital and then completed the initial diagnostic, psychometric and psychophysiologic assessments. Firefighter trainees were recruited from the Lakes Region Community College, Laconia, NH and Fire Academy, Boston Fire Department, Boston, MA. Police trainees were recruited from the Lowell Police Academy, Lowell, MA. Ninety-nine participants reached the project's endpoint, which required exposure to a traumatic event and follow-up testing consisting of diagnostic, psychometric and psychophysiologic assessments. Firefighters comprised 64.9 percent of the sample and the majority was male (91.8 %) and Caucasian (82.2 %). Mean age and education level were 27.0 (SD = 6.5) and 14.1 (SD = 1.8) years, respectively. The average participant fell within the normal range of IQ (Estimated WAIS-R Full Scale IQ: M = 101.8, SD = 10.0) as determined from the Shipley Institute of Living Scale [42,43] and was mentally healthy as measured by depression (Beck Depression Inventory: M = 2.5, SD = 3.2); general psychiatric symptoms (Symptom Checklist-90-Revised Global Severity Index (GSI): M = 0.3, SD = 0.4) and trait anxiety (Speilberger State-Trait Anxiety Inventory: M = 31.2, SD = 8.2). The Structured Clinical Interview for DSM-IV (SCID, [44]) and Clinician-Administered PTSD Scale (CAPS, [45]) were conducted during the pre-trauma assessments at the respective training academies. As determined from the SCID, the percentages of individuals who met DSM-IV criteria for a current diagnosis were as follows: alcohol dependence = 2 %, substance dependence < 1 %, major depression < 1 %, ADHD = 2 %, phobia < 1 %. The percentages of individuals who met DSM-IV criteria for a lifetime diagnosis were as follows: alcohol dependence = 10 %, substance dependence = 3 %, major depression = 3 %, and panic disorder < 1 %. As determined from the CAPS, n = 6 individuals met DSM-IV criteria for a current or lifetime diagnosis of PTSD at the time of the initial assessment and were excluded from the reported study. Trainees who completed the Stressful Life Events Checklist (n = 212) reported experiencing an average of 1.6 (SD = 1.5) different types of traumatic events before the initial assessment, with first exposure at an average age of 10.9 (SD = 8.4) years.

Measures and Procedures

Pre-trauma diagnostic assessment

The SCID Screen Patient Questionnaire (SSPQ) Computer Program for DSM-IV [46] and SCID Overview were administered to each trainee. If a trainee answered yes to any SSPQ items, a diagnostician administered the appropriate SCID module. If the trainee endorsed items that indicated that a traumatic event had occurred and that PTSD-like symptoms were experienced, the CAPS was administered in order to determine whether the participant had current and/or past PTSD and to obtain a continuous score corresponding to overall PTSS/PTSD severity (CAPS total score).

Pre-trauma psychometric assessment

The following instruments were administered: 1) Stressful Life Events Checklist [47], which solicits the frequency of previous traumatic event(s) experienced; 2) NEO-PI-R [41], which measures the dimensions of neuroticism, extraversion, openness to experience, agreeableness, and conscientiousness; 3) SCL-90-R [48] ; 4) STAI [49]; 5) BDI [50]; and 6) Shipley Institute of Living Scale [43], which estimates WAIS-R IQ.

Pre-trauma psychophysiologic assessment

Left orbicularis oculi and corrugator EMG, SC, and HR were recorded using a Coulbourn Lablinc V-series modular instrument system (Coulbourn Instruments LLC, Whitehall, PA). EMG signals were amplified, filtered to include the 90 to 1000 Hz range, and integrated using a 10-msec time constant for orbicularis oculi and a 200-msec time constant for corrugator EMG. For EMG, the skin was abraded and 4-mm (sensor diameter) Invivo Metric Ag/AgCl electrodes filled with electrolyte paste were placed over the left orbicularis oculi and corrugator muscle sites according to published specifications [51]. Skin conductance level was measured directly using a constant 0.5 V through 9-mm (sensor diameter) Invivo Metric Ag/AgCl electrodes placed on the hypothenar surface of the participant's non-dominant hand in accordance with published guidelines [52]. Heart rate was measured through 9-mm (sensor diameter) Invivo Metric Ag/AgCl electrodes filled with electrolytic paste and placed on the inside of each arm; HR was converted from interbeat interval. All psychophysiologic analog signals were digitized at 1000 Hz.

Loud-tones procedure An audiologic screening test was performed to verify that participants could hear a 1000-Hz tone at the 25 dB level in each ear. The stimuli, laboratory assessment procedure and dependent psychophysiologic measures (left orbicularis oculi, SC, & HR) were the same as used in several previous studies of PTSD [17]. The stimuli consisted of 15, 95-dB (sound pressure level), 1000-Hz pure tones presented for 500-ms, with 0-ms rise and fall times generated by a Coulbourn Audio Source Module (V85-05). Stimuli were presented binaurally over headphones. Intertrial intervals were randomly chosen to range between 27 and 52 s.

The psychophysiologic assessment session took place in a humidity- and temperature-controlled room located in quiet areas of the respective training academies. Due to space limitations, the participant, laboratory equipment and technician were located in the same room. A screen prevented the participant from seeing the recording equipment and technician during the testing procedures. The participant was seated in a comfortable chair and, after the recording electrodes had been attached, participants were read the standard instructions as used in our previous research [17]. The technician then placed headphones on the participant, checked that the physiologic measures were being properly recorded, and activated the computer. Following a 5-min resting, baseline-recording period, the series of 15 tones was presented.

Conditioning procedure The conditioning procedure took place after the loud-tone task was completed. The participant was seated approximately 4 feet in front of a monitor that was used to display the CSs. The CS + and CS- were represented by 6-inch diameter blue and white circles, respectively. The UCS was a 500-ms electric shock generated by a Coulbourn Transcutaneous Aversive Finger Stimulator (E13-22) and previously selected by the participant to be "highly annoying but not painful," delivered through electrodes attached to the first and third fingers of the dominant hand. Once the UCS level had been selected, the trainee was given the same instructions as used by [11].

After a 5-min resting period, the three phases of the experiment were initiated. Habituation (Phase I) consisted of five similar presentations each of the to-be CS + and CS- in pseudo-random order, i.e., no more than two consecutive presentations of the same stimulus type. The CS duration was 8 s, with randomly determined intertrial intervals ranging from 15–25 s. Acquisition (Phase II) consisted of five presentations of each stimulus type; a 500-ms shock pulse occurred immediately following each CS + offset. Extinction (Phase III) consisted of 10 similar, non-reinforced presentations each of the CS + and CS-. In each of these three phases, SC, HR, and left corrugator EMG were sampled beginning 4 s prior to CS onset and ending 6 s following CS offset.

Monitoring for a traumatic event

Each trainee who completed the pre-trauma assessment was contacted by mail on a bi-monthly basis to inquire as to the occurrence of a traumatic event during the previous two months that potentially met the DSM-IV PTSD Category A1 criterion. It was not required that an individual also meet the A2 criterion. Those individuals who reported such an "index" event were invited for the post-trauma assessment. The traumatic experiences included: witnessing death or severe injury (n = 59), threat to one's physical integrity (e.g., explosions, fires, high-speed chase, n = 16), motor vehicle accident (n = 4), physical assault (n = 4), and death or serious injury to someone known to the participant (n = 16). The mean amount of time elapsed between the pre-trauma assessment and the reported traumatic event was 19.4 months (SD = 12.2), and between the traumatic event and post-trauma assessment was 12.3 months (SD = 11.5).

Post-trauma assessment

This consisted of two visits separated by approximately one week, the first for psychodiagnostic and psychometric evaluations, and the second for laboratory testing. The CAPS was re-administered during the first visit and was focused on the index traumatic event, and the SCID was re-administered to assess for any new non-PTSD DSM-IV Axis I mental disorders. Participants also completed the Impact of Event Scale-Revised (IES-R, [53]). Script preparation for the script-driven imagery procedure, which took place the following week, was conducted according to our published procedure [1].

Prior to the laboratory testing during the second visit, a urine sample was obtained for drug screening; results indicated negligible drug use.

Psychophysiologic reactivity during script-driven imagery Results from more than 20 studies have provided consistent evidence of heightened psychophysiologic reactivity (SC, HR, or facial EMG responses) to cues reminiscent of a traumatic event in individuals with, compared to without, a diagnosis of current PTSD [54]. Assessment of psychophysiologic responses during imagery of the index traumatic event and other life events was performed according to our published procedure [1]. Personalized "scripts" approximately 30 s in length, composed in the second person, present tense, were created portraying each individual's traumatic events. Scripts related to other types of personal experiences, including stressful, positive, and neutral experiences, were also created. Standard scripts portraying various hypothetical experiences were also used. Scripts were recorded and played back to participants while they vividly imagined each event; HR, SC and facial EMG (left lateral frontalis and corrugator) were measured throughout.

Transcripts of the two personalized traumatic scripts for each individual were reviewed in scrambled order by a highly experienced clinical psychologist who treats patients with PTSD. The clinician rated each script on a 0 – 12 Likert-type scale for the severity of the traumatic event with "12" indicating "the most traumatic event you have encountered in your clinical experience," as we have done previously [2,55]. Ratings of the two traumatic scripts were averaged for each individual to provide a measure of the apparent severity of the traumatic exposure. The average severity rating was M = 7.79, SD = 1.41.

Data reduction

Psychophysiologic response scores for the loud-tone procedure

Each subject's psychophysiological records were reviewed by eye and statistically for aberrant individual response scores. Where a response was clearly aberrant (e.g., a doubling of HR caused by detection of the EKG T-wave), the aberrant value was replaced by the average of responses to the immediately preceding and following trials. We estimate that less than 5 % of data were unusable or imputed. Psychophysiologic responses to the loud tones were quantified in the same manner as in our previous work. An eyeblink EMG response was calculated for each trial by subtracting the average orbicularis oculi level during the 1-s interval immediately preceding tone onset from the highest orbicularis oculi value within 40–200 ms following tone onset. A SC response was calculated for each tone trial by subtracting the average SC level during the 1 s immediately preceding tone onset from the highest SC value within 1–4 s following tone onset. An accelerative HR response was calculated for each tone trial by subtracting the average pre-stimulus HR, as determined from the two heart beats immediately preceding tone onset, from the highest HR value (i.e., shortest IBI) within 1–4 s following tone onset. A square-root transformation was applied to all responses to reduce skewness and heteroscedasticity. Response scores included the mean HR, SC, and eyeblink EMG responses (averaged across the 15 tones). Habituation of responses was measured in two ways. Absolute habituation of SC and EMG responses was assessed by counting the number of trials before reaching a criterion of two successive non-response trials (SC $< .05$ μS; EMG $< .30$ μV). Relative habituation was calculated for all measures from the slope of the regression equation $Y = bx + a$ for Trials 2–15, whereby Y is the square root of the response score, and x is the log trial number.

Psychophysiologic response scores for aversive conditioning

A response score for each acquisition and extinction trial for each measure was calculated by subtracting the average SC, corrugator EMG and HR level for the 2-s interval immediately preceding CS onset from the respective measure's highest value during the 8-s CS interval, as has been previously done [11,56]. "Conditionability" scores for the acquisition and extinction phases were calculated by subtracting the mean SC, corrugator EMG, and HR responses to CS- trials from the respective mean responses to CS + trials. This was done separately for the acquisition and extinction phase.

In addition to examining differential conditioning scores, we included measures that represented SC, corrugator EMG and HR reactivity to only CS + trials during acquisition and extinction. There is evidence suggesting that some individuals with PTSD, while responding strongly to the CS+, respond equally strongly to the CS- thereby producing a small differential conditioning score [e.g., 18]. Thus, a measure that only reflects reactivity to CS + trials might provide a better estimate of reactivity to fear cues. An unconditioned response (UCR) score was calculated by subtracting the average level for the 2-s interval immediately preceding UCS onset from the highest value among those recorded during the UCS interval (0–6 s post-UCS offset).

Psychophysiologic response scores for script-driven imagery

A response score was calculated for each psychophysiologic dependent variable, separately for the two trauma-related scripts, by subtracting the preceding average baseline period value from the average value during imagery. The respective psychophysiologic response scores were then averaged for the two trauma-related scripts. Next, a single index of psychophysiologic reactivity to trauma-related script-driven imagery was obtained using an a priori discriminant function. This function was previously derived using discriminant analysis, a procedure that mathematically determined the optimal weightings for the combination of HR, SC, and lateral frontalis EMG responses during trauma-related imagery of previously studied individuals that maximally distinguished those with versus without current PTSD [1–3,55,57,58]. The sensitivity and specificity of this function are 57 % and 89 %, respectively [59]. Once derived, the discriminant function can be applied to a given individual's HR, SC, and lateral frontalis EMG responses to trauma-related imagery to yield a single score, i.e., "posterior probability" of having PTSD. For the present study, this *a priori* discriminant function was applied to each participant's respective HR, SC, and lateral frontalis EMG responses to trauma-related imagery, thereby providing a single measure of PTSS based solely on their psychophysiological reactivity to trauma-related imagery that can be viewed as an objective measure of emotional reactivity.

Statistical analysis

Variables were summarized using means and SDs or percentages. Study participants who reported experiencing a traumatic event were invited to return to our laboratory to complete the post-trauma assessments. The primary psychologic outcome measures of the study included the CAPS and IES-R total scores. Because no subject met full criteria for PTSD and CAPS total scores were very low (M = 4.1, SD = 8.3, range = 0.0–41.0), i.e., well within the normal range, the IES-R was used as the measure of PTSS severity, as has been done in previous prospective studies that also failed to find cases of PTSD [37,40]. The primary psychophysiologic outcome measure was the posterior probability score derived from the script-driven imagery assessment. Distributions of scores on the outcome measures were highly skewed due to participants' low symptom severity levels. For this reason we dichotomized scores into "high" (upper tertile) and "low" (lower two tertiles) groups to avoid the use of variable transformation and any linearity assumption. The lower two tertiles were combined because scores in the first and second tertiles were comparably low. In order to examine the robustness of results using the aforementioned dichotomization of scores within the current sample, the outcome variables were also tested after being dichotomized into the highest (Q4) and lowest (Q1) quartile groups, as well as into the highest (T3) and lowest (T1) tertile groups, so as to maximize differences between the groups. Results from the three dichotomization strategies were very similar. Consequently, we chose to create the "low" group from the combination of the lower two tertiles (T2, T3) because this strategy used all available data, whereas the other two strategies used only half (Q4 vs. Q1) or two-thirds (T3 vs. T1) of the data.

The list of psychometric, and psychophysiologic pre-trauma predictor variables is presented in Table 1 and, as noted above, were selected primarily on the basis of their having previously been found to discriminate between individuals with and without PTSD. The demographic variables, gender, race, age and education level, were also included as potential predictor variables. Separate logistic stepwise regression analysis using the predictor variables that were found to demonstrate a difference at $p < .20$ for the dichotomized IES-R scores and dichotomized Posterior Probability scores, respectively, were performed. For the regression models, the missing values from the potential predictors were imputed from other available predictor values using the EM algorithm [60] to preserve the sample size.

Results

Relationships between pre-trauma predictor variables and IES-R scores in trauma-exposed individuals

Post-trauma outcome measures

The IES-R served as the primary outcome measure; the overall mean and SD for IES-R scores was: M = 4.8, SD = 9.1, range = 0.0–46.5 and Posterior Probability score (psychophysiologic reactivity during trauma-related imagery), M = 0.35, SD = 0.11, range = 0.15–0.95).

Univariate comparisons for pre-trauma predictors of post-trauma outcome

Relationships between pre-trauma predictors (listed in Table 1) and post-trauma IES-R and Posterior Probability scores (dichotomized as High vs. Low) were examined by means of t-test for unequal variances, a more conservative test than that for equal variances. The following pre-trauma measures produced scores that were significantly different (or nearly so) between the High vs. Low IES-R groups: BDI-II (High: M = 3.6, SD = 4.0; Low: M = 1.9, SD = 2.7; $t(46) = 2.17$, $p = .035$), Shipley Estimated IQ (High: M = 98.4, SD = 13.2; Low: M = 103.5, SD = 7.7; $t(42) = 2.00$, $p = .052$), STAI-Trait (High: M = 33.7, SD = 18.3; Low: M = 29.8, SD = 8.0; $t(60) = 2.17$, $p = .034$), differential corrugator EMG response scores during extinction (High: M = 0.6, SD = 5.1; Low: M = −1.5, SD = 4.0; $t(51) = 2.07$, $p = .043$).

The following pre-trauma measures produced scores that were significantly different (or nearly so) between the High vs. Low Posterior Probability score groups: Shipley Estimated IQ (High: M = 98.4, SD = 11.7; Low: M = 103.9, SD = 7.8; $t(43) = 2.36$, $p = .023$), mean SC response to loud tones (High: M = 0.7, SD = 0.7; Low: M = 0.5, SD = 0.3; $t(53) = 1.99$, $p = .052$), number of trials to reach the SC habituation non-response criterion (High: M = 10.9, SD = 4.1; Low: M = 9.2, SD = 4.2; $t(61) = 1.87$, $p = .066$), mean HR response to CS + trials during acquisition (High: M = 7.1, SD = 3.8; Low: M = 4.9, SD = 4.5; $t(75) = 2.10$, $p = .039$).

Combined pre-trauma predictors of post-trauma outcome

Results of stepwise logistic regression analyses predicting IES-R and Posterior Probability score High vs. Low groups are presented in Table 2. As can be seen in the table, logistic regression identified lower estimated IQ, higher pre-trauma Beck Depression Inventory-II score and a larger differential corrugator EMG response during extinction as the best combination of predictor variables for higher post-trauma IES-R scores. The corresponding c-statistic for the IES-R model derived from the maximized sample was 0.70, indicating that 70 percent of individuals with high IES-R scores were correctly classified, suggesting reasonably good model performance. In order to examine the potential

Table 2 Results of Multiple Logistic Stepwise Regression Predicting Post-trauma Outcome from the Set of Pre-trauma Variables

Maximized Sample						
Outcome Measure	N	Selected Predictor(s)	Odds Ratio	Wald Chi-Square	df	p
IES-R	96	Shipley Est. IQ	0.95	4.28	1	.039
		EMG Diff_E1	1.17	4.46	1	.035
		BDI-II	1.15	3.50	1	.062
Post. Prob.	95	Shipley Est. IQ	0.94	5.72	1	.017
		SC Mean Resp.	4.02	3.70	1	.055

Note: Post. Prob. = Posterior Probability score derived from script-driven imagery assessment; IES-R = Impact of Event Scale-Revised total score; Shipley Est. IQ = Estimated WAIS-R Full Scale IQ from Shipley Institute of Living Scale; EMG Diff_E1 = corrugator electromyogram differential response during extinction, i.e., the averaged CS interval response to the first five CS + trials minus the averaged CS interval response to the first five CS- trials for the extinction phase; BDI-II = Beck Depression Inventory-II score; SC Mean Resp. = Skin conductance mean response to loud-tone presentations.

impact of individual differences in the amount of time elapsed between occurrence of the traumatic event and subsequent laboratory testing and in the clinician-rated severities of the traumatic events, logistic regression analyses were repeated with the amount of time-since-trauma and trauma-severity ratings added to the models. Odds ratios were 1.02 for the time-since-trauma variable and 0.90 for the trauma-severity variable when they were entered into the model; their contributions to the model were non-significant (Wald Chi-Square (1) = 0.84, p = .359 and Wald Chi-Square (1) = 0.33, p = .564, respectively).

Stepwise logistic regression analysis identified lower estimated IQ and larger mean SC responses to the loud tones as the best combination of pre-trauma variables for predicting higher post-trauma Posterior Probability scores. The corresponding c-statistic for the Posterior Probability model derived from the maximized sample was 0.70, indicating that 70 percent of individuals with high Posterior Probability scores were correctly classified. The logistic regression analysis was repeated, adjusting for the amount of time-since-trauma and trauma-severity ratings. Odds ratios were 1.01 for the time-since-trauma variable and 1.04 for the trauma-severity variable when they were entered into the model; their contributions to the models were non-significant (Wald Chi-Square (1) = 0.04, p = .848 and Wald Chi-Square (1) = 0.05, p = .831, respectively).

Discussion

The current study, like those of Guthrie and Bryant [40] and Pole et al. [61], represents a truly *prospective* examination of potential pre-trauma physiologic, psychologic, and demographic predictors of PTSS in firefighters and police, as predictor variables were assessed prior to the occurrence of a traumatic event rather than retrospectively. The present work contributes to findings from previous studies, which have provided indirect evidence for the pre-existing versus acquired nature of psychologic and physiologic markers associated with PTSS [31,36,38].

It is noteworthy that in the present study none of the 99 police and firefighters exposed to a traumatic event met full DSM-IV criteria for PTSD at the post-trauma assessment. The absence of clinical PTSD cases initially surprised us. When the study was originally designed we "conservatively" estimated that the PTSD rate would be about 17 % [4,62,63]. However, recent findings from prospective studies of police and firefighters suggest that a very low rate of PTSD following exposure to a traumatic event is characteristic of these populations. In their study of Australian firefighter recruits, Guthrie and Bryant [40] found that none of the 67 trauma-exposed firefighters met DSM-IV criteria for PTSD at the post-trauma assessment. Pole et al. [61] reported very low levels of PTSD symptom severities in police exposed to at least one traumatic event during the 1-year period following their initial training; only 1 of 138 police met criteria for full PTSD. Thus, the development of PTSD following exposure to a traumatic event appears to be very low in prospectively-studied samples of police and firefighters, likely lower than in the general population and perhaps reflecting a strong self-selection bias or protective benefits from professional training. One might assert that police and firefighters who are still actively engaged in their professions are simply reluctant to endorse symptoms of psychopathology. However, the fact that police and firefighters in the present study also showed normal levels of psychophysiological reactivity while recalling their traumatic events provides some objective support for the absence of significant PTSD symptoms.

The lack of police and firefighters who met full DSM-IV criteria for PTSD precluded our using the categorical diagnosis of PTSD as a post-trauma outcome and necessitated a shift in focus to pre-trauma predictors of PTSS. Despite the relatively low levels of PTSS, the combination of a higher pre-trauma depression score, lower estimated IQ and a larger differential corrugator EMG score during extinction trials of a fear-conditioning procedure significantly predicted higher PTSS. This finding accords well with accumulated evidence indicating that higher IQ appears to be a protective factor against developing PTSD [25] and the recent finding of Guthrie and Bryant [40] that a larger differential corrugator EMG response during extinction is predictive of a higher IES [64] score.

The process(es) underlying impaired extinction of corrugator EMG responses, lower IQ and higher pre-trauma depression symptoms appear to contribute to the pathogenesis of PTSS. Higher pre-trauma depression symptoms could reflect a propensity towards negative emotional affectivity [8]. Corrugator EMG activity is typically interpreted as reflecting emotional valence [65,66]. The persistence of a larger differential corrugator EMG response following fear conditioning, could reflect a pre-trauma propensity towards the *maintenance* of negative emotional responses over time. Greater intellectual ability, as reflected in IQ, likely provides more extensive cognitive resources for managing negative emotional responses [24]. Individuals with lower IQ would have more limited cognitive resources available for coping with negative emotions, which would contribute to their maintenance.

Stepwise logistic regression analysis identified the combination of lower estimated IQ and increased SC reactivity to loud tones as the best predictor of overall psychophysiologic reactivity during script-driven imagery. Guthrie and Bryant [37] and Pole et al. [61] previously reported that pre-trauma SC reactivity to loud tones (or noise) predicted subjective measures of PTSS. Their respective studies did not include a psychophysiologic outcome measure of PTSS. Taken together, findings from the studies of Guthrie and Bryant, Pole et al., and the present work suggest that pre-trauma individual differences in sympathetic nervous system reactivity, as manifest in larger SC responses to loud tones, can be used to predict the development of psychophysiologic and/or subjective PTSS. The inclusion of lower estimated IQ in the predictive model for post-trauma psychophysiologic reactivity suggests that more limited cognitive resources contribute to the maintenance of increased psychophysiological reactivity to trauma reminders, as well as contributing to the persistence of subjective PTSS.

Consideration of the SC and HR findings observed across studies using the loud-tone procedure, which provides an assessment of "unconditioned" responding, suggests that these measures may reflect different involvements of sympathetic and parasympathetic nervous system activity in the development and evolution of PTSS/PTSD. Skin conductance is primarily a measure of sympathetic nervous system activity [67], whereas HR is influenced by the parasympathetic, as well as sympathetic, nervous system. As noted above, there is accumulating evidence that increased SC reactivity to loud tones may be a pre-trauma predictor of PTSS, while there is very strong evidence that increased HR reactivity to loud tones is an acquired feature of PTSS/PTSD [e.g. 36,38]. Across studies of individuals with diagnosable PTSD, increased HR reactivity to loud tones has been reported in all but two studies, whereas increased SC reactivity has been less reliably obtained; interestingly, increased SC reactivity was observed in the two studies that failed to find increased HR reactivity (for review see [54]). This mixed pattern of SC and HR findings in loud-tone studies suggests that, whereas increased sympathetic tone/activity underlies the increased SC reactivity, it is reduced parasympathetic, and not increased sympathetic, tone that is responsible for the heightened HR reactivity to loud tones. This leads to the interesting possibility that heightened sensitivity of the sympathetic nervous system represents a risk factor for, whereas reduced parasympathetic tone is a consequence of, developing PTSS/PTSD.

The present study also observed a significant relationship between the magnitude of the HR response to CS + stimuli during conditioning and the posterior probability score. This provides some limited support for a positive relationship between pre-trauma conditionability and psychophysiologic reactivity to trauma-related imagery. The fact that pre-trauma SC reactivity to loud tones and HR reactivity to CS + stimuli during conditioning predicted post-trauma psychophysiologic reactivity to script-driven imagery but not subjective PTSS (i.e., IES-R) scores raises the possibility that these positive relationships primarily reflect relationships between measures of psychophysiologic reactivity and not with PTSS per se. However, the likelihood that the observed positive relationships simply reflect concordance amongst measures of psychophysiologic reactivity is challenged by the fact that several important measures of psychophysiologic reactivity (e.g., SC orienting response, SC and corrugator EMG responses to CS + trials during conditioning, HR and eyeblink EMG responses to loud tones) did not show relationships with the posterior probability score.

Several limitations of the reported work should be kept in mind. The relatively low, i.e., normal, level of PTSS severity raises the possibility that the relationships observed in the present study between predictor and outcome variables may not extend to clinical levels of PTSD. However, it is also possible that the reported findings underestimate the actual presence and strengths of these relationships, given the restricted ranges of scores and impact this may have had on the correlation estimates. It is possible that the extended time periods between the traumatic event and follow-up assessment for some individuals may have adversely impacted the observed relationships. Although, when the logistic regression analysis was adjusted for the amount of time elapsed between the traumatic event and assessment, the results did not change. Our preference not to correct for multiple t-test comparisons is an additional limitation and caution should be exercised when interpreting the univariate results.

Finally, although the pre-trauma differential corrugator EMG score for extinction contributed to the prediction of IES-R scores in the expected direction, this was due in part to an unexpected pattern of responses in the Low IES-R group. More specifically, the Low IES-R group produced larger corrugator responses to the CS- than to the CS+, resulting in a negative differential score. We believe that the negative mean value for the Low IES-R group is reliable, given the substantial sample size for this subgroup (n = 67); however, the reason for larger corrugator responses to the CS-, compared to CS+, is not clear. As noted above, increased corrugator activity is generally thought to reflect increased negative emotional valence. It may be that when the associative link between CS + and UCS was broken during extinction, participants in the Low IES-R suspected that the experimenter might change the associative relationship such that the CS- would predict the UCS. Why this sort of cognitive processing would be more apparent in the Low IES-R, compared to High IES-R, group is not clear. Regardless of the underlying explanation for this curious pattern of responding to the CS + and CS- during extinction, it is important to acknowledge the potential predictive value of this measure.

Conclusions

The present study successfully identified several predictive relationships between pre-trauma psychological and psychophysiological measures and PTSS. Of particular interest, this study found that lower pre-trauma estimated IQ, a higher depression score and a larger differential corrugator EMG response following fear conditioning predicted higher IES-R scores, suggesting that the processes underlying these indices may contribute to the pathogenesis of PTSS. The combination of lower pre-trauma estimated IQ and increased SC reactivity to loud tones were found to predict greater psychophysiological reactivity (larger posterior probability score) to trauma-related cues, suggesting that processes related to these measures my contribute to the pathophysiology of PTSS. It is important to note that the levels of PTSS and general psychopathology were quite low in our sample of police and firefighters. Even so, the severity of post-trauma symptoms is dimensional and likely is normally distributed across the population. Therefore, it is possible that the predictors of PTSS identified in this study would generalize to a population with greater levels of symptomatology. It is plausible, if not likely, that the reported findings underestimate the actual presence and strengths of relationships between pre-trauma predictor variables and post-trauma outcome measures because of the limited variability in scores.

Prospective studies that identify predictors of emotional sequelae of traumatic events are particularly challenging because they necessitate extensive data collection from a sample wherein only a subset will be exposed to a traumatic event and a relatively small percentage of those exposed to trauma will ultimately develop PTSD. Despite the inherent challenges, these efforts are an important undertaking because of their potential to inform PTSD prevention and early treatment. A primary goal of prospective studies is to discover reliable markers that can aid in identifying individuals who are at highest risk for developing PTSS/PTSD and thereby allow more extensive resiliency training or early interventions to be targeted to those most likely to need them. Such interventions would be cost prohibitive if they were to be provided *en masse* and would be unnecessary for most individuals. Although significant challenges must be overcome when conducting prospective studies of PTSS/PTSD, it is our hope that future research will examine other high-risk populations, incorporate longer follow-up times and recruit larger samples. Such work would contribute substantively to the evolving literature aimed at identifying pre-trauma risk factors for PTSS/PTSD.

Abbreviations

BDI: Beck Depression Inventory; CAPS: Clinician Administered PTSD Scale; CR: Conditioned Response; EMG: Electromyogram; HR: Heart Rate; IES-R: Impact of Event Scale-Revised; NEO-PI-R: NEO Personality Inventory-Revised; PTSD: Post-traumatic Stress Disorder; PTSS: Post-traumatic Stress Symptoms; SC: Skin Conductance; SCID: Structured Clinical Interview for DSM-IV; SCL-90-R GSI: Symptom Checklist 90-Revised; SSPQ: SCID Screen Patient Questionnaire; STAI: State-Trait Anxiety Inventory; UCR: Unconditioned Response; UCS: Unconditioned Stimulus; WAIS-R: Wechsler Adult Intelligence Scale-Revised.

Competing interests

The authors declare no competing interests.

Acknowledgements

This research was supported by U.S. Public Health Service grant R01-MH60315 and Department of Veterans Affairs Merit Review grant to Scott P. Orr. The funding source had no involvement in the study design, collection, analysis or interpretation of the data, writing of the report and decision to submit the paper for publication. We thank Heike Croteau; Sgt. Thomas Fleming, Director, Lowell Police Academy, Lowell, MA; Dr. John Connell and Gary Courtney, Fire Technologies Program, Lakes Region Community College, Laconia, NH; and Captain/Drillmaster Hugh Duffy, Boston Fire Academy, Boston Fire Department, Boston, MA for their invaluable assistance with this project. We would also like to express our appreciation to the police and firefighters for their willingness to participate.

Author details

[1]Department of Psychiatry, Massachusetts General Hospital and Harvard Medical School, Charlestown, MA, USA. [2]Department of Veterans Affairs Medical Center, Manchester, NH, USA. [3]National Center for PTSD, Women's Health Sciences Division, VA Boston Healthcare System, Boston, MA, USA. [4]Department of Psychiatry, Boston University School of Medicine, Boston, MA, USA. [5]General Medicine Division, Massachusetts General Hospital and Harvard Medical School, Boston, MA, USA.

Authors contributions

SPO contributed to the conception and design of the study, oversaw the conduct of the study, oversaw management and scoring of the psychophysiological data, consulted on the data analyses and drafted the manuscript. NBL conducted all diagnostic interviews and assessments and helped edit the final manuscript. MLM recruited all police and firefighter participants, served as liaison with the training academies and followed participants for the occurrence of a traumatic event. SLP contributed to the drafting and editing of the manuscript. RKP contributed to the conception and design of the study and contributed to the drafting and editing of the manuscript. YC performed the statistical analyses and contributed to drafting and editing of the Results section of the manuscript. All authors read and approved the final manuscript.

References

1. Orr SP, Pitman RK, Lasko NB, Herz LR: **Psychophysiologic assessment of posttraumatic stress disorder imagery in World War II and Korean Combat Veterans.** *J Abnorm Psychol* 1993, **102**:152–159.
2. Pitman RK, Orr SP, Forgue DF, de Jong JB, Claiborn JM: **Psychophysiology of PTSD imagery in Vietnam combat veterans.** *Arch Gen Psychiatry* 1987, **44**:970–975.
3. Shalev AY, Orr SP, Pitman RK: **Psychophysiologic assessment of traumatic imagery in Israeli civilian post-traumatic stress disorder patients.** *Am J Psychiatry* 1993, **150**:620–624.
4. Breslau N, Davis G, Andreski P, Peterson E: **Traumatic events and posttraumatic stress disorder in an urban population of young adults.** *Arch Gen Psychiatry* 1991, **48**:216–222.
5. Blanchard EB, Hickling EJ, Forneris CA, Taylor AE, Buckley TC, Loos WR, Jaccard J: **Prediction of remission of acute posttraumatic stress disorder in motor vehicle accident victims.** *J Trauma Stress* 1997, **10**:215–234.
6. McFarlane AC: **The aetiology of post-traumatic stress disorders following a natural disaster.** *Br J Psychiatry* 1988, **152**:116–121.
7. McFarlane AC: **The longitudinal course of posttraumatic morbidity: the range of outcomes and their predictors.** *J Nerv Ment Dis* 1988, **176**:30–40.
8. Clarke LA, Watson D, Mineka S: **Temperament, personality, and the mood and anxiety disorders.** *J Abnorm Psychol* 1994, **103**:103–116.
9. Pitman RK, Orr SP: **Test of the conditioning model of neurosis: differential aversive conditioning of angry and neutral facial expressions in anxiety disorder patients.** *J Abnorm Psychol* 1986, **95**:208–213.
10. Orr SP, Solomon Z, Peri T, Pitman RK, Shalev AY: **Physiologic responses to loud tones in Israeli veterans of the 1973 Yom Kippur War.** *Biol Psychiatry* 1997, **41**:319–326.
11. Orr SP, Metzger LJ, Lasko NB, Macklin ML, Peri T, Pitman RK: ***De novo* conditioning in trauma-exposed individuals with and without post-traumatic stress disorder.** *J Abnorm Psychol* 2000, **109**:290–298.
12. Orr SP, Milad MR, Metzger LJ, Lasko NB, Gilbertson MW, Pitman RK: **Effects of beta blockade, PTSD diagnosis, and explicit threat on the extinction and retention of an aversively conditioned response.** *Biol Psychol* 2006, **73**:262–271.
13. Pitman RK, Lanes DM, Williston SK, Guillaume JL, Metzger LJ, Gehr GM, Orr SP: **Psychophysiologic assessment of posttraumatic stress disorder in breast cancer patients.** *Psychosomatics* 2001, **42**:133–140.
14. Blechert J, Michael T, Vriends N, Margraf J, Wilhelm FH: **Fear conditioning in posttraumatic stress disorder: evidence for delayed extinction of autonomic, experiential, and behavioural responses.** *Behav Res Ther* 2007, **45**:2019–2033.
15. Orr SP, Claiborn JM, Altman B, de Jong JB, Forgue DF, Herz LR, Pitman RK: **Psychometric profile of PTSD, anxious, and healthy Vietnam veterans: Correlations with psychophysiological responses.** *J Consult Clin Psychol* 1990, **58**:329–335.
16. O'Toole BI, Marshall RP, Schureck RJ, Dobson M: **Risk factors for posttraumatic stress disorder in Australian Vietnam veterans.** *Aust N Z J Psychiatry* 1998, **32**:21–31.
17. Orr SP, Lasko NB, Shalev A, Pitman RK: **Physiologic responses to loud tones in Vietnam veterans with PTSD.** *J Abnorm Psychol* 1995, **104**:75–82.
18. Peri T, Ben-Shakhar G, Orr SP, Shalev AY: **Psychophysiologic assessment of aversive conditioning in posttraumatic stress disorder.** *Biol Psychiatry* 2000, **47**:512–519.
19. Shalev AY, Orr SP, Peri P, Schreiber S, Pitman RK: **Physiologic responses to loud tones in Israeli PTSD patients.** *Arch Gen Psychiatry* 1992, **49**:870–975.
20. Bramsen I, Dirkzwager AJE, van der Ploeg HM: **Predeployment personality traits and exposure to trauma as predictors of posttraumatic stress symptoms: a prospective study of former peacekeepers.** *Am J Psychiatry* 2000, **157**:1115–1119.
21. McFarlane AC: **Avoidance and intrusion in posttraumatic stress disorder.** *J Nerv Ment Dis* 1992, **180**:439–445.
22. Fauerbach JA, Lawrence JW, Schmidt CW, Munster AM, Costa PT: **Personality predictors of Injury-related posttraumatic stress disorder.** *J Nerv Ment Dis* 2000, **188**:510–517.
23. Talbert SF, Braswell LC, Albrecht JW, Hyer L, Boudewyns P: **NEO-PI profiles in PTSD as a function of trauma level.** *J Clin Psychol* 1993, **49**:663–669.
24. Gilbertson MW, Paulus LA, Williston SK, Gurvits TV, Lasko NB, Pitman RK, Orr SP: **Neurocognitive function in monozygotic twins discordant for combat exposure: relationship to posttraumatic stress disorder.** *J Abnorm Psychol* 2006, **115**:484–495.
25. Macklin ML, Metzger LJ, Litz BT, McNally RJ, Lasko NB, Orr SP, Pitman RK: **Lower pre-Combat intelligence is a risk factor for post-traumatic stress disorder.** *J Consult Clin Psychol* 1998, **66**:323–326.
26. Pitman RK, Orr SP, Lowenhagen MJ, Macklin ML, Altman A: **Pre-Vietnam contents of PTSD veterans' service medical and personnel records.** *Compr Psychiatry* 1991, **32**:1–7.
27. Vasterling JJ, Duke LM, Brailey K, Constans JI, Sutker PB: **Attention, learning, and memory performances and intellectual resources in Vietnam veterans: PTSD and no disorder comparisons.** *Neuropsychology* 2002, **16**:5–14.
28. Carlier IVE, Lamberts RD, Gersons BPR: **Risk factors for posttraumatic stress symptomatology in police officers: a prospective analysis.** *J Nerv Ment Dis* 1997, **185**:498–506.
29. Zoellner T, Rabe S, Karl A, Maercker A: **Posttraumatic Growth in Accident Survivors: Openness and Optimism as Predictors of Its Constructive or Illusory Sides.** *J Clin Psychol* 2008, **64**:245–263.
30. Davis M: **The mammalian startle response.** In *Neural Mechanisms of Startle.* Edited by Eaton RC. New York: Plenum; 1984:287–351.
31. Griffin MG: **A prospective assessment of auditory startle alterations in rape and physical assault survivors.** *J Trauma Stress* 2008, **21**:91–99.
32. Pole N, Neylan TC, Best SR, Orr SP, Marmar CR: **Fear-potentiated startle and posttraumatic stress symptoms in urban police officers.** *J Trauma Stress* 2003, **16**:471–479.
33. Shalev AY, Peri P, Orr SP, Bonne O, Pitman RK: **Auditory startle responses in help-seeking trauma survivors.** *Psychiatry Res* 1997, **69**:1–7.
34. Carson MA, Metzger LJ, Lasko NB, Paulus LA, Morse AE, Pitman RK, Orr SP: **Physiologic reactivity to startling tones in female nurse veterans with PTSD.** *J Trauma Stress* 2007, **20**:657–666.
35. Metzger LJ, Orr SP, Berry NJ, Ahern CE, Lasko NB, Pitman RK: **Physiologic reactivity to startling tones in women with PTSD.** *J Abnorm Psychol* 1999, **108**:347–352.
36. Orr SP, Metzger LJ, Lasko NB, Macklin ML, Shalev AY, Hu F, Pitman RK: **Psychophysiologic responses to sudden, loud tones in monozygotic twins discordant for combat exposure: relationship to posttraumatic stress disorder.** *Arch Gen Psychiatry* 2003, **60**:283–288.
37. Guthrie RM, Bryant RA: **Auditory startle response in firefighters before and after trauma exposure.** *Am J Psychiatry* 2005, **162**:283–290.
38. Shalev AY, Peri T, Brandes D, Freedman S, Orr SP, Pitman R: **Auditory startle response in trauma survivors with posttraumatic stress disorder: a prospective study.** *Am J Psychiatry* 2000, **157**:255–261.
39. Wessa M, Flor H: **Failure of extinction of fear response in posttraumatic stress disorder: evidence from second-order conditioning.** *Am J Psychiatry* 2007, **164**:1684–1692.
40. Guthrie RM, Bryant RA: **Extinction learning before trauma and subsequent posttraumatic stress.** *Psychosom Med* 2006, **68**:307–311.
41. Costa PT, McCrae RR: ***NEO-PI-R professional manual.*** Odessa, FL: Psychological Assessment Resources, Inc; 1992.
42. Shipley WC: **A self-administering scale for measuring intellectual impairment and deterioration.** *J Psychol* 1940, **9**:371–377.
43. Zachary RA: ***Shipley Institute of Living Scale,*** *Revised Manual.* Los Angeles: Western Psychological Services; 1986.
44. First MB, Spitzer RL, Gibbon M, Williams JBW: ***Structured Clinical Interview for Axis I DSM-IV Disorders,*** *Version 2.0 (May 1994 Draft).* New York: Biometrics Research Department; 1994.
45. Weathers FW, Keane TM, Davidson JR: **Clinician-Administered PTSD Scale: a review of the first ten years of research.** *Depress Anxiety* 2001, **13**:132–156.
46. First MB, Gibbon M, Williams JBW, Spitzer RL: ***SCID Screen Patient Questionnaire Computer Program for DSM-IV,*** *Windows Version.* New York, NY: Multi-Health Systems Inc. & American Psychiatric Press, Inc; 1996.
47. Weathers FW, Pitman RK: ***Stressful Life Events Checklist.*** *Unpublished manuscript, 1996.*: ; 1983.
48. Derogatis LR: ***SCL-90-R: Administration, Scoring & Procedures Manual-II for the R(evised) Version.*** Towson, MD: Clinical Psychometric Research; 1983.
49. Spielberger CD, Gorsuch RL, Lushene RE: ***Manual for the State-Trait Anxiety Inventory (Self-Evaluation Questionnaire).*** Palo Alto: Consulting Psychologists Press; 1990.
50. Beck AT, Rush A, Shaw BF, Emery G: ***Cognitive Therapy of Depression.*** New York: Guilford Press; 1979.
51. Fridlund AJ, Cacioppo JT: **Guidelines for human electromyographic research.** *Psychophysiology* 1986, **23**:567–589.

52. Fowles DC, Christie MJ, Edelberg R, Grings WW, Lykken DT, Venables PH: **Publication recommendations for electrodermal measurements.** *Psychophysiology* 1981, **18**:232–239.
53. Weiss DS, Marmar CR: **The Impact of Event Scale-Revised**. In *Assessing Psychological Trauma and PTSD*. Edited by Wilson JP, Keane TM. New York: Guilford Press; 1997:399–411.
54. Orr SP, Metzger LJ, Miller MW, Kaloupek DG: **Psychophysiological assessment of PTSD**. In *Assessing Psychological Trauma and PTSD*. 2nd edition. Edited by Wilson JP, Keane TM. New York: Guilford Publications; 2004:289–343.
55. Pitman RK, Orr SP, Forgue DF, Altman B, DeJong JB, Herz LR: **Psychophysiologic responses to combat imagery of Vietnam veterans with post-traumatic stress disorder vs. other anxiety disorders.** *J Abnorm Psychol* 1990, **99**:49–54.
56. Pineles SL, Orr MR, Orr SP: **An alternative scoring method for skin conductance responding in a differential fear conditioning paradigm with a long-duration conditioned stimulus.** *Psychophysiology* 2009, **46**:984–995.
57. Carson MA, Paulus LA, Lasko NB, Metzger LJ, Wolfe J, Orr SP, Pitman RK: **Psychophysiologic assessment of post-traumatic stress disorder in Vietnam nurse veterans who witnessed injury or death.** *J Consult Clin Psychol* 2000, **68**:890–897.
58. Orr SP, Lasko NB, Metzger LJ, Berry NJ, Ahern CE, Pitman RK: **Psychophysiologic assessment of women with PTSD resulting from childhood sexual abuse.** *J Consult Clin Psychol* 1998, **66**:906–913.
59. Orr SP, McNally RJ, Rosen GM, Shalev AY: **Psychophysiological reactivity: implications for conceptualizing PTSD**. In *Posttraumatic Stress Disorder: Issues and Controversies*. Edited by Rosen GM. United Kingdom: John Wiley & Sons, Ltd; 2004:101–126.
60. Dempster AP, Laird NM, Rubin DB: **Maximum Likelihood from Incomplete Data via the EM Algorithm.** *Journal of the Royal Statistical Society Ser. B.* 1977, **39**:1–38.
61. Pole N, Neylan TC, Otte C, Henn-Hasse C, Metzler TJ, Marmar CR: **Propsective prediction of posttraumatic stress disorder symptoms using fear potentiated auditory startle responses.** *Biol Psychiatry* 2009, **65**:235–240.
62. Bryant RA, Harvey AG: **Posttraumatic stress reactions in volunteer firefighters.** *J Trauma Stress* 1996, **9**:51–62.
63. Shalev AY, Freedman S, Peri T, Brandes D, Sahar T, Orr SP, Pitman RK: **Prospective study of posttraumatic stress disorder and depression following trauma.** *Am J Psychiatry* 1998, **155**:630–637.
64. Horowitz MJ, Wilner N, Alvarez W: **Impact of Event Scale: A measure of subjective stress.** *Psychosom Med* 1979, **41**:208–218.
65. Fridlund AJ, Izard CE: **Electromyographic studies of facial expressions of emotion and patterns of emotion**. In *Social Psychophysiology: A Sourcebook*. Edited by Cacioppo JT, Petty RE. New York: Guilford Press; 1983:243–286.
66. Larsen JT, Norris CJ, Cacioppo JT: **Effects of positive and negative affect on electromyographic activity over *zygomaticus major* and *corrugator supercilii*.** *Psychophysiology* 2003, **40**:776–785.
67. Lang PJ, Bradley MM, Cuthbert BN: **Emotion, attention and the startle reflex.** *Psychol Rev* 1990, **97**:377–395.

4

Somatic therapies for treatment-resistant depression: ECT, TMS, VNS, DBS

Cristina Cusin* and Darin D Dougherty

Abstract

The field of non-pharmacological therapies for treatment resistant depression (TRD) is rapidly evolving and new somatic therapies are valuable options for patients who have failed numerous other treatments. A major challenge for clinicians (and patients alike) is how to integrate the results from published clinical trials in the clinical decision-making process.

We reviewed the literature for articles reporting results for clinical trials in particular efficacy data, contraindications and side effects of somatic therapies including electroconvulsive therapy (ECT), transcranial magnetic stimulation (TMS), vagal nerve stimulation (VNS) and deep brain stimulation (DBS). Each of these devices has an indication for patients with different level of treatment resistance, based on acuteness of illness, likelihood of response, costs and associated risks. ECT is widely available and its effects are relatively rapid in severe TRD, but its cognitive adverse effects may be cumbersome. TMS is safe and well tolerated, and it has been approved by FDA for adults who have failed to respond to one antidepressant, but its use in TRD is still controversial as it is not supported by rigorous double-blind randomized clinical trials. The options requiring surgical approach are VNS and DBS. VNS has been FDA-approved for TRD, however it is not indicated for management of acute illness. DBS for TRD is still an experimental area of investigation and double-blind clinical trials are underway.

Keywords: Treatment resistant depression, Electroconvulsive therapy, Transcranial magnetic stimulation, Vagal Nerve Stimulation, Deep brain stimulation

Introduction

Major depressive disorder (MDD) affects approximately 18 million people at any one time in the US alone, with a 17.1% lifetime incidence, and is associated with a high rate of morbidity and mortality [1].

Pharmacotherapy is effective in more than half of depressed patients; however, between 20% and 30% of patients suffering from depression may have "treatment-resistant depression" (TRD).

A recent review [2] compared five different models for classifying TRD, evolving from simply rating the adequacy of antidepressant trials to considering a more complex array of factors, including duration of illness, severity and treatment response. However, the validity and reliability of those models have been the focus of only a few studies, and their value for predicting outcome in clinical practice is still unclear.

* Correspondence: ccusin@partners.org
Division of Neurotherapeutics, Department of Psychiatry, Massachusetts General Hospital, 149 13th Street, Rm 2612, Charlestown, MA 02129, USA

The aim of this paper is to review new somatic therapies utilized in the treatment of TRD (defined broadly as failure to respond to two or more adequate trials of antidepressants in the current episode) in comparison with electroconvulsive therapy (ECT), considered the "gold standard" for patients with TRD.

Methods

A literature search was performed using PubMed, Ovid Medline, Cochrane Database of Systematic Reviews and PsychINFO for articles published between 1990 and July 2011 with the following search terms: *ECT* or *electroconvulsive therapy, transcranial magnetic stimulation, TMS, depression, treatment-resistant depression, VNS* or *vagal nerve stimulation, DBS* or *deep brain stimulation, clinical trial.* Out of 807 articles retrieved, we included articles written in English that reported clinical trial results of an original sample, and 98 articles were ultimately reviewed in detail. The reference sections of the articles were checked for cross-references. For ECT, we included only the studies comparing efficacy of ECT with other devices. For DBS, given the absence of randomized controlled trials, we included all clinical trials and case reports.

Results

Electroconvulsive Therapy (ECT)

ECT consists of the application of an electric stimulus to the surface of the head, with the aim of inducing a seizure. The parameters of the stimulus can vary widely (pulsewidth from 0.3 to 1 msec, frequency from 20 to 120 Hz, duration of the stimulus 0.5-8 sec) and are adjusted for each individual patient, according to seizure threshold, clinical efficacy and side effects. The clinical efficacy of ECT in TRD is well established, with 60% to 90% rate of acute response in TRD [3], and it is indicated specifically in severe psychotic depression, catatonia and delirious mania.

ECT is associated with a number of common, but usually temporary, adverse effects such as arrhythmias, headaches, muscle aches, and nausea. Serious medical complications are exceedingly rare, even in patients with severe cardiovascular risk factors. The most common adverse effect of ECT is acute cognitive impairment lasting from few minutes to few days [4] or some form of amnesia, either anterograde or retrograde. More persistent deficits seem to be associated with older age, sine wave stimulation and bitemporal electrode placement [5]. The treatment is administered two to three times per week, and the patient requires an escort, due to driving restrictions after the treatment. ECT is available in academic and community settings, and the cost for each treatment session generally includes fees for the psychiatrist administering the treatment, the anesthesiologist, and the facility where the treatment is delivered. Although these costs vary considerably across centers, a course of 10 outpatient ECT treatments can cost approximately $10,000 to $15,000.

Transcranial Magnetic Stimulation (TMS)

Transcranial magnetic stimulation (TMS) was introduced in 1985 as a technique to stimulate the cerebral cortex non-invasively [6]. A TMS device generates a strong magnetic field, inducing an electric current in a specific area, and this in turn induces intracerebral currents in associated neural circuits. The "single pulse TMS" has been utilized in research on localization of brain functions, while "repetitive TMS" (rTMS) has been used for treatment related studies. It is called "high frequency rTMS" if the stimulus frequency is above 1 Hz, or "low frequency rTM" if stimulus frequency is below 1 Hz. Low frequency rTMS is thought to inhibit cortical firing, while high frequency rTMS is thought to activate it.

The initial application of rTMS for depression was driven by functional imaging data showing reduced activity in the left prefrontal cortex (L DLPF) in patients with depression [7,8]. More recently, the investigators have focused on the idea of an imbalance in the activity of the frontal lobes (hypoactivity in the left frontal lobe and excessive inhibitory activity in the right frontal lobe), therefore leading to an alternative pattern for the treatment of depression combining low-frequency (suppressive) rTMS of the right dorso-lateral prefrontal cortex (R DLPF) with rTMS at high frequency to the L DLPF.

TMS is a non-invasive technique, therefore not requiring anesthesia or driving restrictions, and it is safely performed as an outpatient procedure. In general, TMS is well tolerated, with no evidence of cognitive impairment and with exceedingly rare medical complications. Rare seizures have been reported in the past, but the risk is substantially decreased with current treatment guidelines. The most common adverse effects are headaches and facial pain. A therapeutic TMS course of treatments can be performed by a trained technician, and a typical TMS session lasts between 30 and 60 minutes; sessions take place 5 times a week, usually for a period of 4 to 5 weeks, for a total of 20 to 30 sessions. One of the major obstacles is the time commitment for patients, which entails daily visits of one to two hours to the facility where TMS is provided. The average cost of each session is between $300 and $400, leading to a total cost for an average course of TMS between $6,000 and $12,000.

Efficacy of TMS

Several meta-analyses of rTMS clinical trials have been published in the past ten years, with mixed results. The majority of TMS trials targeted the L DLPC with high-frequency stimulation, while only a few targeted the R DLPC with either low-frequency stimulation [9-11] or both [12-16]. The earliest meta-analysis [17] yielded a positive result for rTMS compared to a sham control; however, it included only five controlled studies and excluded the only negative depression trial for rTMS that had been published at the time [18].

In 2002, Martin and colleagues published a Cochrane review of all the TMS studies available to that date [19]. The authors found that high-frequency (> 1 Hz) prefrontal DLPF rTMS and low-frequency (≤ 1 Hz) R DLPF rTMS were statistically superior to a sham comparison, but only at one time point (immediately after two weeks of treatment), and this difference was not sustained two weeks later. The overall difference between active and sham treatment was not large, though statistically significant, and the authors concluded that there was "no strong evidence to support the benefit of rTMS as an antidepressant treatment." Only one meta-analysis, which included 6 trials, found a negative result for high-frequency prefrontal DLPF rTMS compared to sham [20].

The largest controlled study was sponsored by a TMS equipment manufacturer and involved a double-blind, multisite trial with 301 medication-free patients with MDD who had not benefited from prior treatments. Subjects were randomly assigned to either active (n = 155) or sham TMS (n = 146) conditions [21]. The study found that active TMS was significantly superior to sham TMS at weeks 4 and 6, and its results were the basis for the Food and Drug Administration's (FDA) approval of TMS for patients who had not improved following one antidepressant trial.

The most recent meta-analysis [22] included 34 clinical trials comparing rTMS to sham treatment. This analysis showed a statistically significant difference; however, other papers critically analyzed the methods applied in the clinical trials [23-25] and suggested that though the results showed strong statistical evidence of efficacy, the clinical results were not sufficient to recommend the implementation of TMS in clinical practice because of the methodological limitations and heterogeneity of the studies.

In fact, while the application site of TMS was the L DLPF in more than 90% of the studies, the stimulation parameters were extremely variable and the level of severity of the patients enrolled was generally low, as only 3 out of 34 studies included patients who had failed 2 or more antidepressants in the current episode.

To address those criticisms, the NIH sponsored a large multicenter study in 2009 [26]. In this trial, the parameters of rTMS were standardized to maximize the likelihood of robust antidepressant effect (five times per week with TMS at 10 Hz, 120% of motor threshold, 3000 pulses/session, for 4-6 weeks) and key methodological limitations were addressed (e.g., adequacy of masking, validity of sham treatment, training of raters and reliability of outcome evaluation, magnetic resonance imaging adjustment for proper scalp placement). The results of the primary efficacy analysis revealed a significant difference in the proportion of remitters (14.1% on rTMS versus 5.1% sham, $p = .02$); however, the total number of responders (n = 19) and remitters (n = 18) was overall very low and the number needed to treat (NNT) was 10. It is notable that in this study, as in the previous ones, most of the remitters had low antidepressant treatment resistance at the time of study entry.

Efficacy of TMS IN TRD

A few studies have investigated the use of TMS in patients with TRD specifically, usually in combination with antidepressant drugs. Overall the results reported have been positive, but it is very difficult to draw any conclusion because of small sample sizes, differing inclusion criteria (i.e., inclusion of patients with bipolar depression), variable treatment schedule and high dropout rate. Three were small open-label studies [27-29], and one was double-blind, sham-controlled study of the combination of TMS and escitalopram [30]. In all the aforementioned studies, the level of treatment resistance was low, and only one trial randomized patients with different levels of resistance to unilateral TMS, bilateral or sham [31]. Based on published data, the role for TMS in the treatment of TRD is still unclear.

TMS comparison with ECT

One question that is particularly relevant for the clinician is how TMS compares to ECT in patients with TRD. There have been six prospective studies to date comparing TMS and ECT in patients with a major depressive episode (MDD or bipolar depression) [32-37]. The sample size in each study was usually small, between 25 and 42 patients, and out of those six, three studies indicated superiority for ECT and three found no difference between the two devices. The results were reviewed in a meta-analysis, including a total of 113 TMS patients and 102 ECT patients, yielding a combined 38.0% rate of response or remission rate for TMS versus 58.8% for ECT. This resulted in a highly significant difference in favor of ECT (chi sq = 9.267, $p = 0.0023$) [38]. Major criticisms common to all these studies were that they generally utilized low energy and low frequency for both ECT and TMS, included patients with psychotic features, and did not adequately describe blinding techniques. Despite these limitations, it seems that ECT has superior efficacy, in particular for those patients with severe depression, psychotic features and higher level of treatment-resistance.

TMS summary

In 2008, the U.S. FDA approved rTMS as a treatment for adults with MDD who "have not responded to a single antidepressant medication in the current episode." Since then, one large NIMH-sponsored, multicenter, randomized, sham-controlled study has been conducted [26], and this trial showed a statistically significant difference between the treatments, but overall low rates for both response and remission.

In general, TMS is indicated in adults with MDD who "have not responded to a single antidepressant medication in the current episode." However, numerous questions still persist about the magnitude of the efficacy of TMS in patients with TRD.

Due to concerns that the antidepressant effects of rTMS are not sufficiently robust to be considered "clinically meaningful," insurance companies have often been reluctant to reimburse for TMS treatment

Vagal Nerve Stimulation (VNS)

Vagal Nerve Stimulation (VNS) was approved for treatment-refractory epilepsy in Europe in 1994 and in the US in 1997. Early clinical observations of improvement of mood symptoms in epilepsy patients led to a pilot study of VNS on mood in patients with primary diagnosis of epilepsy. The Cyberonics VNS device currently available on the market consists of a titanium-encased lithium battery, a lead wire system with electrodes, and an anchor tether to secure leads to the vagus nerve. The generator is implanted in the left chest wall and connected with a lead to the left vagus nerve. The device is implanted in a procedure usually lasting 1 to 2 hours, either under local or general anesthesia. Following the surgery, the device is activated telemetrically by a wand connected to a hand-held computerized device. The adjustment of treatment parameters, including selection of stimulus intensity, duration and on/off interval, is non-invasive and is performed using an external telemetric wand. Stimulator settings are programmed to deliver intermittent stimulation with a current of 0.25–3.0 mA, a frequency of 20–50 Hz, a pulse width of 130-500 ms, and duty cycle (e.g. 30 seconds on, 5 minutes off). The mechanism of action of VNS is not completely understood and its effects are thought to be relatively slow, in the order of months; for this reason, VNS is not indicated for the relief of acute depressive exacerbations.

The safety of VNS is well established from its use in the treatment of epilepsy. The side effects of VNS are generally mild and are associated with stimulation (i.e., the "on" phase of the cycle). Because VNS causes stimulation of the superior and recurrent laryngeal nerves, it is frequently associated with problems ranging from alteration of the voice, coughing, throat pain and hoarseness (very common), reversible bradyarrhythmias and obstructive sleep apnea. Infections associated with the hardware are infrequent but possible. Regarding psychiatric adverse effects, the rate of stimulation-induced switch to mania or hypomania in the VNS trials was low in the pivotal trial by Rush and colleagues [39] (<0.01% at one year), and those symptoms subsided with adjustment of stimulation parameters.

VNS Efficacy IN TRD

In psychiatry, VNS has been developed primarily as adjunctive therapy for patients with TRD who have failed to respond or have declined ECT; therefore, no comparison with ECT is available. The first open-label trial of VNS in depression enrolled 30 patients with a major depressive episode (MDD or bipolar depression) who had failed at least two adequate antidepressant trials (the average number of failed trials was 4.8 ± 2.7). VNS was used as augmentation strategy, and the subjects received 10 weeks of stimulation in combination with their medication regimen. The results at 10 weeks were a response rate of 40% and a remission rate of 17% [40].

The second pilot study combined the initial study cohort with another sample of 30 patients, followed for 12 weeks, and obtained a response rate of 30% and remission of 15% [41]. The higher degree of treatment resistance in the second pilot study may have been a significant factor in the less favorable outcome. Similar results were reported by Schlaepfer and colleagues in an open-label European study including 74 patients [42]. The striking finding in the long-term follow-up of both those studies was the apparent increase over time in response and remission rates [43,44].

The largest (n =235) randomized, sham-controlled, multicenter study of adjunctive VNS, which enrolled patients with higher level of treatment-resistance (failed to respond to two or more monotherapies and two augmentations, failure to respond to ECT), did not find a significant difference between active and sham groups at 12 weeks (15% and 10%, for response and remission respectively) [39]. However, follow-up observations of this cohort suggested a cumulative beneficial effect of treatment over time, reaching response rates between 27% and 34% and remission of 15% at one year [45], with similar outcomes for patients with MDD and BP depression [46]. It is very interesting that in the long term follow-up, the authors reported a decline in suicide attempts, diminished levels of suicidal ideation, and fewer hospitalizations for depression in patients with VNS compared with patients with the same level of symptom severity but taking medications [47].

Overall the number needed to treat (NNT) for VNS ranged from 4 to 10, which, given the level of treatment resistance in this population, is clinically significant. In 2005, based on the clinical trial data, the FDA approved the use of VNS as an adjunctive therapy for treatment-resistant depression in adult patients who have failed 4 or more medications. Unfortunately the same data were deemed insufficient for approval of reimbursement under Medicare/Medicaid, therefore seriously limiting the access of patients to VNS.

The estimated cost for the surgical implantation of VNS in day surgery is on the order of $40,000 to $45.000. Furthermore, this estimate does not include the cost of post-operative device adjustments ($350-$620), which are rather frequent at the beginning of treatment and may significantly impact the total costs of the treatment.

VNS summary

The safety of VNS is well established from its use in the treatment of epilepsy for almost two decades, and it appears to be effective in patients with MDD or Bipolar II disorder with low to moderate, but not extreme, antidepressant resistance. VNS is usually considered as an adjunct to pharmacologic treatment, and it can safely be combined with ECT in case of an acute relapse. Because its effects take much longer to appear compared to antidepressants or ECT, VNS cannot be considered a treatment for acute TRD. The major barriers preventing its diffusion in clinical practice of this device are the elevated cost and the lack of reimbursement by insurance providers in the US at present.

Deep Brain Stimulation (DBS)

DBS is a reversible neurosurgical procedure, consisting of implanting electrodes at specific anatomical locations and delivering an electrical impulse of variable intensity and frequency through those electrodes. DBS is thought to induce an electrical field that alters complex firing patterns of the neurons and thus modifies activity in the neuronal circuits. DBS has been utilized for treatment-refractory essential tremor and is approved for Parkinson's disease [48] and dystonia. In 2009, DBS was approved for treatment of otherwise intractable obsessive-compulsive disorder (OCD) in Europe and in US.

Since the early 1960s, it has been observed that both acute and chronic stimulation could induce mood changes, including hypomania, dysphoria, and anhedonia. These observations led to the development of clinical trials to test the possible efficacy of DBS in treatment-refractory mood disorders. A number of research groups are currently investigating different sites for implantation of electrodes (for a complete review see [49]).

1. Subcingulate –Broadmann area 25 (SCG 25) - Mayberg and colleagues have demonstrated the integral role of the subgenual cingulate cortex in both normal and pathological shifts in mood [50]. Moreover, other studies have indicated an association between a clinical response to antidepressants and decrease in metabolism in limbic and striatal areas (subgenual cingulate cortex, hippocampus, insula, and pallidum) and increase in metabolism in dorsal cortical areas (prefrontal, parietal, anterior, and posterior cingulate cortex).
2. Ventral anterior internal capsule/ventral striatum (VC/VS) - The dorsal and ventral prefrontal cortex (PFC) have been found to be dysfunctional in neuroimaging studies of patients with MDD. These regions are nodes in a corticostriatalthalamocortical (CSTC) circuit that also includes components of the striatum and thalamus. The VC/VS target for DBS was developed following studies of gamma-knife capsulotomy for obsessive-compulsive disorder (OCD) and investigated in early studies by Nuttin [51] and Greenberg [52]. In those patients with primary OCD, a significant improvement was noticed in depressive symptoms, leading to the investigation of this target in MDD. Functional neuroimaging studies in DBS subjects showed activation of the ventral pre-frontal cortex, striatum, and thalamus during acute stimulation of the VC/VS target [53].
3. Nucleus accumbens (NAC) and ventral striatum - The reward circuitry of the ventral striatum and NAC has been associated with drug addiction and depression. The NAC and ventral striatum receive projections primarily from the anterior cingulate cortex, insular cortex, and orbitofrontal cortex. The NAC then projects to the dorsomedial nucleus of the thalamus by way of the ventral tegmental area, ventral pallidum, and substantia nigra—which in turn projects back to the prefrontal cortex, orbitofrontal cortex, anterior cingulate cortex, amygdala, and hypothalamus; this forms the limbic loop of the basal ganglia [54].
4. Inferior thalamic peduncle (ITP) - The ITP is a bundle of fibers that connects the thalamic system to the orbitofrontal cortex. This system is thought to induce electrocortical synchronization and to allow the inhibition of irrelevant stimuli, thus allowing selective attention. The ITP has been identified by Velasco and colleagues [55] as a potential stimulation target for TRD. At present there is only one case report of successful DBS electrode implantation in the ITP for refractory depression [56].
5. Lateral habenula (LH) - The LH has been proposed as a putative target for DBS. The habenular nuclear complex projects to the locus ceruleus, medial dorsal frontal cortex, orbitofrontal cortex, insula and mesolimbic areas, and ventral tegmentum/brainstem. At present there is one case report of DBS at the LH for MDD [57].

Implantation of DBS

The implantation of DBS electrodes and batteries is a complex neurosurgical procedure. Under stereotactic guidance, two electrodes are placed in deep structures of the brain, relative to a set of anatomical landmarks. Two programmable neurostimulators are implanted in the chest area under the clavicle and are connected to the corresponding electrode by extension wires under general anesthesia. Systematic outpatient adjustment of stimulation parameters (active contacts, amplitude, duration, frequency) and frequent follow-ups are necessary, especially during the first 6-12 months after implantation. The rates of surgical complications are quite variable and include intracranial hemorrhage, infections, and rarely stroke, lead erosion and lead migration.

From the psychiatric point of view, there is a risk of developing manic or hypomanic symptoms, anxiety, or worsening depression, but those symptoms are in general transient and respond to modification in parameters of stimulation. Suicides have been reported in patients with movement disorders and depression implanted with DBS at different targets.

DBS in treatment-resistant patients requires a dedicated multidisciplinary team of neurosurgeons, psychiatrists, neuropsychologists and support staff. The estimated cost of the implant is approximately $200,000 -$250,000, including device implantation and hospital stay but not including preoperative assessments, travel expenses, or costs possibly related to surgical complications. Replacements of the batteries add to the total burden for the patient, being necessary every 12-24 months on average, with an estimated cost of approximately $95,000 each time for hardware replacement and surgery. It is difficult to estimate the total additional cost of the sessions necessary to adjust the parameters, between $350 and $650 with an initial frequency of every two weeks, then every month on average for the first year. A more comprehensive evaluation of costs of DBS in patients with Parkinson's disorder outlined the importance of using broader outcome measures of quality of life to calculate the true impact of DBS on patients and their caregivers [58].

DBS Efficacy IN TRD

To our knowledge, preliminary double-blind, randomized, sham-controlled studies are being conducted for two targets, SC25 and VC/VS, and the results have not been published yet. In literature, open-label studies have been published for three targets: SC25, VC/VS and NAC.

1. SCG25
   The early open-label study recruited 20 patients [59] with an MDE and a level of treatment-resistance of 4 or 5. For this cohort, the follow-up has reached a mean duration of 42 months [60]. The percentage of patients who responded was 62.5% after 1 year, 46.2% after 2 years, 75.0% after 3 years, and 64.3% at last follow-up visit. Remission rates over time also remained consistent with rates of 18.8% after year 1, 15.4% after year 2, 50% after year 3, and 42.9% at last follow-up visit. More recently, a Spanish group published the results of another independent open-label trial of DBS implanted at SCG25 in 8 patients with a level of TRD of 5 [61]. In this sample, the response and remission rates were respectively 87.5% and 37.5% at 6 months and 62.5% and 50% at one year.
2. VC/VS
   In a sample of 26 patients with intractable OCD who received VC/VS DBS treatment, the majority also had comorbid depression. In this cohort, after 36 months of VC/VS DBS stimulation, average HAM-D scores decreased by 43.2%, and 14 of the 26 patients met criteria for remission. Based on previous experience with OCD patients[62], an open-label, multicentric trial of VC/VS DBS for severe TRD was conducted with 15 patients with level of treatment resistance of 5 and mean duration of illness of 21 ± 11 years [63]. The results were extremely positive, with response rates of 40% at 6 months and 53.3% at 24 months, while remission rates were respectively 20% and 40%. In general, the DBS treatment was well tolerated, and no patients withdrew from the study.
3. NAC
   In 2008, Schlaepfer and colleagues described bilateral implantation in the shell and core of the NAC in 3 patients with TRD [64]. In 2010, the same group published the results for open-label 1-year study including 10 patients [65]. All of the patients enrolled in the study had a history of recurrent or chronic TRD and a high level of treatment-resistance. The results were similar to those obtained with DBS at other targets, with 50% of the patients reaching the threshold for response at 12 months.

DBS summary

DBS for TRD is an experimental area of investigation. Given the elevated costs and the risks related to the surgical procedure, DBS has been limited to the most treatment-refractory cases of depression. The data on efficacy in TRD are limited to a series of open-label studies, and rigorous double-blind trials are being conducted to establish its role in the management of patients with moderate to severe illness. DBS is not a treatment indicated for acute worsening, as the effects of stimulation can take weeks to months to manifest. Moreover the interactions between stimulation and medications need to be carefully managed. In the case of relapse, DBS can be combined successfully with previously ineffective antidepressant treatments, including medications, ECT and psychotherapies.

Review and conclusions

Treatment-resistant depression has been associated with poor clinical outcomes, impaired long- term social functioning, and high rates of medical comorbidity and mortality.

Device-based therapy can be successfully integrated into the algorithm for management of TRD, in conjunction with the continuation of antidepressant regimens. Each device has specific indications according to the level of the patient's treatment resistance. A summary of

Table 1 Comparison of devices for Treatment Resistant Depression (TRD). ECT : Electroconvulsive Therapy; TMS Transcranial Magnetic Stimulation; VNS : Vagal Nerve Stimulation, DBS; Deep Brain Stimulation

	ECT	TMS	VNS	DBS
FDA status	"Gold standard" in TRD	Approved for TRD after failure of one AD	Approved	Not approved – under investigation
Reimbursed by insurance	Yes	Few cases	No	No
Requires surgery/multidisciplinary team	General anesthesia	no	Yes	Yes
Acute clinical efficacy	yes	yes	No	no
Approximate costs (USD)	10-15,000 for 3-4 weeks	6-12,000 for 3-4 weeks	40-45,000 for surgery + device	200-250,000 for surgery + device
Follow-up adjustments / maintenance (per visit, USD)	200-800	200-400	350-620	350-620

the features of each device as compared to ECT is presented in Table 1.

TMS is safe and well tolerated, and it has been approved by the FDA for adults with depression who have failed to respond to one antidepressant. Given its favorable side effect profile, it may also be indicated for patients who are intolerant of medications. Its use in TRD is currently not firmly supported by clinical trials.

VNS and DBS have much higher costs and require a surgical approach; therefore they have been utilized primarily in patients with high, or extremely high, level of treatment-resistance, usually after the patient has failed a course of ECT. VNS has a well-established safety record deriving from its use in the treatment of epilepsy; it is FDA-approved for TRD and appears to be most effective in patients with MDD or bipolar disorder with low to moderate, but not extreme, antidepressant resistance.

DBS for TRD is an experimental area of investigation for which the optimal neuroanatomical targets and stimulation parameters have yet to be determined. Given the elevated costs and the risks related to surgical implantation, DBS has been utilized in the most treatment-refractory cases. Future directions for the clinical development of TMS involve designing double-blind randomized controlled trials of augmentation of antidepressant therapy in patients who are drug-naïve or have moderate depression severity and designing protocols for long-term maintenance. For VNS, papers about its long-term benefits and limited adverse effects are being published, but it is unclear whether more controlled trials in depression will be pursued. For DBS, a series of open-label studies on DBS for TRD have been published, and double-blind research trials are underway.

As the number of patients treated with new devices increases, the ideal candidates and target population for each device will likely be established.

Competing interest
The author(s) declare that they have no competing interests.

Authors' contributions
Dr. Dougherty receives funding from Medtronic (research and consulting/honoraria), Northstar (research), and Cyberonics (research).

CC and DD participated to the review of the literature and drafting of the manuscript. All authors read and approved the final manuscript.

Acknowledgments
The authors thank Alexandra Rodman and Trina Chang, MD for the help in reviewing the manuscript.

References

1. Kessler RC, Berglund P, Demler O, Jin R, Koretz D, Merikangas KR, Rush AJ, Walters EE, Wang PS: **The epidemiology of major depressive disorder: results from the National Comorbidity Survey Replication (NCS-R).** *JAMA* 2003, **289**:3095–3105.
2. Ruhe HG, van Rooijen G, Spijker J, Peeters FP, Schene AH: **Staging methods for treatment resistant depression. A systematic review.** *J Affect Disord* 2012, **137**:35–45.
3. UK ECT Review Group: **Efficacy and safety of electroconvulsive therapy in depressive disorders: a systematic review and meta-analysis.** *Lancet* 2003, **361**:799–808.
4. Semkovska M, McLoughlin DM: **Objective cognitive performance associated with electroconvulsive therapy for depression: a systematic review and meta-analysis.** *Biol Psychiatry* 2010, **68**:568–577.
5. Sackeim HA, Prudic J, Fuller R, Keilp J, Lavori PW, Olfson M: **The cognitive effects of electroconvulsive therapy in community settings.** *Neuropsychopharmacology* 2007, **32**:244–254.
6. Barker AT, Jalinous R, Freeston IL: **Non-invasive magnetic stimulation of human motor cortex.** *Lancet* 1985, **1**:1106–1107.
7. Videbech P: **PET measurements of brain glucose metabolism and blood flow in major depressive disorder: a critical review.** *Acta Psychiatr Scand* 2000, **101**:11–20.
8. Barrett J, Della-Maggiore V, Chouinard PA, Paus T: **Mechanisms of action underlying the effect of repetitive transcranial magnetic stimulation on mood: behavioral and brain imaging studies.** *Neuropsychopharmacology* 2004, **29**:1172–1189.
9. Klein E, Kreinin I, Chistyakov A, Koren D, Mecz L, Marmur S, Ben-Shachar D, Feinsod M: **Therapeutic efficacy of right prefrontal slow repetitive transcranial magnetic stimulation in major depression: a double-blind controlled study.** *Arch Gen Psychiatry* 1999, **56**:315–320.
10. Kauffmann CD, Cheema MA, Miller BE: **Slow right prefrontal transcranial magnetic stimulation as a treatment for medication-resistant depression: a double-blind, placebo-controlled study.** *Depress Anxiety* 2004, **19**:59–62.
11. Januel D, Dumortier G, Verdon CM, Stamatiadis L, Saba G, Cabaret W, Benadhira R, Rocamora JF, Braha S, Kalalou K, *et al*: **A double-blind sham controlled study of right prefrontal repetitive transcranial magnetic stimulation (rTMS): therapeutic and cognitive effect in medication free unipolar depression during 4 weeks.** *Prog Neuropsychopharmacol Biol Psychiatry* 2006, **30**:126–130.
12. Hoppner J, Schulz M, Irmisch G, Mau R, Schlafke D, Richter J: **Antidepressant efficacy of two different rTMS procedures. High frequency over left versus low frequency over right prefrontal cortex**

compared with sham stimulation. *Eur Arch Psychiatry Clin Neurosci* 2003, **253:**103–109.

13. Fitzgerald PB, Brown TL, Marston NA, Daskalakis ZJ, De Castella A, Kulkarni J: **Transcranial magnetic stimulation in the treatment of depression: a double-blind, placebo-controlled trial.** *Arch Gen Psychiatry* 2003, **60:**1002–1008.
14. Garcia-Toro M, Salva J, Daumal J, Andres J, Romera M, Lafau O, Echevarria M, Mestre M, Bosch C, Collado C, *et al*: **High (20-Hz) and low (1-Hz) frequency transcranial magnetic stimulation as adjuvant treatment in medication-resistant depression.** *Psychiatry Res* 2006, **146:**53–57.
15. Fitzgerald PB, Huntsman S, Gunewardene R, Kulkarni J, Daskalakis ZJ: **A randomized trial of low-frequency right-prefrontal-cortex transcranial magnetic stimulation as augmentation in treatment-resistant major depression.** *Int J Neuropsychopharmacol* 2006, **9:**655–666.
16. Stern WM, Tormos JM, Press DZ, Pearlman C, Pascual-Leone A: **Antidepressant effects of high and low frequency repetitive transcranial magnetic stimulation to the dorsolateral prefrontal cortex: a double-blind, randomized, placebo-controlled trial.** *J Neuropsychiatry Clin Neurosci* 2007, **19:**179–186.
17. McNamara B, Ray JL, Arthurs OJ, Boniface S: **Transcranial magnetic stimulation for depression and other psychiatric disorders.** *Psychol Med* 2001, **31:**1141–1146.
18. Loo C, Mitchell P, Sachdev P, McDarmont B, Parker G, Gandevia S: **Double-blind controlled investigation of transcranial magnetic stimulation for the treatment of resistant major depression.** *Am J Psychiatry* 1999, **156:**946–948.
19. Martin JL, Barbanoj MJ, Schlaepfer TE, Clos S, Perez V, Kulisevsky J, Gironell A: **Transcranial magnetic stimulation for treating depression.** *Cochrane Database Syst Rev* 2002, **2:**CD003493.
20. Couturier JL: **Efficacy of rapid-rate repetitive transcranial magnetic stimulation in the treatment of depression: a systematic review and meta-analysis.** *J Psychiatry Neurosci* 2005, **30:**83–90.
21. O'Reardon JP, Solvason HB, Janicak PG, Sampson S, Isenberg KE, Nahas Z, McDonald WM, Avery D, Fitzgerald PB, Loo C, *et al*: **Efficacy and safety of transcranial magnetic stimulation in the acute treatment of major depression: a multisite randomized controlled trial.** *Biol Psychiatry* 2007, **62:**1208–1216.
22. Slotema CW, Blom JD, Hoek HW, Sommer IE: **Should we expand the toolbox of psychiatric treatment methods to include Repetitive Transcranial Magnetic Stimulation (rTMS)? A meta-analysis of the efficacy of rTMS in psychiatric disorders.** *J Clin Psychiatry* 2010, **71:**873–884.
23. Loo CK, Mitchell PB: **A review of the efficacy of transcranial magnetic stimulation (TMS) treatment for depression, and current and future strategies to optimize efficacy.** *J Affect Disord* 2005, **88:**255–267.
24. Ridding MC, Rothwell JC: **Is there a future for therapeutic use of transcranial magnetic stimulation?** *Nat Rev Neurosci* 2007, **8:**559–567.
25. Brunoni AR, Fregni F: **Clinical trial design in non-invasive brain stimulation psychiatric research.** *Int J Methods Psychiatr Res* 2011, **20:**e19–e30.
26. George MS, Lisanby SH, Avery D, McDonald WM, Durkalski V, Pavlicova M, Anderson B, Nahas Z, Bulow P, Zarkowski P, *et al*: **Daily left prefrontal transcranial magnetic stimulation therapy for major depressive disorder: a sham-controlled randomized trial.** *Arch Gen Psychiatry* 2010, **67:**507–516.
27. Jhanwar VG, Bishnoi RJ, Singh L, Jhanwar MR: **Utility of repetitive transcranial magnetic stimulation as an augmenting treatment method in treatment-resistant depression.** *Indian J Psychiatry* 2011, **53:**145–148.
28. Dell'Osso B, Mundo E, D'Urso N, Pozzoli S, Buoli M, Ciabatti M, Rosanova M, Massimini M, Bellina V, Mariotti M, Altamura AC: **Augmentative repetitive navigated transcranial magnetic stimulation (rTMS) in drug-resistant bipolar depression.** *Bipolar Disord* 2009, **11:**76–81.
29. Hadley D, Anderson BS, Borckardt JJ, Arana A, Li X, Nahas Z, George MS: **Safety, tolerability, and effectiveness of high doses of adjunctive daily left prefrontal repetitive transcranial magnetic stimulation for treatment-resistant depression in a clinical setting.** *J ECT* 2011, **27:**18–25.
30. Bretlau LG, Lunde M, Lindberg L, Unden M, Dissing S, Bech P: **Repetitive transcranial magnetic stimulation (rTMS) in combination with escitalopram in patients with treatment-resistant major depression: a double-blind, randomised, sham-controlled trial.** *Pharmacopsychiatry* 2008, **41:**41–47.
31. Blumberger DM, Mulsant BH, Fitzgerald PB, Rajji TK, Ravindran AV, Young LT, Levinson AJ, Daskalakis ZJ: **A randomized double-blind sham-controlled comparison of unilateral and bilateral repetitive transcranial magnetic stimulation for treatment-resistant major depression.** *World J Biol Psychiatry*, (in press) published online July 2011.
32. Pridmore S, Bruno R, Turnier-Shea Y, Reid P, Rybak M: **Comparison of unlimited numbers of rapid transcranial magnetic stimulation (rTMS) and ECT treatment sessions in major depressive episode.** *Int J Neuropsychopharmacol* 2000, **3:**129–134.
33. Grunhaus L, Dannon PN, Schreiber S, Dolberg OH, Amiaz R, Ziv R, Lefkifker E: **Repetitive transcranial magnetic stimulation is as effective as electroconvulsive therapy in the treatment of nondelusional major depressive disorder: an open study.** *Biol Psychiatry* 2000, **47:**314–324.
34. Janicak PG, Dowd SM, Martis B, Alam D, Beedle D, Krasuski J, Strong MJ, Sharma R, Rosen C, Viana M: **Repetitive transcranial magnetic stimulation versus electroconvulsive therapy for major depression: preliminary results of a randomized trial.** *Biol Psychiatry* 2002, **51:**659–667.
35. Grunhaus L, Schreiber S, Dolberg OT, Polak D, Dannon PN: **A randomized controlled comparison of electroconvulsive therapy and repetitive transcranial magnetic stimulation in severe and resistant nonpsychotic major depression.** *Biol Psychiatry* 2003, **53:**324–331.
36. Rosa MA, Gattaz WF, Pascual-Leone A, Fregni F, Rosa MO, Rumi DO, Myczkowski M, Silva MF, Mansur C, Rigonatti SP, *et al*: **Comparison of repetitive transcranial magnetic stimulation and electroconvulsive therapy in unipolar non-psychotic refractory depression: a randomized, single-blind study.** *Int J Neuropsychopharmacol* 2006, **9:**667–676.
37. Eranti S, Mogg A, Pluck G, Landau S, Purvis R, Brown RG, Howard R, Knapp M, Philpot M, Rabe-Hesketh S, *et al*: **A randomized, controlled trial with 6-month follow-up of repetitive transcranial magnetic stimulation and electroconvulsive therapy for severe depression.** *Am J Psychiatry* 2007, **164:**73–81.
38. Rasmussen KG: **Some considerations in choosing electroconvulsive therapy versus transcranial magnetic stimulation for depression.** *J ECT* 2011, **27:**51–54.
39. Rush AJ, Marangell LB, Sackeim HA, George MS, Brannan SK, Davis SM, Howland R, Kling MA, Rittberg BR, Burke WJ, *et al*: **Vagus nerve stimulation for treatment-resistant depression: a randomized, controlled acute phase trial.** *Biol Psychiatry* 2005, **58:**347–354.
40. Rush AJ, George MS, Sackeim HA, Marangell LB, Husain MM, Giller C, Nahas Z, Haines S, Simpson RK Jr, Goodman R: **Vagus nerve stimulation (VNS) for treatment-resistant depressions: a multicenter study.** *Biol Psychiatry* 2000, **47:**276–286.
41. Sackeim HA, Rush AJ, George MS, Marangell LB, Husain MM, Nahas Z, Johnson CR, Seidman S, Giller C, Haines S, *et al*: **Vagus nerve stimulation (VNS) for treatment-resistant depression: efficacy, side effects, and predictors of outcome.** *Neuropsychopharmacology* 2001, **25:**713–728.
42. Schlaepfer TE, Frick C, Zobel A, Maier W, Heuser I, Bajbouj M, O'Keane V, Corcoran C, Adolfsson R, Trimble M, *et al*: **Vagus nerve stimulation for depression: efficacy and safety in a European study.** *Psychol Med* 2008, **38:**651–661.
43. Nahas Z, Marangell LB, Husain MM, Rush AJ, Sackeim HA, Lisanby SH, Martinez JM, George MS: **Two-year outcome of vagus nerve stimulation (VNS) for treatment of major depressive episodes.** *J Clin Psychiatry* 2005, **66:**1097–1104.
44. Bajbouj M, Merkl A, Schlaepfer TE, Frick C, Zobel A, Maier W, O'Keane V, Corcoran C, Adolfsson R, Trimble M, *et al*: **Two-year outcome of vagus nerve stimulation in treatment-resistant depression.** *J Clin Psychopharmacol* 2010, **30:**273–281.
45. Rush AJ, Sackeim HA, Marangell LB, George MS, Brannan SK, Davis SM, Lavori P, Howland R, Kling MA, Rittberg B, *et al*: **Effects of 12 months of vagus nerve stimulation in treatment-resistant depression: a naturalistic study.** *Biol Psychiatry* 2005, **58:**355–363.
46. Nierenberg AA, Alpert JE, Gardner-Schuster EE, Seay S, Mischoulon D: **Vagus nerve stimulation: 2-year outcomes for bipolar versus unipolar treatment-resistant depression.** *Biol Psychiatry* 2008, **64:**455–460.
47. Burke WJ, Moreno FA: **Suicidality in treatment-resistant depression: results from a 24-month trial of vagus nerve stimulation.** In *Proceedings of 156th American Psychiatric Association Annual Meeting.*; 2006. Toronto. Canada: May 20-25.
48. Deep-Brain Stimulation for Parkinson's Disease Study Group: **Deep-brain stimulation of the subthalamic nucleus or the pars interna of the globus pallidus in Parkinson's disease.** *N Engl J Med* 2001, **345:**956–963.

49. Hauptman JS, DeSalles AA, Espinoza R, Sedrak M, Ishida W: **Potential surgical targets for deep brain stimulation in treatment-resistant depression.** *Neurosurg Focus* 2008, **25:**E3.
50. Mayberg HS, Liotti M, Brannan SK, McGinnis S, Mahurin RK, Jerabek PA, Silva JA, Tekell JL, Martin CC, Lancaster JL, Fox PT: **Reciprocal limbic-cortical function and negative mood: converging PET findings in depression and normal sadness.** *Am J Psychiatry* 1999, **156:**675–682.
51. Nuttin B, Cosyns P, Demeulemeester H, Gybels J, Meyerson B: **Electrical stimulation in anterior limbs of internal capsules in patients with obsessive-compulsive disorder.** *Lancet* 1999, **354:**1526.
52. Greenberg BD, Price LH, Rauch SL, Friehs G, Noren G, Malone D, Carpenter LL, Rezai AR, Rasmussen SA: **Neurosurgery for intractable obsessive-compulsive disorder and depression: critical issues.** *Neurosurg Clin N Am* 2003, **14:**199–212.
53. Rauch SL, Dougherty DD, Malone D, Rezai A, Friehs G, Fischman AJ, Alpert NM, Haber SN, Stypulkowski PH, Rise MT, *et al*: **A functional neuroimaging investigation of deep brain stimulation in patients with obsessive-compulsive disorder.** *J Neurosurg* 2006, **104:**558–565.
54. Kopell BH, Greenberg BD: **Anatomy and physiology of the basal ganglia: implications for DBS in psychiatry.** *Neurosci Biobehav Rev* 2008, **32:**408–422.
55. Velasco F, Velasco M, Jimenez F, Velasco AL, Salin-Pascual R: **Neurobiological background for performing surgical intervention in the inferior thalamic peduncle for treatment of major depression disorders.** *Neurosurgery* 2005, **57:**439–448. discussion 439-448.
56. Jimenez F, Velasco F, Salin-Pascual R, Hernandez JA, Velasco M, Criales JL, Nicolini H: **A patient with a resistant major depression disorder treated with deep brain stimulation in the inferior thalamic peduncle.** *Neurosurgery* 2005, **57:**585–593. discussion 585-593.
57. Sartorius A, Kiening KL, Kirsch P, von Gall CC, Haberkorn U, Unterberg AW, Henn FA, Meyer-Lindenberg A: **Remission of major depression under deep brain stimulation of the lateral habenula in a therapy-refractory patient.** *Biol Psychiatry* 2010, **67:**e9–e11.
58. McIntosh ES: **Perspective on the economic evaluation of deep brain stimulation.** *Front Integr Neurosci* 2011, **5:**19.
59. Lozano AM, Mayberg HS, Giacobbe P, Hamani C, Craddock RC, Kennedy SH: **Subcallosal cingulate gyrus deep brain stimulation for treatment-resistant depression.** *Biol Psychiatry* 2008, **64:**461–467.
60. Kennedy SH, Giacobbe P, Rizvi SJ, Placenza FM, Nishikawa Y, Mayberg HS, Lozano AM: **Deep brain stimulation for treatment-resistant depression: follow-up after 3 to 6 years.** *Am J Psychiatry* 2011, **168:**502–510.
61. Puigdemont D, Perez-Egea R, Portella MJ, Molet J, de Diego-Adelino J, Gironell A, Radua J, Gomez-Anson B, Rodriguez R, Serra M, *et al*: **Deep brain stimulation of the subcallosal cingulate gyrus: further evidence in treatment-resistant major depression.** *Int J Neuropsychopharmacol* 2012, **15:**1–13.
62. Greenberg BD, Gabriels LA, Malone DA Jr, Rezai AR, Friehs GM, Okun MS, Shapira NA, Foote KD, Cosyns PR, Kubu CS, *et al*: **Deep brain stimulation of the ventral internal capsule/ventral striatum for obsessive-compulsive disorder: worldwide experience.** *MolPsychiatry* 2010, **15:**64–79.
63. Malone DA Jr, Dougherty DD, Rezai AR, Carpenter LL, Friehs GM, Eskandar EN, Rauch SL, Rasmussen SA, Machado AG, Kubu CS, *et al*: **Deep brain stimulation of the ventral capsule/ventral striatum for treatment-resistant depression.** *Biol Psychiatry* 2009, **65:**267–275.
64. Schlaepfer TE, Cohen MX, Frick C, Kosel M, Brodesser D, Axmacher N, Joe AY, Kreft M, Lenartz D, Sturm V: **Deep brain stimulation to reward circuitry alleviates anhedonia in refractory major depression.** *Neuropsychopharmacology* 2008, **33:**368–377.
65. Bewernick BH, Hurlemann R, Matusch A, Kayser S, Grubert C, Hadrysiewicz B, Axmacher N, Lemke M, Cooper-Mahkorn D, Cohen MX, *et al*: **Nucleus accumbens deep brain stimulation decreases ratings of depression and anxiety in treatment-resistant depression.** *Biol Psychiatry* 2010, **67:**110–116.

5

Is there less to social anxiety than meets the eye? Behavioral and neural responses to three socio-emotional tasks

Michal Ziv*, Philippe R Goldin, Hooria Jazaieri, Kevin S Hahn and James J Gross

Abstract

Background: Social anxiety disorder (SAD) is widely thought to be characterized by heightened behavioral and limbic reactivity to socio-emotional stimuli. However, although behavioral findings are clear, neural findings are surprisingly mixed.

Methods: Using functional magnetic resonance imaging (fMRI), we examined behavioral and brain responses in *a priori* emotion generative regions of interest (amygdala and insula) in 67 patients with generalized SAD and in 28 healthy controls (HC) during three distinct socio-emotional tasks. We administered these socio-emotional tasks during one fMRI scanning session: 1) looming harsh faces (Faces); 2) videotaped actors delivering social criticism (Criticism); and 3) written negative self-beliefs (Beliefs).

Results: In each task, SAD patients reported heightened negative emotion, compared to HC. There were, however, no SAD versus HC differential brain responses in the amygdala and insula. Between-group whole-brain analyses confirmed no group differences in the responses of the amygdala and insula, and indicated different brain networks activated during each of the tasks. In SAD participants, social anxiety symptom severity was associated with increased BOLD signal in the left insula during the Faces task.

Conclusions: The similar responses in amygdala and insula in SAD and HC participants suggest that heightened negative emotion responses reported by patients with SAD may be related to dysfunction in higher cognitive processes (e.g., distorted appraisal, attention biases, or ineffective cognitive reappraisal). In addition, the findings of this study emphasize the differential effects of socio-emotional experimental tasks.

Keywords: Social anxiety, Amygdala, Insula, Emotion reactivity, fMRI, Socio-emotional tasks

Background

Social anxiety disorder (SAD) is defined by a marked and persistent fear of social or performance situations in which the person is exposed to unfamiliar people, or possible scrutiny by others [1]. When interacting with others, people with SAD experience intense anxiety accompanied by physical symptoms such as blushing, heart racing, sweating, trembling, and nausea, as well as stuttering and trouble concentrating [2]. SAD is one of the most common anxiety disorders, with a lifetime prevalence of up to 13% [3]. When untreated, SAD can lead to elevated social isolation, depression, anxiety, and alcohol and/or substance abuse [4].

Models of SAD have highlighted the role of emotional hyper-reactivity in feared social situations. Exaggerated emotional responses are thought to arise from maladaptive appraisals of the social situation that transform innocuous social cues into interpersonal threats [5]. This hyper-reactivity often leads to attempts to escape from or avoid the anxiety-provoking object or situation [2].

To study the behavioral and brain aspects of this emotional hyper-reactivity, most studies have employed negatively valenced facial expressions as socio-emotional probes. Behaviorally, these studies show hyper-arousal and increased emotional distress in patients with SAD

* Correspondence: michalz@stanford.edu
Department of Psychology, Stanford University, Jordan Hall, Bldg. 420, Stanford, CA, USA

when exposed to negative face stimuli [2]. Neurally, however, the findings are less clear.

The amygdala, which plays a critical role in the recognition of fear in facial expressions [6], was a natural target in studies of the neural basis of emotional reactivity in SAD. It was suggested that the heightened emotional responses in SAD patients were associated with increased amygdala activity [7]. Amaral [8] proposed a model based on lesion studies in monkeys, which suggested that the amygdala performs a protective function, namely, allowing the organism to detect and avoid danger. This model provided a rationale for theories implicating the amygdala in the neuropathology of SAD.

Many studies have indeed demonstrated heightened amygdala responses in patients with SAD when viewing angry, fearful and even neutral facial expressions [7,9-12]. However, other studies, some using stimuli other than faces, failed to detect differential amygdala activation between patients with SAD and HC [13-17]. For example, Quadflieg and colleagues (2008) have found that both SAD patients and HC recruit the amygdala when listening to angry compared to neutral prosody [17]. Similarly, Goldin and colleagues (2009) found increased amygdala responses to harsh facial expressions with longer stimulus presentation times (6 seconds) in both SAD patients and healthy controls [16]. Other studies have even found *decreased* amygdala responses in SAD patients compared to HC. For example, Kilts and colleagues (2006) have found decreased amygdala responses during both script-driven imagery of anxiety-provoking social situations and a mental arithmetic task in SAD [14].

A second limbic region that is thought to play a prominent role in SAD neuropathology is the insula. The insula is interconnected with the amygdala, thalamus, and orbitofrontal cortex [18], regulates the autonomic nervous system [19], and is involved in the recognition and experience of aversive states [20] and threat processing [21]. Thus, hyper-reactivity of the insula in SAD patients might be responsible for the generation of fear responses to social aversive stimuli.

A recent meta-analysis identified four functionally distinct sub-regions in the human insula implicated in social-emotional, sensorimotor, olfacto-gustatory, and cognitive brain networks [22]. The ventral part of the insula was associated with the social-emotional domain. This ventral region was active in 195 experiments of emotion generation (paradigms of "induction, imagination or recall of own happiness, fear, anxiety, anger, sadness, or disgust") and 120 empathy related experiments (paradigms of judging emotions in faces or attending to pain in others). This differentiation matches previous cytoarchitectonic studies in non-human primates that found differences between the anterior-basal agranular, allocortical, and posterior granular parts of the insula [23]. The anterior-ventral region is involved in the generation and mediation of feeling as a response to environmental stimuli and affective states [24], and in the recognition of emotions in faces [25]. In SAD, increased activity in this insula region was associated with visualization of angry and disgusted faces [13,26], viewing of images with negative emotional content [27], and anticipation of a public speaking task [28]. However, several studies did not find such activity differences [17,29] and others found *decreased* activity in the insula during a public speaking task [30] and during an implicit learning test [31].

Thus, despite the clear focus of neuroimaging studies on the amygdala and insula as key regions in SAD pathology, findings are mixed. One explanation for these mixed findings might be related to factors such as different stimuli and experimental designs used to elicit emotional responses (mainly emotional faces until a few years ago, and images, written words, and auditory stimuli more recently), small patients groups, differences in exclusion criteria (e.g., different psychiatric co-morbidity), and other experimental parameters.

However, another explanation could be a lack of concordance between the behavioral and physiological components of anxiety. This idea was raised by Mauss and colleagues in a study of non-clinical social anxiety [32]. In this study, anxiety experience, subjectively perceived physiological activation, and objectively measured physiological activation were assessed in high and low trait social anxiety participants using an impromptu speech paradigm. The study found no differences in physiological responding between high and low trait social anxiety, despite clear differences between the two groups in their subjective experience of anxiety and their perceived physiological activation. Although this study did not measure brain responses, and did not employ a clinical sample, it did raise an important question about the widely assumed link between behavioral and physiological responses in the context of social anxiety.

In light of the mixed literature on the neural correlates of emotion reactivity in SAD, the goal of the present study was to examine both behavioral responses and BOLD signal changes in SAD compared to HC when reacting to distinct types of socio-emotional stimuli. To test whether behavior and brain responses vary by context, we used three different socio-emotional tasks: 1) viewing looming harsh faces (Faces), 2) watching dynamic videos of actors delivering social criticism (Criticism), and 3) reading negative self-beliefs (Beliefs). These tasks mirror the specific types of interpersonal evaluations and negative thoughts that are especially salient in patients with SAD. As suggested by the literature, we focused on the amygdala and the insula regions, but also performed whole-brain analyses to examine the involvement of other brain networks in SAD.

We hypothesized that, compared to HC, patients with SAD would have (1) greater self-reported negative emotion reactivity for each of the three tasks; and (2) greater BOLD responses in the amygdala and insula. In secondary analyses, we examined the differential effect of each socio-emotional task on negative emotion reactivity and neural responses in SAD and HC, and whether – among SAD participants – negative emotion reactivity and neural responses were associated with social anxiety symptom severity.

Methods

Participants

Participants included 67 (32 females) adults who met *DSM-IV-TR* [1] criteria for primary generalized SAD and 28 (13 females) healthy controls (HC) with no lifetime history of psychiatric disorders (Table 1). Patients were recruited through clinician referrals and advertisements on community and online bulletin boards. Two PhD-level clinical psychologists assessed each potential participant using the Anxiety Disorders Interview Schedule for *DSM-IV-TR Lifetime version (ADIS-IV-L)* [33]. We invited into the study only patients who met clinical diagnostic criteria for a principal diagnosis of current generalized SAD (defined as greater than moderate anxiety/fear for 5 or more distinct social situations) or healthy controls (with no current or past history of DSM-IV disorders).

Both SAD and HC had a mean age of 33 years (range: SAD 21–53 years; HC 21–52 years, see Table 1) and were right-handed as assessed by the Edinburgh Handedness Inventory [34]. Potential patients were excluded if they reported current pharmacotherapy or psychotherapy, history of neurological disorders, and current psychiatric disorders (other than SAD, generalized anxiety disorder, agoraphobia without a history of panic attacks, dysthymia, or specific phobia). HC were not permitted to meet criteria for any current or past psychiatric disorders.

Table 1 Demographic and clinical variables

	SAD n = 67	HC n = 28	*t*-value	Partial eta^2
Females (n)	32	13		
Age (Mean years ± SD)	33.0 ± 8.8	32.6 ± 9.5	0.2	
Education (Mean years ± SD)	16.7 ± 2.4	17.5 ± 1.5	1.6	
EDI (Mean ± SD)	9.9 ± 0.3	9.8 ± 0.4	0.30	
Ethnicity				
- Caucasian	38	17		
- Asian	17	8		
- Latino	8	2		
- Native American	1	1		
- Native Hawaiian	1	0		
- Filipino	1	0		
LSAS-SR (Mean ± SD)	84.1 ± 17.5	15.3 ± 9.1	19.3 *	.85

Note: EDI = Edinburgh Handedness Inventory, LSAS-SR = Liebowitz Social Anxiety Scale–Self-Report.
* $P < .0001$.

Among patients, *current* Axis-I co-morbidity included 3 with panic attacks, 13 with generalized anxiety disorder, 3 with dysthymia and 5 with specific phobia. *Past* Axis-I co-morbidity included 13 with major depression, 4 with substance abuse, 1 with panic attacks, 1 with dysthymia, and 1 with eating disorder. Thirty-three patients reported past (i.e., ended more than 1 year ago) non-cognitive-behavioral psychotherapy, and 20 reported past pharmacotherapy. All participants provided informed consent in accordance with Stanford University Human Subjects Committee rules.

Clinical assessment

To asses social anxiety symptom severity, participants completed the Liebowitz Social Anxiety Scale-Self-Report (LSAS-SR) [35]. This questionnaire assesses both fear and behavioral avoidance of social situations, and is widely used in the research of SAD [36].

Experimental tasks

Prior to scanning, patients were trained on the three socio-emotional tasks programmed in Eprime (Psychology Software Tools, Inc). The stimuli used in the pre-fMRI training were not the same stimuli used in the MR scanner. All three tasks were composed of "React", "Asterisks" and "Reframe" conditions. In the present study, we report on data from the React condition, contrasting it with the Asterisks condition. The results for the Reframe condition will be published elsewhere.

During the "React" condition, participants were instructed to react normally without any attempt to control, modify, or regulate any reactions. After each React condition, participants provided a negative emotion rating using a button response pad positioned in the participant's right hand inside the magnet by responding to "How negative do you feel?" (1 = not at all to 5 = very much).

The Asterisks condition served as a low-level comparison condition, during which one to five white asterisks were displayed over a black background. Participants were asked to count how many asterisks were on the screen during the Faces and Criticism tasks, and were not given any counting instructions during the Beliefs task. There were 13 trials for this condition in the Faces task, 18 trials in the Criticism task, and 7 trials in the Beliefs task.

Harsh looming faces (Faces task)

The task consisted of 24 trials during which the participant viewed color photos of Ekman's facial action coded [37] faces displaying anger and contempt. The length of the entire task was 516 TRs, which is 12 minutes and 54 sec (774 sec). Each trial consisted of a cue to look (1.5 sec), a single harsh facial stimulus (9 sec) presented in color and appearing to move closer to the participant every 3 sec to simulate looming, and a negative emotion rating after the face stimulus terminated (3 sec) (Figure 1a). Participants were trained prior to the baseline scan to react to the faces by engaging in the picture ("Just let yourself feel") and thinking: "This person is upset with me; angry with me".

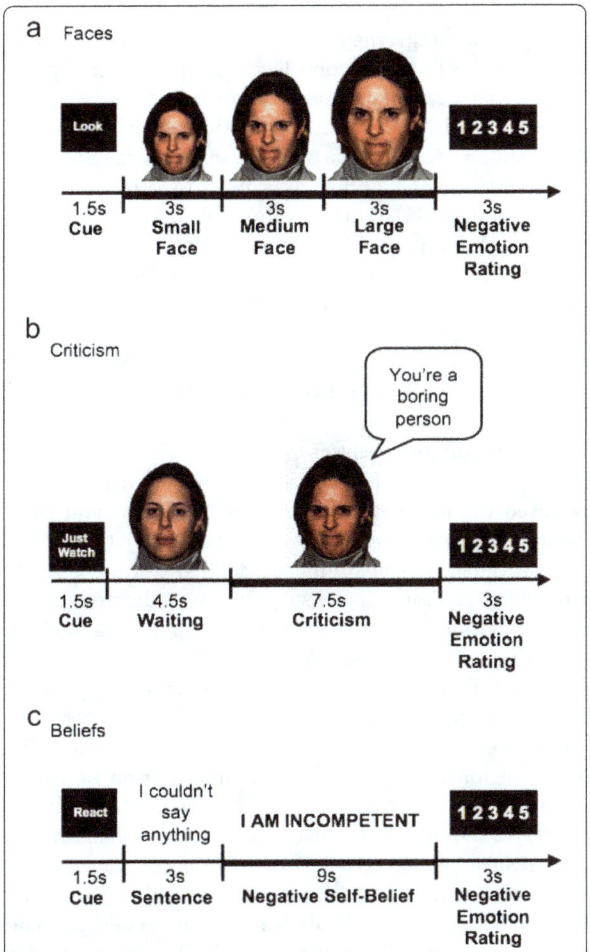

Figure 1 The three socio-emotional tasks. (**a**) Harsh looming faces (Faces); (**b**) social criticism (Criticism); (**c**) negative self-beliefs (Beliefs). For each task, a "React" trial consisted of: 1) a 1.5 seconds "Cue"; 2) a socio-emotional stimulus (a harsh looming face/ a video-clip of an actor delivering social criticism/ an autobiographical sentence + NSB); and 3) a negative emotion rating scale. Participants were instructed to react normally to the stimuli without any attempt to control, modify or regulate their reactions.

Dynamic social criticism (Criticism task)

The task consisted of videotaped actors delivering social criticism and social praise and harsh or happy evaluation-congruent facial expressions (Figure 1b). The stimuli were delivered by five male and five female actors (seven Anglo-Americans and three Asian-Americans) with an age range of 23–50. Each condition consisted of 16 trials delivered across two runs of 342 TRs, 8 min 35 sec each (513 sec). Each 13.5 sec trial consisted of a cue to "Just Watch" (1.5 sec), followed by a video clip of an actor delivering social evaluation (12 sec). Each 12 sec video clip had a 4.5 sec waiting period during which the actor silently maintained a neutral facial expression followed by a 7.5 sec evaluation period in which the actor delivered a social criticism or praise statement while displaying a harsh or positive facial expression. For the current study, only social criticism trials were included in the analysis (see examples in Table 2). After each video clip, participants were cued to rate their current negative emotion (3 sec). Participants were trained prior to scanning to react to the social criticism by reflecting on how the statement represents something true about themselves.

Negative self-beliefs (Beliefs task)

This task consisted of five situations. The first was an experimenter-composed neutral situation about cleaning a car that was used to obtain baseline emotion ratings for reading neutral statements. Then, four participant-generated autobiographical social anxiety situations characterized by

Table 2 Examples of social criticism and negative self-beliefs

Social criticism statements	Negative self beliefs
You don't seem very smart	I ALWAYS MESS UP
You've lost my interest	OTHERS SEE MY FAULTS
I feel uncomfortable being with you	I FELT HUMILIATED
You would not make a good leader	OTHERS THINK I'M A FOOL
You don't seem courageous	I AM INCOMPETENT
You're a boring person	OTHERS DO NOT LIKE ME
Do you always look so run down?	I AM WEIRD
You haven't accomplished much	OTHERS THINK I AM NOT NORMAL
Everyone thinks you are so weird	I AM STUPID
You never know what to say	OTHERS KNOW SOMETHING IS WRONG WITH ME

social anxiety, humiliation, and embarrassment were presented. Three situations were presented in a first run lasting 374 TRs, 9 min 21 sec (561 sec), followed by two situations in a second run of 256 TRs, 6 min 24 sec (534 sec). For each situation, participants composed a single paragraph describing the events, thoughts, and feelings and provided situation specific negative self-beliefs (NSBs, see examples in Table 2).

Each situation consisted of an instruction to React (1.5 sec), 16 sentences in white font against a black background describing the situation (3 sec each), 10 NSBs (9 sec each) embedded in the unfolding story in uppercase letters that flashed 9 times (850 msec on + 150 msec off), and a negative emotion rating after each NSB (3 sec) (Figure 1c). Negative self-beliefs were flashed to maintain attention. Participants were trained prior to scanning to react to NSBs by reflecting on how the NSB represents something that is true about themselves.

Image acquisition

Imaging was performed on a General Electric 3-T Signa magnet with a T2*-weighted gradient echo spiral-in/out pulse sequence [38] and a custom-built quadrature "dome" elliptical bird cage head-coil (GE Healthcare, Milwaukee, Wisconsin). Head movement was minimized using a bite-bar and foam padding. Functional volumes (516 for faces, 684 for criticism, 630 for belief tasks) were obtained from 22 sequential axial slices (repetition time = 1500 milliseconds, echo time = 30 milliseconds, flip angle = 60°, field of view = 22 cm, matrix = 64x64, single-shot, resolution = 3.438 mm^2 x 4.5 mm). Three-dimensional high-resolution anatomical scans were acquired using a fast spin-echo spoiled gradient recall (resolution = .8594 mm^2 x 1.5 mm; field of view = 22 cm, frequency encoding = 256).

fMRI data pre-processing

Analysis of Functional Neuroimages (AFNI) software [39] was used for preprocessing and statistical analysis. Each functional run was subjected to preprocessing steps to maximize signal-to-noise contrast. This included an analysis of potential outliers, volume registration to a base image, motion correction, 4 mm^3 isotropic Gaussian spatial smoothing, high-pass filtering (.011 Hz), linear detrending, and conversion into BOLD signal percentage change in each voxel. In addition, to allow for T2* equilibration effects, the first four images of each functional run were excluded. For the Criticism and Beliefs tasks, the two functional runs were concatenated prior to statistical analysis. No volumes demonstrated motion in the x, y, or z directions in excess of ±1 mm. There was no evidence of stimulus-correlated motion, as assessed by correlations between condition specific reference functions and x, y, z motion correction parameters.

fMRI statistical analysis

Multiple-regression implemented with AFNI 3dDeconvolve included baseline parameters to remove mean, linear, and quadratic trends, and motion-related variance in the BOLD signal. For each task, the React condition was defined as: for Faces, the 9 sec single face stimulus; for Criticism, the 7.5 sec. evaluation period; and for the beliefs the 9 sec. of NSBs (see bold lines in Figures 1a,b,c). Regressors for the Asterisks and React conditions were convolved with the Cohen's gamma variate model of the hemodynamic response function [40]. Functional MRI BOLD signal intensity was computed as percentage of signal change, an effect size measure [(MR signal per voxel per time point / mean MR signal in that voxel for the entire functional run) x 100].

Individual brain maps were converted to Talairach atlas space [41] and second-level group statistical parametric maps were produced according to a random-effects model. To correct for multiple comparisons, AlphaSim, a Monte Carlo simulation bootstrapping program in the AFNI library, was used to protect against false positives [42]. This method uses a voxel-wise and cluster volume joint-probability threshold to establish a cluster-wise false positive cluster detection level. The cluster statistical threshold for the between group analyses consisted of a voxel-wise $P < .005$ and cluster volume higher than 162 mm^3 (4 voxels x 3.438 mm^3) to protect against false-positive cluster detection at $P < .01$.

Regions of interest analyses

To examine emotion reactivity related brain responses, we used the left and right amygdala, and left and right insula as *a priori* regions of interest (ROIs) (Figure 2). The amygdala was anatomically defined using the AFNI Talairach Daemon. The insula ROI was defined as the social-emotional sub-region identified in a meta-analysis by Kurth et al. ([22], see Additional file 1: Table S1 for peak xyz Talairach coordinates). We created spherical masks (radius = 7 mm, volume = 1,437 mm^3) centered on the peak xyz Talairach coordinates in left and right insula regions, separately. The volume of each ROI was: left amygdala: 81 voxels = 3,292 mm^3, right amygdala: 81 voxels = 3,292 mm3, left insula: 237 voxels = 9,631 mm3, right insula: 244 voxels = 9,915 mm. We examined BOLD responses within these ROIs with a SAD versus HC between-group ANOVA of React versus Asterisks. The mean and standard deviations per ROI, per group, per task, were calculated. We removed outliers defined as greater than 3 standard deviations from the mean per ROI per group per task.

To examine the relationship between social anxiety symptom severity and brain responses in SAD patients, we computed Pearson correlation coefficients using SPSS. To correct for Type 1 error, the statistical threshold was

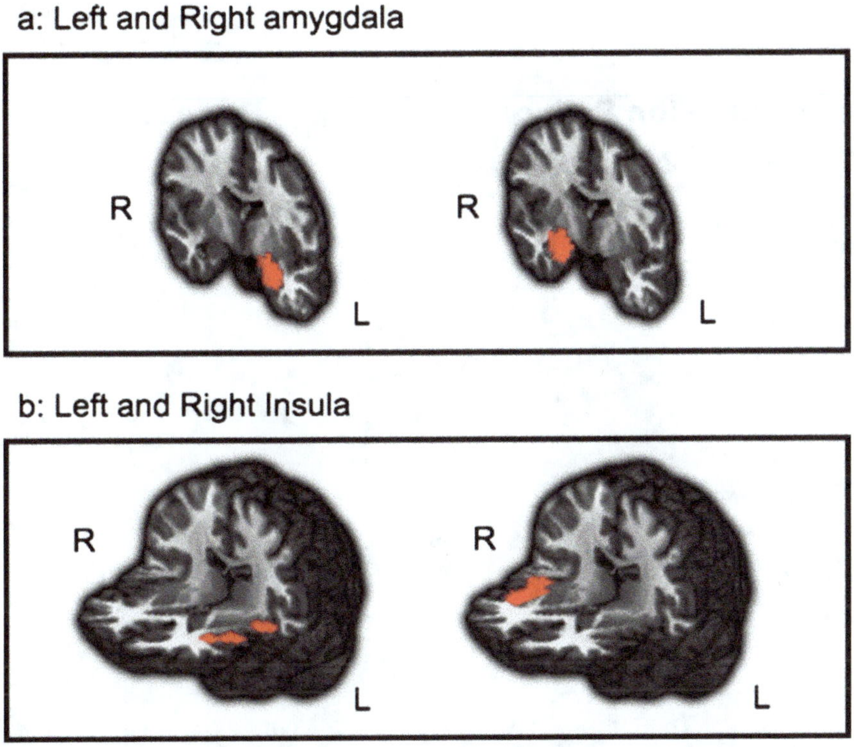

Figure 2 The a priori regions of interest. a: Left and right amygdala. **b**: Left and right insula.

set at $P < .02$ ($P = .05/3$), to adjust for the three correlations that were tested (symptom severity and brain responses during Faces, symptom severity and brain responses during Criticism, and symptom severity and brain responses during Beliefs).

Whole-brain analyses

For whole-brain analyses, we identified a sub-group of the 27 SAD patients with the highest social anxiety symptom severity (LSAS-SR scores between 85–102) and compared them to the 27 HC using a between-group ANOVA of React versus Asterisk. We selected the SAD participants with the highest levels of symptom severity to provide the most sensitive test possible of our hypothesis that groups would differ in behavior and brain responses.

Results

Primary analyses

Faces

Negative emotion ratings A between-group t-test revealed greater negative emotion ratings for SAD (n = 63, mean = 2.94, SD = 0.69) than HC (n = 28, mean = 2.11, SD = 0.82; $t_{89} = 4.98$, $P < .0001$) when reacting to harsh faces (Figure 3a).

Brain responses For react faces versus asterisks counting, between-group t-tests of BOLD responses showed no differences between SAD and HC in left and right amygdala (all *Ps* > .74), and in the left and right insula (all *Ps* > .07, Figure 3b). In supplementary analyses, between-group whole brain t-tests showed that, compared to HC, patients had *greater* BOLD responses in the medial frontal gyrus, left middle frontal gyrus, superior frontal gyrus, right superior temporal gyrus, and left middle temporal gyrus/inferior frontal gyrus (Table 3).

Criticism

Negative emotion ratings A between-group t-test revealed greater negative emotion ratings for SAD (n = 66, mean = 3.15, SD = 0.81) than HC (n = 28, mean = 2.16, SD = 0.73; $t_{92} = 5.57$, $P < .0001$) when reacting to criticism (Figure 4a).

Brain responses There were no differences between SAD and HC in left and right amygdala (all *Ps* > .28), and left and right insula (all *Ps* > .40, Figure 4b). A between-group whole-brain t-test for react to criticism versus asterisks counting showed that, compared to HC, patients had *greater* BOLD responses in the left lingual gyrus, bilateral middle temporal gyrus, and the right parahippocampal gyrus (Table 3).

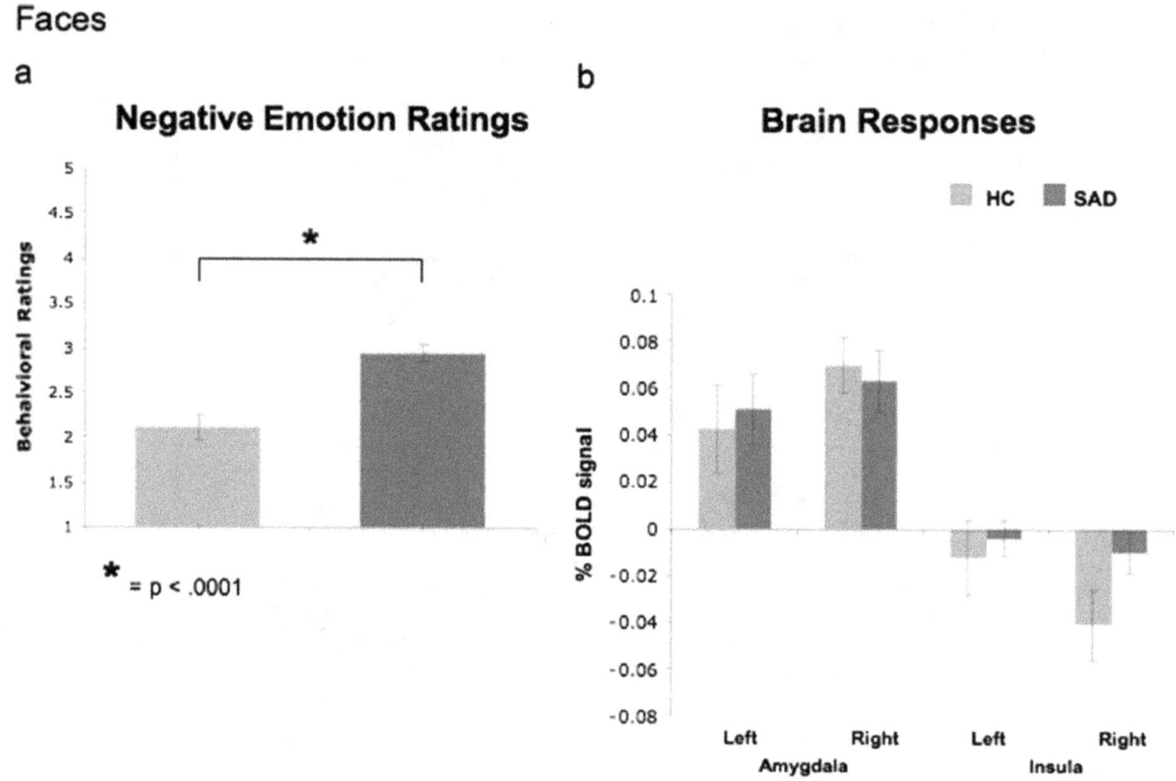

Figure 3 Faces task. Between groups differences in negative emotion ratings (**a**) and in % BOLD signal changes in the left and right amygdala and left and right insula (**b**).

Beliefs

Negative emotion ratings A between-group t-test revealed greater negative emotion ratings for SAD (n = 65, mean = 3.70, SD = 0.60) than HC (n = 25, mean = 2.69, SD = 1.04; $t_{88} = 5.76$, $P < .0001$) when reacting to negative self-beliefs (Figure 5a).

Brain responses There were no differences between SAD and HC in left and right amygdala (all *P*s > .12), and left and right insula (all *P*s > .69, Figure 5b). A between-group whole-brain t-test showed that, compared to HC, patients had *lesser* BOLD responses in the right middle frontal gyrus and left superior frontal gyrus when reacting to beliefs versus asterisks (Table 3).

Secondary analyses

Negative emotion ratings

Between-group differences A 2 Group (SAD, HC) x 3 Task (Faces, Criticism, Beliefs) repeated-measures ANOVA of negative emotion ratings yielded main effects of group (SAD > HC, $F_{1,85} = 35.34$, $P < .0001$, partial eta^2 (η_p^2) = .29) and task ($F_{2,170} = 42.80$, $P < .0001$, $\eta_p^2 = .34$, Belief > Criticism > Faces for SAD; Belief > Criticism = Faces for HC), with no group by task interaction (Figure 6).

Association with social anxiety symptoms In patients with SAD, no correlation was found between social anxiety symptom severity (LSAS-SR) and negative emotion ratings when reacting to faces ($P > .08$), criticism ($P > .05$), and beliefs ($P > .54$).

Brain responses

Between group differences To examine the differential responses to each of the tasks in SAD and HC, we conducted a 2 Group (SAD, HC) x 3 Task (Faces, Criticism, Beliefs) repeated-measures ANOVA of BOLD responses in the left and right amygdala and insula.

Amygdala For the left amygdala, there were no main effects of task or group, and no group by task interaction (all *P*s > .05) (Figure 7a). For the right amygdala, there was a main effect of task ($F_{2,154} = 4.61$, $P < .011$, $\eta_p^2 = .06$), and no main effect of group or group by task interaction (all *P*s > .28). Follow-up paired-samples t-tests indicated that in SAD, there were greater BOLD responses when reacting to criticism, and when reacting to faces, compared to beliefs, with no significant difference between criticism and faces (Criticism = Faces > Beliefs, all *P*s < .0001). In HC, no significant differences were found

Table 3 Between-group differential BOLD responses for React versus Asterisks in 27 patients with SAD versus 27 HC

Brain regions	x y z	Vol (mm^3)	*t*-value
Faces			
SAD > HC			
Medial Frontal Gyrus	0, 62, 8	2235	4.4
Superior Medial Frontal Gyrus	0, 52, 36	447	3.2
Left Medial Frontal Gyrus	−7, 59, -2	244	3.33
	−14, 52, 1	203	3.21
Left Middle Frontal Gyrus	−28, 52, 5	162	3.12
	−28, 49, 12	284	3.11
Left Middle Temporal Gyrus	−52, 14, -12	325	3.6
Right Superior Temporal Gyrus	52, -61, 19	406	3.03
Criticism			
SAD > HC			
Left Lingual Gyrus	−24, -75, -9	244	3.13
	−17, -82, 5	162	2.96
Left Middle Temporal Gyrus	−52, 0, -16	203	3.45
Right Middle Temporal Gyrus	48, -10, -16	203	3.71
Right Parahippocampus	14, -10, -16	162	3.23
Beliefs			
SAD > HC - none			
HC > SAD			
Right Middle Frontal Gyrus	52, 38, 36	244	3.19
Left Superior Temporal Gyrus	−69, -27, 12	162	3.46

Note. *t*-value threshold ≥ 2.932, voxel $P < 0.005$, minimum cluster volume threshold ≥162 mm^3 (4 voxels x 3.438 mm^3), cluster $P < 0.01$.
BA = Brodmann area, xyz = Talairach and Tournoux coordinates of maximum BOLD signal intensity voxel.

in the response to criticism, beliefs, and faces (Criticism = Faces = Belief, all *P*s > .21) (Figure 7b).

Insula For the left insula, there was a main effect of task ($F_{2,172} = 76.51$, $P < .0001$, $\eta_p^2 = .47$), and no main effect of group or group by task interaction (all *P*s > .28). Follow-up paired-samples t-tests indicated greater BOLD responses when reacting to criticism, compared to beliefs, and a significant difference between beliefs and faces, in both patients and HC (Criticism > Beliefs > Faces, all *P*s < .0001) (Figure 8a).

For the right insula, there was a main effect of task ($F_{2,174} = 122.31$, $P < .0001$, $\eta_p^2 = .58$), and a group by task interaction ($F_{2,174} = 3.97$, $P < .021$, $\eta_p^2 = .04$), with no main effect of group ($P > .41$). Follow-up paired samples t-tests indicated greater BOLD responses when reacting to criticism, compared to beliefs, and a significant difference between beliefs and faces, in both SAD and HC (Criticism > Belief > Faces, all *P*s < .0001) (Figure 8b).

Association with social anxiety symptoms In patients with SAD, there was an association of social anxiety symptom severity and BOLD responses in the left insula during the Faces task (r = .40, *P* = .001; Figure 9).

Discussion

The goal of the present study was to investigate behavioral and brain responses in patients with SAD versus HC when reacting to three socio-emotional tasks (faces, criticism, beliefs). As we expected, at the behavioral level all three tasks induced heightened negative reactivity in SAD versus HC participants. However, we found no evidence of between-group differences in amygdala and insula BOLD responses. Both SAD and HC had increased left and right amygdala responses in all three tasks, and increased left and right insula responses in 2 of the 3 tasks (Criticism and Beliefs).

How might this discrepancy between our current results and previous work on emotion-related brain responses in SAD be explained? One possibility is that differences in the experimental tasks used played a crucial role [43]. To date, most studies have used static facial expression stimuli to examine neural processing of interpersonal threat cues. Studies that have investigated social stimuli other than faces have yielded mixed results [16,17,44,45]. For example, no differential recruitment of the amygdala and insula in SAD and HC were found when listening to angry versus neutral voices [17], when performing a social situation task [44], or when playing a 'decision making' game with others [45].

In our study, we used three distinct types of socio-emotional tasks with relatively high levels of complexity. The Faces task used a static emotional facial expression with the addition of looming (i.e., the appearance of approaching the perceiver). The Criticism task used dynamic videos of an actor delivering socially critical comments. The Beliefs task used participant-generated negative self-beliefs embedded in an autobiographical script about a socially painful interpersonal situation. In addition, all three tasks paradigms had longer stimulus presentation durations (9–12 sec) than have been used in most prior studies.

It is possible that the increased stimulus complexity and presentation durations in our study increased the likelihood that healthy subjects would evaluate the stimuli as threatening, and thus may have yielded emotion reactivity related brain responses similar to those generated by the patients with SAD. In addition to the stimuli used to elicit emotional responses, other design parameters such as whether the participants are instructed to simply look at the stimuli, or whether they have to perform a task, and whether the task is implicit or explicit, may have contributed to the observed findings [46].

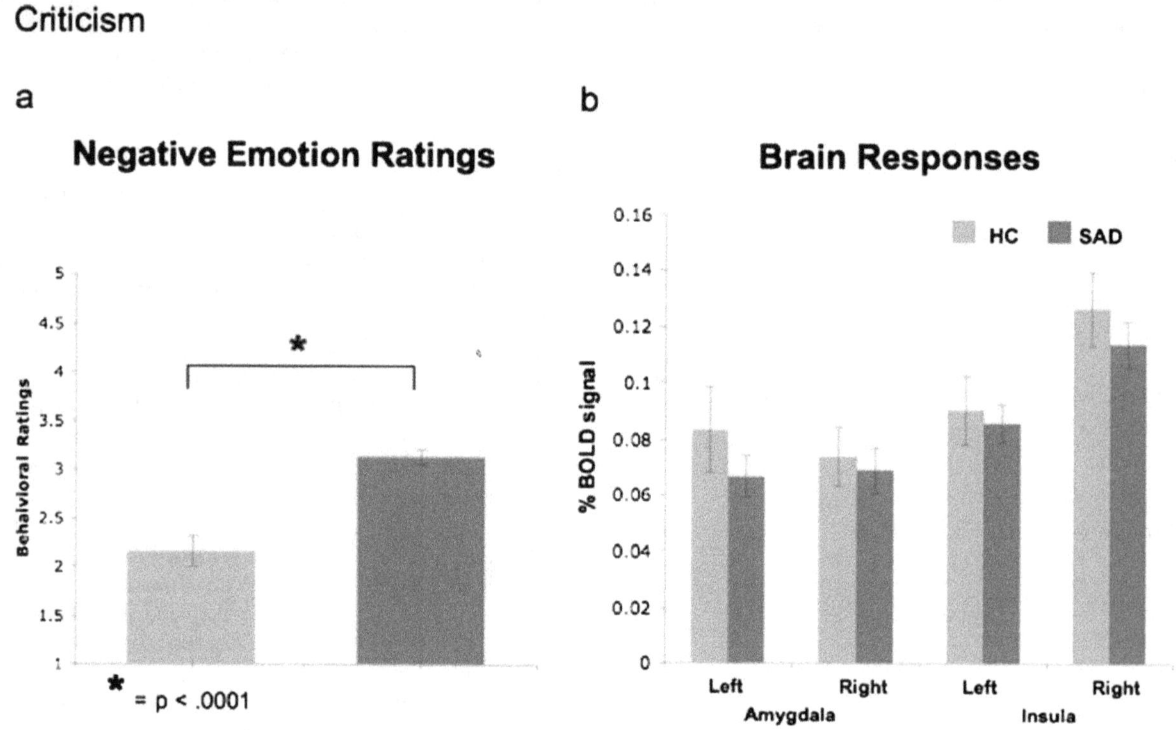

Figure 4 Criticism task. Between groups differences in negative emotion ratings (**a**) and in % BOLD signal changes in the left and right amygdala and left and right insula (**b**).

A second possible explanation of our findings builds upon the first, and suggests that at least in the complex socio-emotional contexts we employed in our study (and which characterize many everyday life contexts), increased negative emotion ratings in SAD may be related to exaggerated cognitive biases, including negative self-reflective and ruminative processes. It is also possible that there are differential tendencies to implement spontaneous (uninstructed) emotion regulation directed at the emotion experience in HC versus SAD patients. This could have yielded lower levels of negative emotion ratings in HC. Thus, if the normative pattern shown in HC is to engage in automatic emotion regulation, then one feature of SAD is the absence of such un-cued, automatic activation of emotion regulation. Therefore, maladaptive cognitive processes, such as rumination, suppression, and self-criticism, and ineffective emotion regulation, in SAD may lead to exaggerated negative emotion experience.

If such accounts are correct, we might expect other brain regions (in addition to amygdala and insula) to show differential response patterns between SAD and HC when exposed to socio-emotional stimuli. Indeed, whole brain analyses revealed SAD versus HC differences in several brain regions, specifically, increased frontal, occipital, and temporal cortical activity in SAD versus HC during the Faces and Criticism tasks, and decreased frontal activity in SAD versus HC during the Beliefs task (Table 3). These regions have been shown to be involved in emotion regulation (middle frontal gyrus) [47], recognition of faces (middle temporal gyrus) [48], language processing (superior temporal gyrus), memory (lingual gyrus, parahippocampus), and social cognition (medial frontal gyrus, superior temporal gyrus) [49]. In SAD, though not much discussed, abnormal activity in these regions has been related to difficulties in reasoning [28], mentalizing abilities [45], and impaired perception of self and others [50-52]. Additionally, the whole brain analyses further support our findings of no between-group differences in amygdala and insula activity when reacting to the socio-emotional tasks.

Congruent with these findings, in a recent study, Doehrmann and colleagues (2012) examined the association between responses to cognitive-behavioral therapy for SAD and pre-treatment brain activations to social (facial) and nonsocial (scene) stimuli [53]. They found pre-treatment activity in visual cortical regions correlated with treatment outcome, and no association with treatment outcome in the amygdala, despite its robust activation to all experimental conditions. The authors explained these

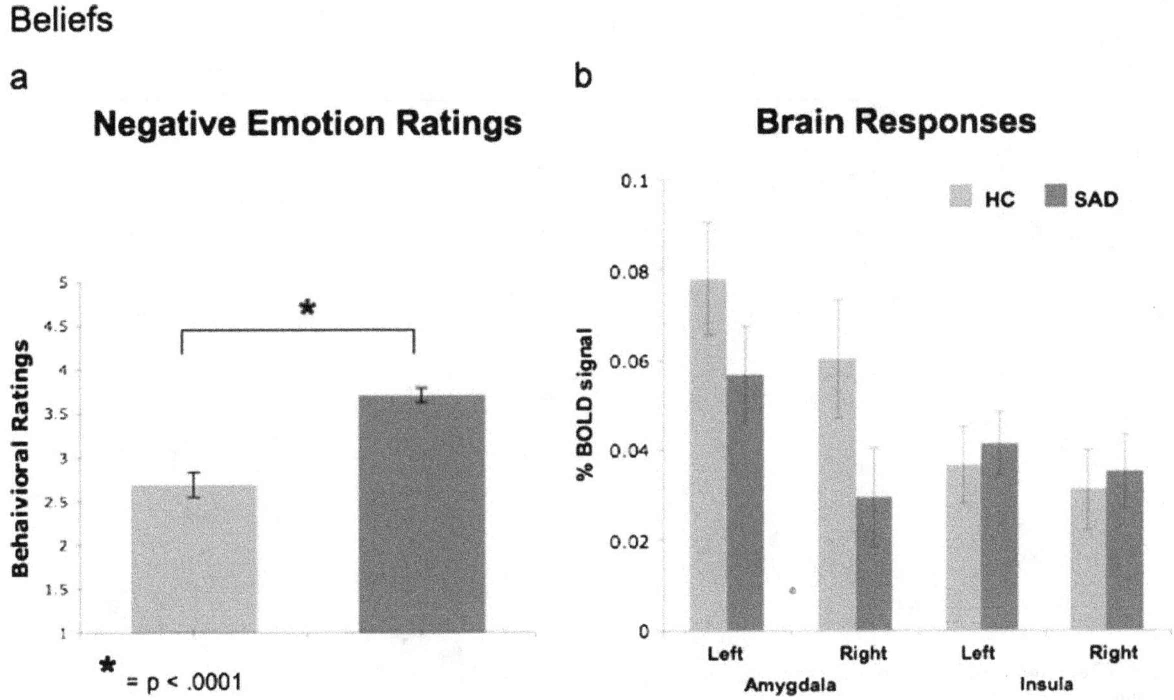

Figure 5 Beliefs task. Between groups differences in negative emotion ratings (**a**) and in % BOLD signal changes in the left and right amygdala and left and right insula (**b**).

results by emphasizing dysfunctional emotion regulation, and specifically attentional deployment, in SAD. They suggested that CBT is perhaps particularly successful in patients with better emotion regulation capacities, which is correlated with already stronger responses to angry faces in visual regions. Thus, in addition to showing no abnormality in baseline amygdala response in SAD, this study suggests that brain regions more related to emotion regulation and not to emotion reactivity, might be the core deficit in SAD, and the focus of change during treatment.

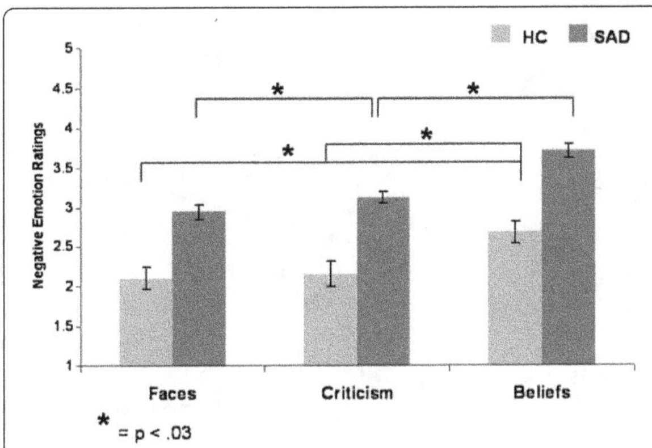

Figure 6 Task effects within each group - negative emotion ratings. For SAD, ratings were the highest for Beliefs, and lowest for the Faces task (Beliefs > Criticism > Faces). For HC, ratings were the highest for Beliefs, with no difference between Criticism and Faces (Beliefs > Criticism = Faces).

More generally, our finding of increased negativity in SAD compared to HC when facing emotional stimuli, with no such SAD versus HC differences in the amygdala and insula responses, could suggest that self-report of negative emotion is less tightly coupled with increased limbic activity than is typically thought, at least in the context of social anxiety. This hypothesis accords with the findings of Mauss and colleagues [32], namely, a decoupling of subjective emotion and physiological measures and objective physiological responses in high and low socially anxious participants when giving an impromptu speech. The authors suggested that the findings of increased physiological activation during the speech in all participants (and not only in participants who reported increased experience of anxiety) leaves open the possibility that physiological activation might be necessary for the experience of anxiety, but such activation is clearly not sufficient to explain inter-individual variation in anxiety experience. The results of the current study strengthen the conclusions of Mauss and her colleagues.

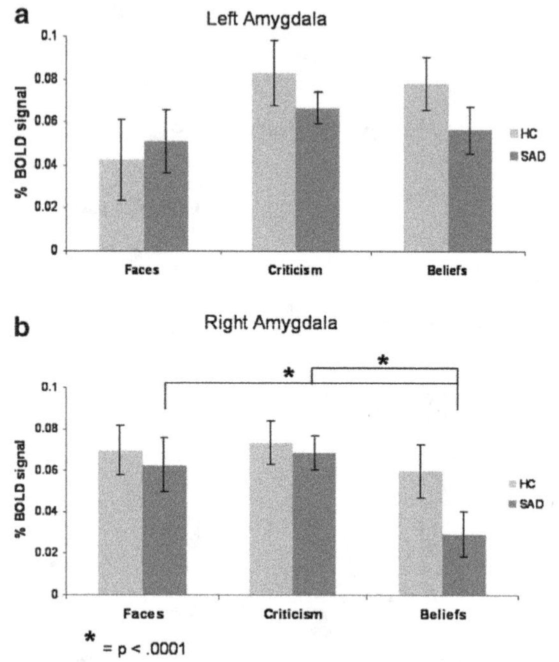

Figure 7 Task effects within each group – amygdala BOLD Responses. For the left amygdala, there was no main effect of task in SAD and in HC. For the right amygdala, there were greater BOLD responses when reacting to criticism, and when reacting to faces, compared to beliefs (Criticism = Faces > Beliefs) in SAD, and no significant between tasks differences in HC (Criticism = Faces = Beliefs).

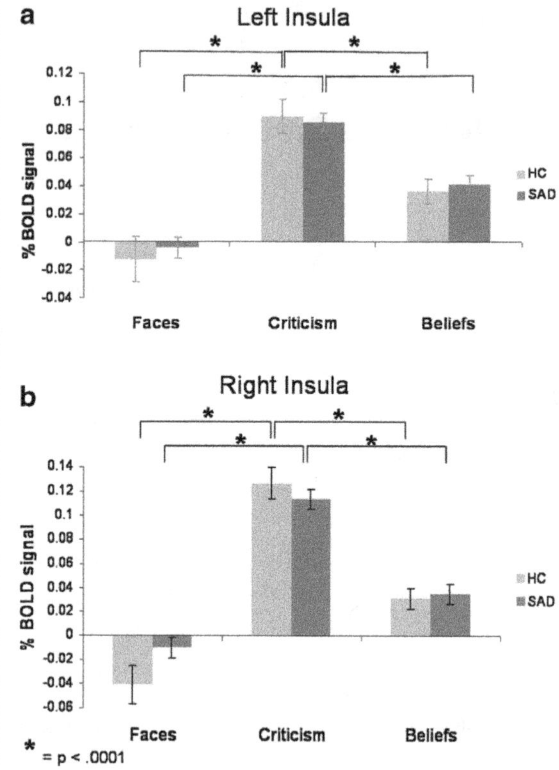

Figure 8 Task effects within each group – insula BOLD responses. For both left and right insula, there were greater BOLD responses when reacting to criticism, compared to beliefs, and a significant difference between beliefs and faces, in SAD and HC (Criticism > Beliefs > Faces).

It might be that the relation between subjective feeling and physiological response is more complex than a simple 'amygdala = emotion' equation would suggest.

It also bears comment that in the current study, examination of between task effects enabled us to examine whether the behavioral and neural results were related to a particular type of socio-emotional stimuli. Although all three tasks were successful in terms of inducing higher emotional responses in SAD, compared to HC, it seems that no task activated all emotion generation brain regions consistently. Our results indicate that different contexts, i.e. different "anxiety-inducing" experimental probes may have quite different effects, behaviorally and neurally. Behaviorally, the Beliefs task yielded the highest negative emotion reactions in both SAD and HC. Thus, the idiographic, participant-generated negative self-beliefs were the most potent emotional probe, most likely because of their self-relevance or personal salience. These probes were also the most ecologically valid type of stimuli in our study, as negative self-focused automatic thoughts are usually the focus of most forms of psychological interventions for SAD. Interestingly, the Beliefs task, which elicited the greatest negative emotion responses,

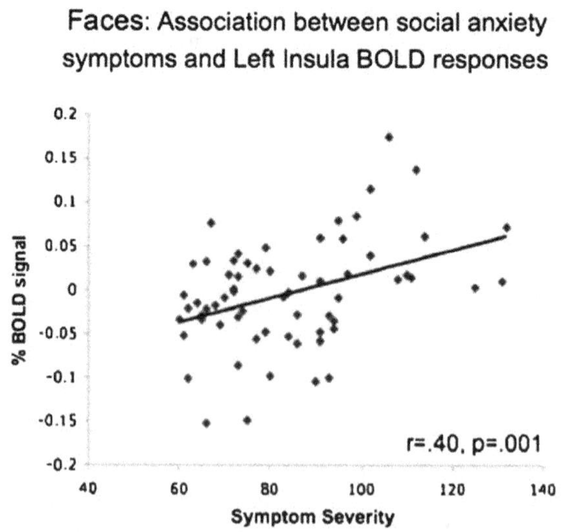

Figure 9 Faces - association with social anxiety symptoms. During the Faces task, social anxiety symptom severity was associated with BOLD responses in the left insula.

did not elicit the greatest brain responses. Specifically, right amygdala responses were equally high for Criticism and Faces, and lower for Beliefs (with no differential task effects in the left amygdala) in SAD patients. BOLD responses in the left and right insula were highest when reacting to Criticism > Beliefs > Faces in both SAD and HC.

Contrary to our hypothesis, social anxiety symptom severity was not correlated with negative emotion ratings, and was associated only with greater left insula activation during the Faces task, with no association with amygdala response. This finding accords with the findings of Schmidt and colleagues [46] of a positive correlation between insula activity and symptom severity in SAD patients, despite no differential effect in the insula between SAD and HC, during explicit processing of verbal threat-related stimuli. The association with symptom severity suggests that within patients with SAD, symptom severity matters. Thus, during the Faces task, even though as a group SAD patients had insula responses comparable to the HC group, greater social anxiety symptom severity within patients was found to be associated with increased neural responses. A recent study by Furmark and colleagues further supports the importance of looking beyond only meeting diagnostic criteria for SAD. They found that both patients with SAD and HC had increased left amygdala activation in response to angry compared with neutral faces, but that genotype (serotonergic polymorphisms) and not diagnosis explained a significant portion of the variance in amygdala responsiveness [54].

Conclusions

This is the first study to specifically assess three distinct types of socio-emotional experimental tasks in a large sample of patients with SAD at a single time point. Our main finding is similar increased amygdala and insula responses when reacting to socio-emotional stimuli, despite increased emotional responses in SAD, compared to HC. The fact that we obtained the same result using three different tasks provides strong validation of our findings. To test our hypothesis of deficits in emotion regulation processes in SAD, future studies should investigate regulation processes, both explicit (when instructed to regulate) and implicit (spontaneous), in SAD and in HC. A direct examination of emotion regulation processes and their association with neural activity in limbic and cortical brain regions could help in understanding the deficient appraisal processes in SAD.

Methodologically, more studies are needed to further examine different kinds of tasks/contexts, which might help to evaluate the influence of different variables, such as the degree of personal salience, the intensity of the emotional stimuli, and the modality of the stimuli, on the behavioral and neural responses. Also, in addition to examination of negative emotional stimuli, an interesting venue could be the investigation of positive emotional stimuli, such as social praise, or positive self-related thoughts.

In this study, in order to be able to compare between the different tasks, we contrasted the React condition to an Asterisks condition. However, in the future, it will be important to examine the results when contrasting reactivity to negative stimuli with reactivity to neutral stimuli as well.

Finally, an interesting question arising from the current results is whether other clinical populations such as major depression, generalized anxiety, or mixed anxiety-depression, show the same dissociation between heightened emotional reactivity and similar limbic responses, compared to HC. In the future, it will be important to compare behavioral and BOLD responses during negative emotional contexts in SAD group versus other clinical populations, in order to examine the specificity of the results reported here.

Additional file

Additional file 1: Table S1. Peak XYZ Talairach Coordinates for the Left and Right Insula, as Defined by Kurth's Meta Analysis [22].

Competing interests

The authors of this manuscript do not have any direct or indirect conflicts of interest to disclose.

Authors' contributions

MZ participated in the study's design and coordination, contributed to data acquisition, conducted the fMRI sessions, conducted the data analyses, and took lead on writing the manuscript. PRG helped conceive of the design of the study, participated in the study's design and coordination, contributed to data acquisition, conducted the fMRI sessions, consulted on data analyses, and contributed to writing the manuscript. HJ participated in the study's design and coordination, contributed to data acquisition, conducted the fMRI sessions, consulted on data analyses, and contributed to writing the manuscript. KSH consulted on data analyses, and contributed to writing the manuscript. JJG helped conceive of the design of the study, consulted on data analyses, and contributed to writing the manuscript. All authors have read and approved the final manuscript.

Acknowledgments

We wish to thank Gary Glover, Ph.D. for his technical assistance with magnetic resonance imaging. This research was supported by an NIMH Grant R01 MH076074, awarded to James Gross. Michal Ziv had full access to all of the data in the study and takes responsibility for the integrity of the data and the accuracy of the data analysis.

References

1. DSM-IV-TR: *Diagnostic and Statistical Manual of Mental Disorders*. 4th edition. Washington, DC: American Psychiatric Association; 2000.
2. Stein MB, Stein DJ: **Social anxiety disorder.** *Lancet* 2008, **371:**1115–1125.
3. Heimberg L: *Hope, Schneier: Social Phobia: Diagnosis, Assessment, and Treatment*. New York: Guilford Press; 1995.
4. Rapee RM: *Descriptive Psychopathology of Social Phobia*. New York, NY: Guilford Press; 1995.

5. Rapee RM, Heimberg RG: **A cognitive-behavioral model of anxiety in social phobia.** *Behav Res Ther* 1997, **35:**741–756.
6. Adolphs R, Tranel D, Damasio H, Damasio AR: **Fear and the human amygdala.** *J Neurosci* 1995, **15:**5879–5891.
7. Stein MB, Goldin PR, Sareen J, Zorrilla LT, Brown GG: **Increased amygdala activation to angry and contemptuous faces in generalized social phobia.** *Arch Gen Psychiatr* 2002, **59:**1027–1034.
8. Amaral DG: **The primate amygdala and the neurobiology of social behavior: implications for understanding social anxiety.** *Biol Psychiatr* 2002, **51:**11–17.
9. Straube T, Mentzel HJ, Miltner WH: **Common and distinct brain activation to threat and safety signals in social phobia.** *Neuropsychobiology* 2005, **52:**163–168.
10. Birbaumer N, Grodd W, Diedrich O, Klose U, Erb M, Lotze M, Schneider F, Weiss U, Flor H: **fMRI reveals amygdala activation to human faces in social phobics.** *Neuroreport* 1998, **9:**1223–1226.
11. Phan KL, Fitzgerald DA, Nathan PJ, Tancer ME: **Association between amygdala hyperactivity to harsh faces and severity of social anxiety in generalized social phobia.** *Biol Psychiatr* 2006, **59:**424–429.
12. Cooney RE, Atlas LY, Joormann J, Eugene F, Gotlib IH: **Amygdala activation in the processing of neutral faces in social anxiety disorder: is neutral really neutral?** *Psychiatr Res* 2006, **148:**55–59.
13. Amir N, Klumpp H, Elias J, Bedwell JS, Yanasak N, Miller LS: **Increased activation of the anterior cingulate cortex during processing of disgust faces in individuals with social phobia.** *Biol Psychiatr* 2005, **57:**975–981.
14. Kilts CD, Kelsey JE, Knight B, Ely TD, Bowman FD, Gross RE, Selvig A, Gordon A, Newport DJ, Nemeroff CB: **The neural correlates of social anxiety disorder and response to pharmacotherapy.** *Neuropsychopharmacology* 2006, **31:**2243–2253.
15. Van Ameringen M, Mancini C, Szechtman H, Nahmias C, Oakman JM, Hall GB, Pipe B, Farvolden P: **A PET provocation study of generalized social phobia.** *Psychiatr Res* 2004, **132:**13–18.
16. Goldin PR, Manber-Ball T, Werner K, Heimberg R, Gross JJ: **Neural mechanisms of cognitive reappraisal of negative self-beliefs in social anxiety disorder.** *Biol Psychiatr* 2009, **66:**1091–1099.
17. Quadflieg S, Mohr A, Mentzel HJ, Miltner WH, Straube T: **Modulation of the neural network involved in the processing of anger prosody: the role of task-relevance and social phobia.** *Biol Psychol* 2008, **78:**129–137.
18. Mesulam MM, Mufson EJ: **Insula of the old world monkey. III: efferent cortical output and comments on function.** *J Comp Neurol* 1982, **212:**38–52.
19. Oppenheimer SM, Gelb A, Girvin JP, Hachinski VC: **Cardiovascular effects of human insular cortex stimulation.** *Neurology* 1992, **42:**1727–1732.
20. Phan KL, Wager T, Taylor SF, Liberzon I: **Functional neuroanatomy of emotion: a meta-analysis of emotion activation studies in PET and fMRI.** *Neuroimage* 2002, **16:**331–348.
21. Paulus MP, Stein MB: **An insular view of anxiety.** *Biol Psychiatr* 2006, **60:**383–387.
22. Kurth F, Zilles K, Fox PT, Laird AR, Eickhoff SB: **A link between the systems: functional differentiation and integration within the human insula revealed by meta-analysis.** *Brain Struct Funct* 2010, **214:**519–534.
23. Mesulam MM, Mufson EJ: **Insula of the old world monkey. I. Architectonics in the insulo-orbito-temporal component of the paralimbic brain.** *J Comp Neurol* 1982, **212:**1–22.
24. Dolan RJ: **Emotion, cognition, and behavior.** *Science* 2002, **298:**1191–1194.
25. Phillips ML, Drevets WC, Rauch SL, Lane R: **Neurobiology of emotion perception I: the neural basis of normal emotion perception.** *Biol Psychiatr* 2003, **54:**504–514.
26. Straube T, Kolassa IT, Glauer M, Mentzel HJ, Miltner WH: **Effect of task conditions on brain responses to threatening faces in social phobics: an event-related functional magnetic resonance imaging study.** *Biol Psychiatr* 2004, **56:**921–930.
27. Shah SG, Klumpp H, Angstadt M, Nathan PJ, Phan KL: **Amygdala and insula response to emotional images in patients with generalized social anxiety disorder.** *J Psychiatr Neurosci* 2009, **34:**296–302.
28. Lorberbaum JP, Kose S, Johnson MR, Arana GW, Sullivan LK, Hamner MB, Ballenger JC, Lydiard RB, Brodrick PS, Bohning DE, George MS: **Neural correlates of speech anticipatory anxiety in generalized social phobia.** *Neuroreport* 2004, **15:**2701–2705.
29. Blair K, Geraci M, Devido J, McCaffrey D, Chen G, Vythilingam M, Ng P, Hollon N, Jones M, Blair RJ, Pine DS: **Neural response to self- and other referential praise and criticism in generalized social phobia.** *Arch Gen Psychiatr* 2008, **65:**1176–1184.
30. Tillfors M, Furmark T, Marteinsdottir I, Fischer H, Pissiota A, Langstrom B, Fredrikson M: **Cerebral blood flow in subjects with social phobia during stressful speaking tasks: a PET study.** *Am J Psychiatr* 2001, **158:**1220–1226.
31. Sareen J, Campbell DW, Leslie WD, Malisza KL, Stein MB, Paulus MP, Kravetsky LB, Kjernisted KD, Walker JR, Reiss JP: **Striatal function in generalized social phobia: a functional magnetic resonance imaging study.** *Biol Psychiatr* 2007, **61:**396–404.
32. Mauss IB, Wilhelm FH, Gross JJ: **Is there less to social anxiety than meets the eye? Emotion experience, expression, and bodily responding.** *Cognit Emotion* 2004, **18:**631–662.
33. DiNardo PA, Brown TA, Barlow DH: *Anxiety Disorders Interview Schedule for DSM-IV: Lifetime Version (ADIS-IV-L).* Albany, NY: Graywind Publications Inc; 1994.
34. Oldfield RC: **The assessment and analysis of handedness: the Edinburgh inventory.** *Neuropsychologia* 1971, **9:**97–113.
35. Liebowitz MR: **Social phobia.** *Mod Probl Pharmacopsychiatr* 1987, **22:**141–173.
36. Fresco DM, Coles ME, Heimberg RG, Liebowitz MR, Hami S, Stein MB, Goetz D: **The Liebowitz Social Anxiety Scale: a comparison of the psychometric properties of self-report and clinician-administered formats.** *Psychol Med* 2001, **31:**1025–1035.
37. Ekman P, Friesen W: *Facial Action Coding System: A Technique for the Measurment of Facial Movement.* Palo Alto: Consulting Psychologists Press; 1978.
38. Glover GH, Law CS: **Spiral-in/out BOLD fMRI for increased SNR and reduced susceptibility artifacts.** *Magn Reson Med* 2001, **46:**515–522.
39. Cox RW: **AFNI: software for analysis and visualization of functional magnetic resonance neuroimages.** *Comput Biomed Res* 1996, **29:**162–173.
40. Cohen MS: **Parametric analysis of fMRI data using linear systems methods.** *Neuroimage* 1997, **6:**93–103.
41. Talairach J, Tournoux P: *Co-Planar Stereotaxic Atlas of the Human Brain.* New York: Thieme; 1988.
42. Forman SD, Cohen JD, Fitzgerald M, Eddy WF, Mintun MA, Noll DC: **Improved assessment of significant activation in functional magnetic resonance imaging (fMRI): use of a cluster-size threshold.** *Magn Reson Med* 1995, **33:**636–647.
43. Freitas-Ferrari MC, Hallak JE, Trzesniak C, Filho AS, Machado-de-Sousa JP, Chagas MH, Nardi AE, Crippa JA: **Neuroimaging in social anxiety disorder: a systematic review of the literature.** *Prog Neuropsychopharmacol Biol Psychiatr* 2010, **34:**565–580.
44. Nakao T, Sanematsu H, Yoshiura T, Togao O, Murayama K, Tomita M, Masuda Y, Kanba S: **fMRI of patients with social anxiety disorder during a social situation task.** *Neurosci Res* 2011, **69:**67–72.
45. Sripada CS, Angstadt M, Banks S, Nathan PJ, Liberzon I, Phan KL: **Functional neuroimaging of mentalizing during the trust game in social anxiety disorder.** *Neuroreport* 2009, **20:**984–989.
46. Schmidt S, Mohr A, Miltner WH, Straube T: **Task-dependent neural correlates of the processing of verbal threat-related stimuli in social phobia.** *Biol Psychol* 2010, **84:**304–312.
47. Diekhof EK, Geier K, Falkai P, Gruber O: **Fear is only as deep as the mind allows: a coordinate-based meta-analysis of neuroimaging studies on the regulation of negative affect.** *Neuroimage* 2011, **58:**275–285.
48. Haxby JV, Hoffman EA, Gobbini MI: **The distributed human neural system for face perception.** *Trends Cogn Sci* 2000, **4:**223–233.
49. Adolphs R: **The social brain: neural basis of social knowledge.** *Annu Rev Psychol* 2009, **60:**693–716.
50. Warwick JM, Carey P, Jordaan GP, Dupont P, Stein DJ: **Resting brain perfusion in social anxiety disorder: a voxel-wise whole brain comparison with healthy control subjects.** *Prog Neuropsychopharmacol Biol Psychiatr* 2008, **32:**1251–1256.
51. Guyer AE, Lau JY, McClure-Tone EB, Parrish J, Shiffrin ND, Reynolds RC, Chen G, Blair RJ, Leibenluft E, Fox NA, *et al*: **Amygdala and ventrolateral prefrontal cortex function during anticipated peer evaluation in pediatric social anxiety.** *Arch Gen Psychiatr* 2008, **65:**1303–1312.
52. Blair KS, Geraci M, Otero M, Majestic C, Odenheimer S, Jacobs M, Blair RJ, Pine DS: **Atypical modulation of medial prefrontal cortex to self-referential comments in generalized social phobia.** *Psychiatr Res* 2011, **193:**38–45.

53. Doehrmann O, Ghosh SS, Polli FE, Reynolds GO, Horn F, Keshavan A, Triantafyllou C, Saygin ZM, Whitfield-Gabrieli S, Hofmann SG, *et al*: **Predicting treatment response in social anxiety disorder from functional magnetic resonance imaging.** *Arch Gen Psychiatr* 2013, **70**:87–97.
54. Furmark T, Henningsson S, Appel L, Ahs F, Linnman C, Pissiota A, Faria V, Oreland L, Bani M, Pich EM, *et al*: **Genotype over-diagnosis in amygdala responsiveness: affective processing in social anxiety disorder.** *J Psychiatr Neurosci* 2009, **34**:30–40.

6

Criteria of validity for animal models of psychiatric disorders: focus on anxiety disorders and depression

Catherine Belzung[1*] and Maël Lemoine[2]

Abstract

Animal models of psychiatric disorders are usually discussed with regard to three criteria first elaborated by Willner; face, predictive and construct validity. Here, we draw the history of these concepts and then try to redraw and refine these criteria, using the framework of the diathesis model of depression that has been proposed by several authors. We thus propose a set of five major criteria (with sub-categories for some of them); homological validity (including species validity and strain validity), pathogenic validity (including ontopathogenic validity and triggering validity), mechanistic validity, face validity (including ethological and biomarker validity) and predictive validity (including induction and remission validity). Homological validity requires that an adequate species and strain be chosen: considering species validity, primates will be considered to have a higher score than drosophila, and considering strains, a high stress reactivity in a strain scores higher than a low stress reactivity in another strain. Pathological validity corresponds to the fact that, in order to shape pathological characteristics, the organism has been manipulated both during the developmental period (for example, maternal separation: ontopathogenic validity) and during adulthood (for example, stress: triggering validity). Mechanistic validity corresponds to the fact that the cognitive (for example, cognitive bias) or biological mechanisms (such as dysfunction of the hormonal stress axis regulation) underlying the disorder are identical in both humans and animals. Face validity corresponds to the observable behavioral (ethological validity) or biological (biomarker validity) outcomes: for example anhedonic behavior (ethological validity) or elevated corticosterone (biomarker validity). Finally, predictive validity corresponds to the identity of the relationship between the triggering factor and the outcome (induction validity) and between the effects of the treatments on the two organisms (remission validity). The relevance of this framework is then discussed regarding various animal models of depression.

Introduction

In recent years, the translational approach, which aims at bridging the gaps between basic animal research and medical practice, has gained much popularity. This concept, although not new in medicine, became popular with its introduction in the National Institutes of Health Roadmap initiative [1,2]. It applies also to the field of psychiatry, and particularly to the one of affective disorders, a nosographical entity including depression and anxiety disorders. In the framework of translational medicine, a robust approach should include both research going from the bench to the bedside (from animals to humans, or from basic to clinical research) but also 'back translation research' (from humans to animals). Most efforts have been devoted to the former, focusing on the design of animal models (particularly using rodents) that would be relevant to study the human disorder and to predict the therapeutic outcomes of future treatments. Unfortunately, little research follows the opposite direction, using the back-translational approach and thus going from the bedside to the bench. However, this method is crucial when trying to assess the function of some mechanisms discovered in animal models in the pathophysiology of human disorders and when trying to discover new treatments for these conditions. For example, the contribution of hippocampal neurogenesis in the pathophysiology of depression and in the therapeutic efficacy of pharmacological treatments

* Correspondence: catherine.belzung@univ-tours.fr
[1]U930, UFR Sciences et Techniques, Parc Grandmont, Rue Monge, Tours, 37200, France
Full list of author information is available at the end of the article

has been shown using rodent models [3-6], and then confirmed in human studies [7,8]. In any case, these approaches require that these rodent models are suitable to study the clinical condition.

Two opposite attitudes exist. The first is one of skepticism: animal models already have limited interest even in the case of diseases affecting largely shared physiological systems among mammals. How could they be reliable in the case of largely specific features of the human species, such as diseases involving mostly disorders of the higher cognitive abilities? For instance, how could one distinguish a rodent model for autism from a rodent model for schizophrenia? Is there a relevant difference between rodent models of depressive disorders and rodent models of anxiety disorders? The second attitude is constructive, and consists of trying to elevate the quality of our models, regardless of general and theoretical objections. Instead of falling into evolutionary or even philosophical debates, the question then focuses on methodological concerns. This paper takes the second attitude. More specifically, the improvement of the validity of animal models has been addressed through the proposal of quality criteria since the 1960s. These criteria have continued to evolve. It seems timely to reassess them and possibly recast the standards of this core part of translational research. After having outlined the traditional standard criteria, the present paper thus propounds an up-to-date set of such criteria of animal models' validity.

A review of the classic criteria of validity for animal models of psychiatric disorders

According to several authors, an animal model of a psychiatric condition should fulfill a multidimensional set of criteria of validity to be considered relevant for human pathology. Many authors have proposed a list of such criteria, focusing on models of depression and models of anxiety (see Table 1). Interestingly, since the 1960s, authors have felt increasingly concerned with criteria of external validity and less with criteria of internal validity (with exceptions such as [9-11]). Internal validity addresses the consistency of the experimental design: reproducibility, inter-observer reliability, randomization, multicentric design, design (test-control), blind experimentation, and so on. These questions are indeed not specific to animal studies, but are widely shared across all fields of experimental science [11]. On the other hand, external validity concerns the general question of the applicability of the results of a study on a sample to the target population: it obviously raises supplemental concern in the case of animal models because of the necessity to resort to analogical arguments. It is these concerns that led to the need for specific criteria for ensuring the external validity of animal studies. To our knowledge, the first attempt to define such criteria of validity for animal models was elaborated in 1964 by Janssen [12]. This author proposed eight criteria to decide whether a procedure was relevant or not:

Table 1 Criteria for animal models of depression and of anxiety disorders

Reference	N	Predictive validity	Face validity	Construct validity	Others
[12]	8	Specificity			Efficiency Speed Simplicity Reproducibility Adequate design Adequate data processing Correlation with other tests
[13]	5	Similar response to treatments	Analogy of symptoms		Observable and measurable behavioral changes Interobserver agreement Reproducibility of the system
[14]	4	Is the model thorough in describing features of its cures? Similarity of cure	Symptoms similarity	Is the model thorough in describing features of its cause? Similarity of physiology, cause	Does model describe the disorder or a sub-category? Is the model thorough in describing features of its prevention? Similarity of prevention
[17]	3	Predictability	Isomorphism	Homology	
[9]	6	Predictive validity	Face validity	Construct validity	Reliability Etiological validity Convergent validity Discriminant validity
[28]	3	Predictive	Face	Construct	
[18]	6	Predictive	Face	Etiological validity Construct validity	Convergent validity Reliability
[19]	3	Predictive	Face	Construct	

The criteria proposed by various authors are compared to the three criteria elaborated by Willner (1994) [15]. N: number of proposed criteria.

efficiency, speed, simplicity, reproducibility, specificity, adequate design and data processing and correlation with other tests. These criteria did mainly apply to screening tests, and were rather pragmatic, as researchers were mainly interested in finding a device and/or protocol enabling them to rapidly test new compounds. It is to be noticed also that these criteria are not really relevant to translational research, as they did not refer to the clinical condition: the idea here was not to model a disorder, but to find a reproducible, reliable and rapid method to test compounds. Interestingly, this list mostly focused on criteria of internal validity. The first paper that explicitly proposed criteria for 'animal models', focusing on external validity, was published 5 years later by McKinney and Bunney [13] and focused on depression. The literature in the field of animal models of affective disorders frequently cites this paper, claiming that McKinney and Bunney proposed four validity criteria (same etiology, same symptoms, same response to treatments and same biochemistry). As a matter of fact, this article presents the available methods to induce depressive-like symptoms and then proposes five requirements for an animal model: analogy of symptoms, existence of observable and measurable behavioral changes, interobserver agreement, same response to treatments and reproducibility of the system. However, these criteria were not well defined at that time, as their description was limited to one sentence in this original paper. Interestingly, these authors propose the criterion of similarity in symptoms and in response to treatments, which recapitulates two of the four criteria that are usually attributed to these authors. Concerning the two remaining criteria of the list of four (same etiology and same biochemistry), they cannot be recapitulated under the three remaining concepts they propose. For example, similarity in etiology is not really explicitly mentioned in that list, even if in the paper the authors describe social loss as one of the factors that can be used to elicit depressive-like symptoms. In 1977, additional criteria were added by Abramson and Seligman [14]; they mentioned the similarity of etiology, but also an interesting criterion that was unfortunately abandoned: the precision of the sub-nosographic entity ('Does the laboratory model describe (...) a naturally occurring psychopathology or only a subgroup?'). However, most of the researchers working in the field of animal models of depression rely on the proposal made by Willner in 1984 of three criteria of validity: face validity, predictive validity and construct validity [15]. Willner (personal communication) was inspired by the latter criterion as proposed 30 years earlier by Cronbach and Meehl [16] in the field of psychology. Note that these criteria are still used by the European Federation of Psychologists' Association, albeit under different terminology. Willner's article can really be considered seminal in the field of animal models of psychiatric disorders (it is cited 547 times in March 2011), and most authors now refer to it, either by changing some of the criteria of that list or by adding a hierarchy between these criteria. Soubrié and Simon [17] for example rather use the French terms for 'homology', 'isomorphism' and 'predictability' while Koob *et al.* [18] do not include predictive validity but add etiological validity and convergent validity. Geyer and Markou [9] include etiological validity, convergent and discriminant validity, and claim that predictive validity is the crucial aspect. Koob *et al.* consider reliability and predictive validity to be essential criteria, while face, convergent, etiological and construct validity are more secondary. For Sarter and Bruno [19], on the other hand, construct validity is much more important than face and predictive validity. For Robbins [20], homology is central for construct validity. However, it is possible that these diverging points of view also stem from different definitions of the various criteria. We thus will first try to carefully examine the definition of the various criteria, by focusing on the three criteria proposed by Willner [15] or their equivalents.

Predictive validity

According to Willner [15], predictive validity relies on five sub-criteria: 'whether a model correctly identifies (1) antidepressant treatments of pharmacologically diverse types (2), without making errors of omission (3) or commission (4), and whether potency in the model correlates with clinical potency (5).' According to this definition, this criterion really relies on a pharmacological correlation (non-pharmacological treatments are not mentioned). It is clear from these examples that this criterion is not at all intended to translate aspects of human pathology in animals, as it is only concerned with pharmacological effects. In another paper by the same authors [21], the criterion has been extended to include response to all available treatments (for example, in the case of depression, not only pharmacological antidepressants but also electroconvulsive therapy), so that one can conclude that it can correspond to a human-animal correlation of therapeutic outcomes. This concept is similar to one of the criteria proposed by McKinney and Bunney [13], as the description given by these authors ('The treatment modalities effective in reversing depression in humans should reverse the changes seen in animals') more or less recapitulates Willner's sub-criteria 1, 2 and 3. It is, however, not convergent with the 'specificity' criteria of Janssen [12] who claimed, 'Specificity, a given drug effects being characteristic for a well-defined class of chemicals and indicative of a specific mode of action.' There is no reference to psychiatric disorder, that is, to the idea that the treatment should reverse disease-related symptoms. However, the definition employed by Koob *et al.* [18] is quite different, in their paper focusing on anxiety, predictive validity is defined as 'the ability to make consistent predictions about anxiety based on an animal's performance in the model.' Definitions convergent with this proposal can also be found in Geyer and Markou's paper [9], as these authors extend this criterion to what 'allows one to make predictions about the human phenomenon based on the performance of the model.' It is clear that their use of the term 'prediction' is not limited to the ability to predict the efficacy of treatments. So, this criterion of predictive validity is, in most cases, limited to the ability of the model to accurately respond to the treatments that are employed, but some authors also use it in a broader sense, including the model's aptitude to predict some specific markers of the disease.

Face validity

For Willner [15], 'Face validity is assessed by whether antidepressant effects are only present on, or are potentiated by, chronic administration (1), and whether the model resembles depression in a number of respects (2), which are specific to depression (3), and do actually coexist in a specific sub-group of depressions (4); also, the model should not show features which are not seen clinically (5).' By this definition, face validity interestingly encompasses both some treatment features and symptomatic aspects. Examples that Willner uses to illustrate this criterion include reserpine reversal, amphetamine potentiation, 5-hydroxytryptophan-induced depression, bulbectomy, isolation-induced hyperactivity, exhaustion stress and disturbance of circadian rhythms. The discussion about the fact that face validity applies to these models makes it clear that, according to this author, face validity includes both pharmacological similarity and phenomenological identity. For example, he mentions that in the unpredictable chronic mild stress (UCMS) model, antidepressants are effective after chronic, but not acute, treatment. He also notes that reserpine induces similar behavioral effects in animals and in humans, that hyperactivity and heightened glucocorticoid levels are observed both in depressed people and in rodents subjected to bulbectomy or to unpredictable chronic stress, and that elevation of the threshold for intracranial self-stimulation resembles the anhedonia displayed by depressed people. Later on, the same author claims that face validity corresponds to 'the extent of similarity between the model and the disorder is examined, on as wide as possible a range of symptoms and signs' [21]. Here, therapeutic outcomes are not explicitly mentioned anymore and the definition rather shifts toward requiring the identity of symptoms. This is reminiscent of McKinney and Bunney proposing that, the symptoms of the depression so induced should be reasonably analogous to those seen in human depression' [13]. Geyer and Markou [9], as well as Sarter and Bruno [19], define face validity as 'the degree of phenomenological similarity between the model and the disorder to be modeled.' It should be noted that this phenomenological identity, as formulated here, encompasses the behavioral and/or cognitive aspects only, not their physiological and/or neural bases. This suggests that, in fact, face validity corresponds to an attempt to mimic diagnostic criteria of the psychiatric conditions, such as those listed in the tenth revision of the World Health Organization's International Statistical Classification of Diseases and Related Health Problems (ICD-10) or the American Psychiatric Association's Diagnostic and Statistical Manual of Mental Disorders (DSM-IV); indeed, these criteria are generally behavioral and/or cognitive only, without referring to any etiology or biological basis. Another aspect should be considered here. In recent years, a debate has emerged (see, for example, [2,22-24]) between the view that a relevant model should in fact apply to the disorder (depression, for example) or rather to dimensions, symptoms and/or endophenotypes (a model of anhedonia for example). In the first case, the phenomenon to be mimicked corresponds to a set of probably interdependent variables, while in the second case, there is no attempt to model a disorder, but rather to model one particular dimension of a disorder, which is possible if the various symptoms of a given pathology are independent from the others. In the first case, the changes observed in the animal should include several dimensions. For example, a model of depression should include anhedonia, but also changes in mood, in appetite, in sleep, and so on.

Construct validity

Concerning construct validity, the picture is rather complex and the views defended by various authors are summarized in Table 2. In his seminal paper on animal models of depression, Willner [15] proposed that construct validity correspond to the fact that 'both the behavior in the model (1) and the features of depression being modeled (2) can be unambiguously interpreted, and are homologous (3), and whether the feature being modeled stands in an established empirical (4) and theoretical (5) relationship to depression.' The paper then describes several animal models of depression, discussing the fact that these models may or may not fulfill the construct validity requirement. Willner then discusses six methods for their potential ability to fulfill the construct validity criterion: learned helplessness, behavioral despair, UCMS, maternal separation, incentive

Table 2 Definitions for "construct validity"

Definition	Reference
'Whether both the behavior in the model (1) and the features of depression being modeled (2) can be unambiguously interpreted, and are homologous (3), and whether the feature being modeled stands in an established empirical (4) and theoretical (5) relationship to depression.'	[15]
'a theoretical account of the disordered behavior in the model, a theoretical account of the disorder itself, and a means to bring the two theories into alignment'	[26]
'Construct validity of a test is commonly defined as the accuracy with which the test measures what it is intended to measure'	[9]
'the accuracy with which the model measures what it is intended to measure'	[18]
'bring the theoretical accounts of both the disorder itself and the disordered behavior exhibited by the model into alignment'	[21]
'a theory-driven, experimental substantiation of the behavioral and/or neuronal components of the model' '(...) map a theory about the biopsychological mechanisms of a human disorder on to a biopsychotheory of a particular animal behavior'	[19]

disengagement and intracranial self-stimulation (updated list to be found in [25] for anxiety models). This discussion indicates that sub-criterion 5, theoretical relationship to depression, is understood in a very broad and polysemic sense. It includes theories about the nature of the depressive state, the crucial impact of some dysfunctional processes (for example, that helplessness or anhedonia are central symptoms in depression), the dynamic of the disorder (for example, its biphasic course) and its etiology. The etiology, in turn, includes theories about the part some external events take in the triggering of a depressive-like state (stress or separation may cause depression in humans and depressive-like symptoms in non-human mammals), the central importance of some specific characteristics of these events (uncontrollability or unpredictability of the stressors as central mechanisms) and the involvement of underlying biological processes (for example, the participation of a dysfunction of the brain reward system).

These aspects could be considered different sub-dimensions of this criterion. The same concept, in which construct validity is seen as an attempt to establish a theoretical rationale of animal models both at the level of a similarity of the behavioral and/or cognitive dysfunctional processes and at the level of a similarity of the etiology, was developed in later papers by Willner [21]. In a book chapter on animal models of depression [26], the same author explicates two additional facts; firstly, that similarity between the biological dysfunctions in the clinical population and in the animal model is an essential aspect of this criterion; secondly, that homology between the modeled processes is not only required in addition to a similarity in the etiology and the cause of the abnormalities seen, but the link between these two levels should be translated as well: 'a theoretical account of the disordered behavior in the model, a theoretical account of the disorder itself, and a means to bring the two theories into alignment.'

In other terms, this means that if one considers that anhedonia, for example, is a crucial feature of depression (the first requirement above) and should be present in the animal model, and that anhedonia is caused by a dysfunction of the brain reward system including the nucleus accumbens (the second requirement), then the relationship between anhedonia and the function of the nucleus accumbens should be the same in animals and humans and its dysfunction should be similar in the depressed subjects and in the animal subjected to the model. A close assumption is found by Sarter and Bruno [19]. However, in the paper by Geyer and Markou [9], construct validity is also defined in relation to theoretical constructs, but it is clearly separated from etiological validity. Having given the example of the UCMS model, they claim that this protocol draws from theories on the link between 'stress and consummatory behavior', and assume that the role of stress in depression and anhedonia is a core symptom of depression. However, when trying to discuss this criterion, many authors ignore the first aspect (the similarity of the theoretical construct about the dysfunctional cognitive, behavioral and/or psychological processes) and thus mention only the second aspect, that is, the similarity of the etiology, either when theorizing about the external events causing the depressive state or focusing on the underlying biological basis (see [25] for an exception). For example, concerning the first aspect, UCMS translates the diathesis theory of depression, as stress in vulnerable rodents may induce depressive-like behaviors. The diathesis theory of depression claims that depression relates to a predisposition that has been acquired during the developmental period, resulting both from genetic and from environmental factors and rendering the subject more vulnerable to triggering factors such as stress. The second aspect can be illustrated with the example of the model consisting of corticosterone administration in mice [27], which in fact relies on the theory that depression is related to a dysfunction of the hypothalamus-pituitary-adrenal axis. Interestingly, when discussing a given animal model of affective disorder with regard to this criterion of construct validity, most authors only focus on one of these aspects, insisting either only on theories about the dysfunctional process (for example, focusing on helplessness for the learned helplessness model), on the biological etiology (a defect in glucocorticoid release regulation in the corticosterone administration model) or on the early environmental etiology (maternal separation). In some cases, such as the unpredictable mild stress model, the construct validity criterion can be discussed according to several of these sub-dimensions, including the importance of stress in triggering the depressive episode, the crucial nature of the unpredictability of these stressors in the etiology of the disorder and the centrality of anhedonia. However, the crucial importance of this construct validity criterion is not emphasized by all authors. For example, according to Weiss and Kilts, 'although theoretically based models are likely to provide interesting and valuable information about the relation of certain behaviors to physiological changes, they face no fewer fundamental problems in establishing their validity as models of diagnostic categories than did the psychodynamic formulation they have replaced' [28]. Tables 1 and 2 recap the results of this review.

A reformulation of the classic criteria of validity

These criteria would benefit from being defined more precisely. For instance, Treit *et al.* [29] have very critically assessed the precision and the applicability of the three traditional criteria. An animal model can be thought of as a three-stage input-output process intended to resemble the original path to disease (see Figure 1). On this basis, nine criteria on the overall validity of an animal model, whatever the disorder is, can be proposed. These include five major criteria, from which four (homological validity, pathogenic validity, face validity and predictive validity) can be sub-divided into two sub-criteria each. It is necessary to compare these new criteria with the traditional criteria presented earlier. As a matter of fact, this new proposal is not intended to simply subdivide and sharpen Willner's original three criteria of validity, but rather consists of an integration of Willner's criteria into a broader framework. By so doing, although part of his terminology is salvaged, the meaning is not necessarily the same. In the end, it will also be clarifying to apply these new criteria to well-known models.

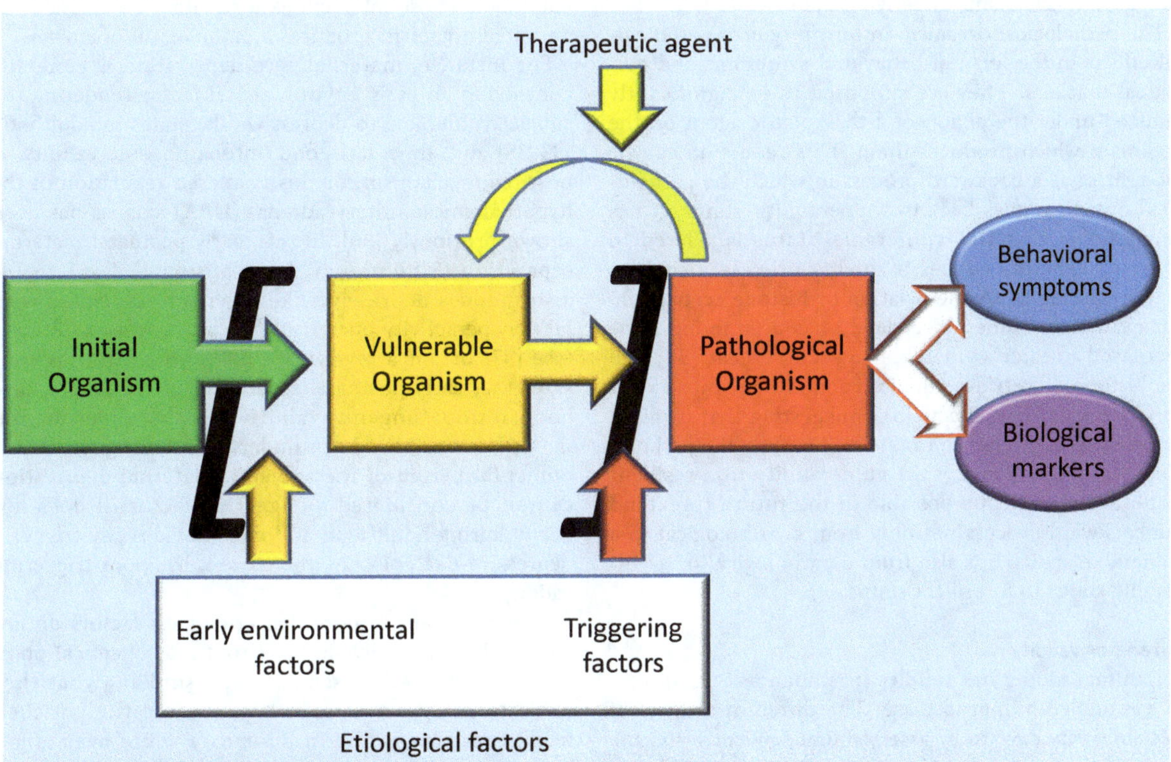

Figure 1 A framework for animal models. Animal models are not just organisms supposed to resemble a human dysfunction: the processes by which both animal and humans fall into this state must also be similar. Here is a simplified representation of how this occurs.

General framework of animal studies

An animal model of a disease is not just a model of the action of a therapeutic agent at time *t*. It has to draw from the comparison between two pathological organisms [25] but possibly should also mimic the temporal and etiological process of transformation from a healthy organism to a pathological one via the state of vulnerability. The field of biological psychiatry has been dramatically improved lately thanks to the concept of diathesis.

Figure 1 represents the proposed general framework. The initial organism consists of a set of mechanisms mainly defined by genetic properties. It is then exposed to etiological factors. First, early environmental factors transform it, mainly through epigenetic mechanisms, into a vulnerable organism. The initial organism can be either vulnerable or non-vulnerable from a genetic point of view. Therefore some models aim directly at the transformation of an initial, vulnerable organism into a pathological organism; however on most models this defines the second step. Second, triggering factors occurring in adulthood transform the vulnerable organism into a pathological organism. This third state of the organism is considered to be significantly different from the first one. The difference defines the cognitive and biological mechanisms underlying the disease.

The pathological organism in turn produces pathological effects in the form of behavioral symptoms and biological markers. They are supposed to be significantly reduced under the action of a therapeutic agent on the organism which produces them. This reduction can be thought of as a backward process in which the pathological organism goes back to 'vulnerability' status. It has been shown that the 'vulnerable' status is related to some epigenetic changes involving processes such as region-specific DNA-methylation or histone acetylation. For example, histone deacetylase 2 has been found to be increased in mice vulnerable to social defeat [30] and the histone deacetylase inhibitor, sodium butyrate, exerts antidepressant-like effects [31], suggesting that it might be possible in the future to reverse not only the pathological state, but also to shift vulnerability to a resilient state. So, it might be possible in the future to extend the backward process not only from a pathological to a vulnerable status, but also from a pathological or a vulnerable status to a resilient status.

Criteria of validity

An animal model has validity inasmuch as it is similar to a modeled human disease. The different aspects of this similarity have to be assessed independently. On the basis of the model of animal models presented above, we propose five major criteria (with sub-categories for some of them). Figure 2 recaps the criteria.

Homological validity

The homological validity of an animal model assesses two choices - that of the species and that of a particular strain of the species. For instance, *Caenorhabditis elegans* is a poor choice to model the reduction of the hippocampal volume in depression, but a better one to model basic serotonergic phenomena under stress (see [22] for both a discussion of the concept of homology and a thorough analysis of the difficulties of the choice of a particular species for an animal model). The choice of a particular strain is also part of the homological validity of an animal model. For example, the Flinders Sensitive Line of rat would be a more relevant choice than the Flinders Resistant Line when trying to model depression, as they have been suggested to be prone to display depressive-like states, both at the behavioral and biological levels (see [32] for a review).

Pathogenic validity

The pathogenic validity of a model assesses the similarity of the processes that lead to disease. It thus seems useful to contrast *ontopathogenic validity*, that is, early environmental factors whose interaction with the initial organism produces a vulnerable organism according to the theory of diathesis, with *triggering validity*, that is, the similarity of triggering factors occurring during adulthood whose interactions with either a vulnerable or an initial organism produces a pathological organism.

For instance, maternal care deprivation is generally considered an early environmental factor rendering the subject vulnerable to depressive-like states in adulthood [33-35] and, thus, has good ontopathogenic validity. A possible mechanism for this is altered regulation of the hypothalamic-pituitary-adrenal (HPA) axis, as has been shown previously [36]. In rats, early postnatal maternal separation (3 hours/day, from postnatal day 1 to 14) also induces depressive-like behavior associated with HPA hyperactivity once the offspring reaches adulthood (see [37] or, for a review, see [38]). One can thus consider that early postnatal separation in rats might have good ontopathogenic validity (as the experimental manipulations have been undertaken during the developmental period of the subject). Maternal deprivation cannot be considered a triggering factor (it does not occur during adulthood and does not directly trigger a depressive-like episode); therefore it has poor triggering validity.

It is important to note that etiological factors do not have to be materially similar (from a biochemical point of view), but rather semantically similar (what they mean to an organism). For example, a cat might elicit fear in rodents, while in humans a white bear might induce the same state. The two stimuli (cat and bear) are not materially identical, but have the same meaning (threat) in the rodents and the humans world. The same

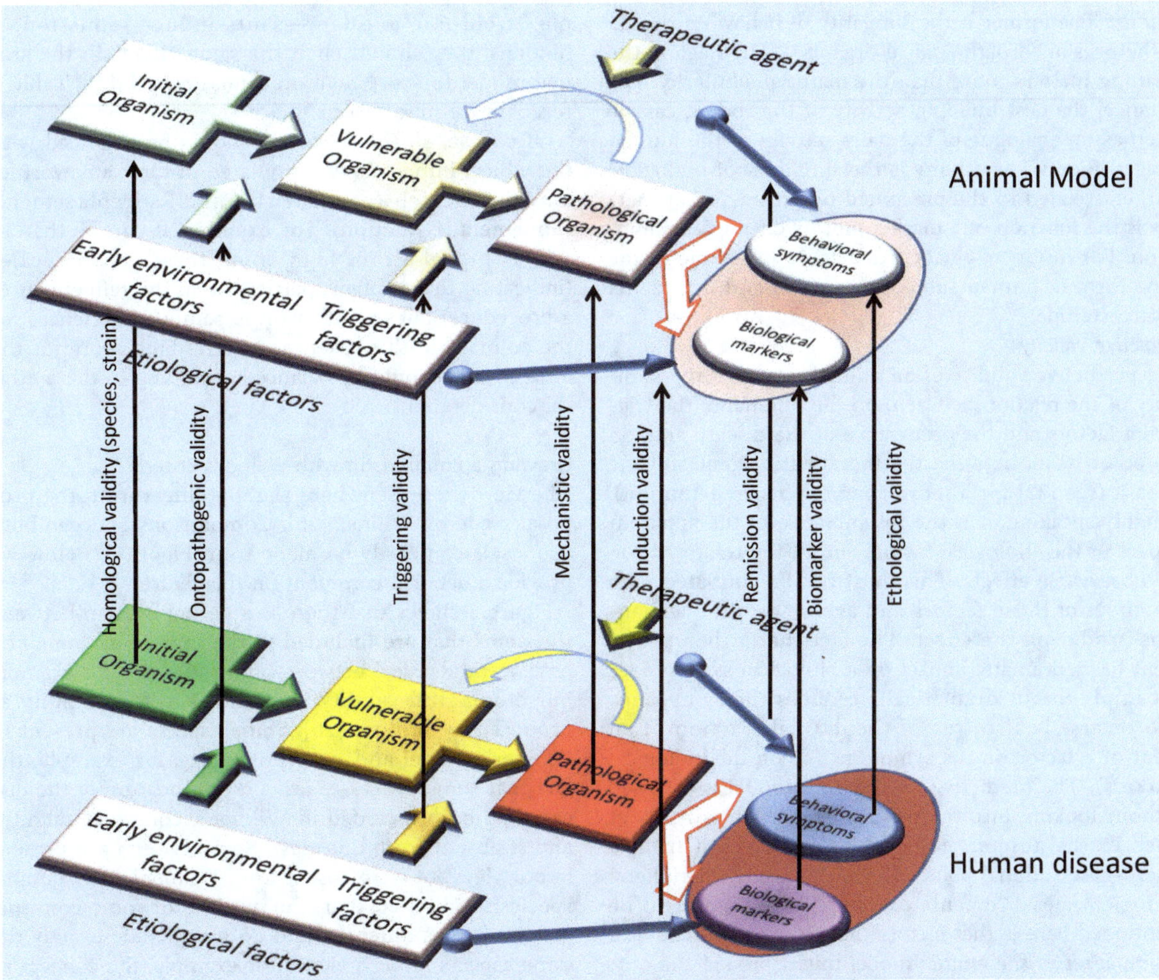

Figure 2 Criteria of validity for animal models. A comparison between the general process of the human disease (on the lower plane) and its animal model (on the higher plan). The orthogonal black arrows link the crucial points of similarity between the parallel processes and represent the different criteria of overall validity for animal models (or the various kinds of validity according to which an animal model ought to be designed).

meaning can thus supervene on different physical stimuli for different species, and the same physical stimulus can have different meanings for different species.

Mechanistic validity

The mechanistic validity of an animal model assesses the similarity of the mechanism we suppose or know is working in the animal disease to the mechanism that is or is presumed to be working in the human disease. It refers at the same time to the mechanism that we think is producing the symptoms and biological markers, and to the mechanism we think is sensitive to the action of effective therapeutic agents. This mechanism can be either cognitive or neurobiological. This similarity of mechanism is quite independent from the similarity of the effects of the mechanisms. For instance, even if the serotonergic organism is impaired in the same manner in both depressed animal subjects and depressed human patients, neither the symptoms nor the biological markers are necessarily the same. Indeed, what is observed is not the direct effect of the mechanism, but rather the result of the interaction of this mechanism with a lot of other mechanisms in the organism. Therefore, mechanistic validity and face validity have to be assessed independently.

Face validity

The face validity of an animal model is the similarity of what is observed in the animal model to what is observed in the human modeled organism. Face validity has to do with both *ethological validity* and *biomarker validity*. The former is the similarity of behaviors related to the presumed pathological organism. Here again, the meaning matters more than the material similarity. For instance, the nest building activity of the rodent can be taken as an analogue of the daily activity of the human subject. Biomarker validity is the similarity of biological markers related to the presumed organism. What matters is the function of a marker, not its chemical composition. For instance, glucocorticoids do not come in the same form in human subjects (cortisol) and in rodents (corticosterone).

Predictive validity

The predictive validity of an animal model is the similarity of the relation between, on the one hand, the triggering factors and the occurrence of the disease and, on the other hand, between the therapeutic agent and the disease (see [22] for a more comprehensive definition). Roughly speaking, it is the resemblance of the apparent impact of the etiological factors and of the treatment on the observable effects. This must not be conflated with the effect of those factors and agents on the mechanisms producing the effect. The fact that a therapeutic agent has a dramatic impact on a biological system does not imply that it dramatically reduces the symptoms. The reverse is also true of the dramatic action of an agent or a factor on the symptoms (or on the biological markers). The predictive validity of a model is assessed without looking into the mechanism which is really at work in the animal: generally it is assessed from a macro-observational point of view or through peripheral biological measurements (biomarkers). A point to be mentioned here is that factors that alter the outcome of a biomarker in the animal model might predict the outcome of the same challenge in humans. For example, if increasing the stimulus intensity induces a linear change in the outcome in the animal, this should also be found in the clinical situation. On the other hand, the mechanistic validity is assessed through direct observation of what is really happening inside the pathological organism. So, one needs to assess the validity of this direct link between 'input' and 'output' separately from the resemblance of the mechanisms which presumably transform the input into the output. Of course, one must also distinguish *induction validity* from *remission validity*. The former suggests that the action of the etiological factors on the observable effects of the model disease resemble its action on the observable effects of the human disease. For example, if chronic stress triggers depression-related biomarkers both in humans and in animals, an animal model based on the chronic application of stressors may have good induction validity. In the latter, the action of the treatment on the observable effects in the animal model may resemble its action on the observable effects in the human disease. For example, if chronic antidepressants induce remission in humans, they should elicit the same effects in the animal model to score high on remission validity. Table 3 recaps these nine criteria.

Of course, all these criteria should be balanced with the ethical implications formulated in the framework of animal research (particularly the 3Rs: replacement, refinement, reduction). For example, it can be that an animal model scores high on all these validity scales (indicating that it might participate in the refinement of a procedure) but that it involves painful experiences for the animals: in this case, the general high score for the nine criteria should be balanced according to these ethical considerations.

Drawing a comparison with Willner's criteria

The view we present here slightly differs from the proposal made by Willner [26]. Comparisons between both proposals can easily be made from Figure 3. Below we provide a detailed comment on this figure.

Figure 3 shows that there is a partial overlap between the items that are included in the criteria as some criteria seem identical between both the views, for example our ethological validity is identical to face validity as proposed by Willner [26]. Some aspects are present in Willner's model and not in our view; for example, the fact that some processes are a crucial feature of the disease had been included in Willner's 'construct validity', and is absent from our view. Some criteria are present in our view but were absent from Willner's, for example, species validity. Further, the outlines of some concepts are sometimes different, and do not include exactly the same aspects in both views (for example, the concept of face validity). More precisely:

1. Our concept of species validity was not explicitly mentioned in the initial proposal by Willner. However, it overlaps with the concept of homological validity that has been extensively discussed previously [20] for its relevance to animal models of psychiatric disorders (particularly those characterized by a deficit of high order cognitive processing).

2. The concept of strain validity, as it corresponds to a human-animal similarity of the genetic predisposition that participates in the etiology of the disease, could be included in Willner's 'construct validity' concept, as the similarity of the theories about the causes of the disorder was mentioned in his definition of construct validity. The same applies to ontopathogenic validity and to triggering validity. Here we propose to carefully disentangle these different dimensions, as they might correspond to very different constructs.

3. Our description of mechanistic validity only partially overlaps with Willner's conception of construct

Table 3 The criteria of validity for animal models.

Kind of validity	*Aspect of validity*	*Object of validity (animal/human similarity of...)*
homological validity	species validity	Species
	strain validity	strain
pathogenic validity	ontopathogenic validity	interaction transforming an initial organism into a vulnerable organism.
	triggering validity	interaction transforming an initial or a vulnerable organism into a pathological organism.
mechanistic validity		theoretical cognitive or neurobiological mechanisms producing the observable effects of the disease.
face validity	ethological validity	behavioral symptoms of the disease
	biomarker validity	biomarkers associated with the disease
predictive validity	induction validity	relation between the triggering factor and the observable effects of the disease.
	remission validity	relation between the therapeutic agent and the observable effects of the disease.

validity. Indeed, in our proposal, it corresponds to the biological and cognitive mechanisms that produce the pathological outcomes. In Willner's view, the cognitive mechanisms were not explicitly included. Further, Willner also included many other dimensions that are clearly separate in our proposal. This was done to account for the very different nature of the items that were included in Willner's view of construct validity, as it included constructs about etiology, about the course of the disease, and so on.

4. Ethological validity corresponds more or less to Willner's face validity, which was defined as the

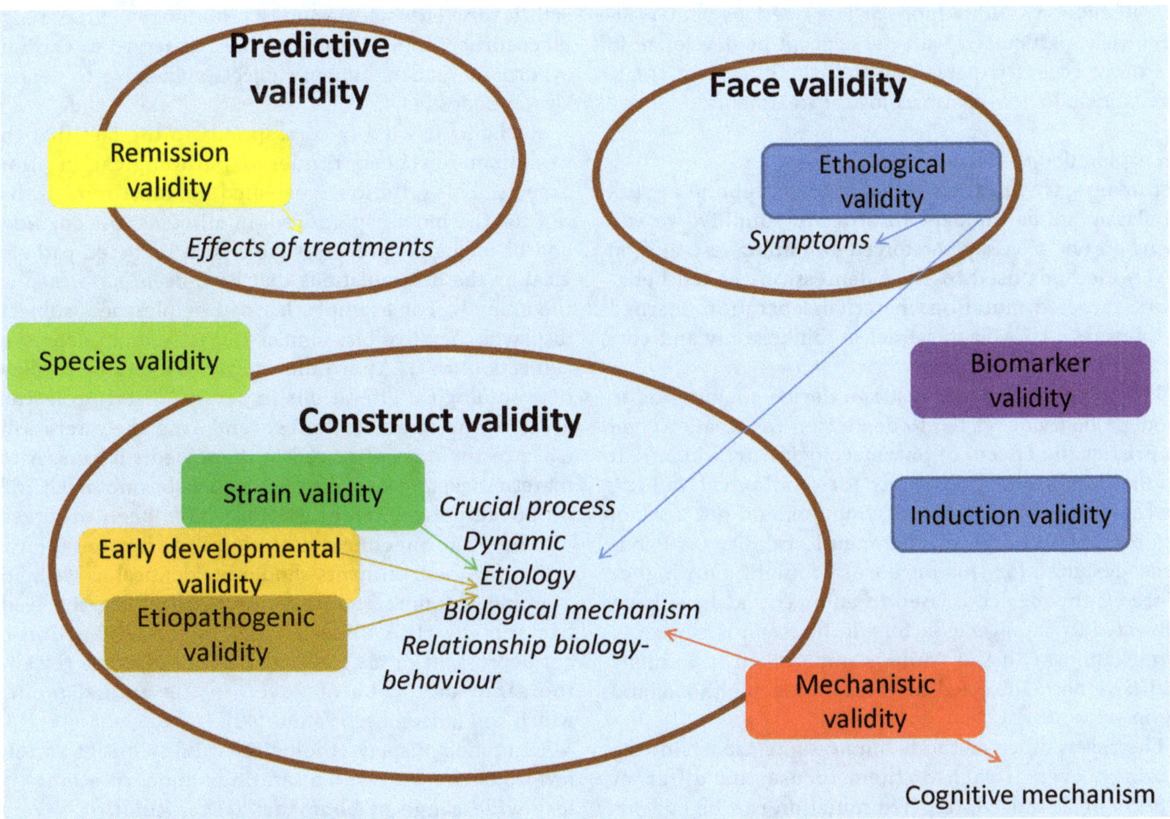

Figure 3 A comparison between Willner's criteria and the present proposal. Willner's criteria are represented by the brown circles and our nine criteria are represented by squares with the same color code as in Figures 1 and 2. Where a square fully overlaps with one of Willner's criteria (or with one aspect of one of Willner's criteria) it is represented inside the corresponding circle. Where it partially overlaps, it sits astride the circle. Where the criterion (or an aspect of it) has not been described by Willner, it stands outside the circles. Arrows indicate which sub-aspect of Willner's criteria corresponds to our proposed criteria.

symptomatic similarity. However, it might extend somewhat beyond that view, including also some aspects that were previously included in construct validity, such as the similarity in the course of the disease or its dynamic, (for example, in the case of an animal model of bipolar disorder, this would correspond to an alternation of manic and depressive-like states).

5. The biomarker validity, corresponding to a similarity of the biological markers, was not present *per se* in Willner's initial view. Indeed, he included an identity of the biological mechanisms underlying the disease, but the mechanisms were not separated from the markers. However, this aspect was later included in face validity [21].

6. Induction validity was not explicitly mentioned by Willner. Rather, he focused on the identity of the relationship between the biological mechanism and the symptoms (an item that was included in his conception of construct validity and that is absent in our model) while we focus on the relationship between the causes of the pathological outcome.

7. Remission validity more or less overlaps with Willner's view, particularly with the concept he developed in his more recent papers, in which the effects of treatments include non-pharmacological treatments.

An exploration of classic models

Let us now try to explore whether our proposal applies to classic animal models. In order to simplify, we will focus on one bioassay, the forced swimming test, and on seven methods used to elicit depression-related behaviors: targeted mutation, maternal separation, learned helplessness, UCMS, social defeat, bulbectomy and corticosterone administration.

The forced swimming test is a device enabling us to model a behavior related to depression (resignation) and to predict the effects of pharmacological treatments. It might thus score moderately for ethological validity (because it only mimics one symptom, and not a set of symptoms) and high on therapeutic validity (as it has been designed for this purpose). It might gain higher scores if this device is used in animals that have been subjected to pathogenic factors, if the strain is chosen in a relevant way, if the study is undertaken in animals that have been subjected to stress during adulthood, and so on.

The seven other methods mimic some aspects of the etiology, even if each of them focuses on different aspects of it. Indeed, targeted mutation can be considered to score highly on strain validity, while maternal separation rather focuses on ontopathogenic validity. Learned helplessness, social defeat and UCMS all manipulate triggering factors. Therefore, each of these methods might gain validity if combined with other dimensions of etiology (or lose validity in the opposite case). For example, if UCMS is performed in BALB/c mice, a strain exhibiting a polymorphism for genes rendering the subject vulnerable to stress and displaying poor maternal care, it might score not only for triggering validity, but also for strain and ontopathogenic validity. The same reasoning applies to social defeat and learned helplessness. It will score lower if applied to invertebrates than if applied to rodents, even if observations have shown that learned helplessness also evokes behavioral alterations in invertebrates (see [39] for a review). Concerning bulbectomy, it does not really mimic an etiology of depression, because, in humans, the loss of olfaction does not provoke self-rated depression [40] and as the olfactory dysfunctions seen in depressed subjects mainly concern an alteration in the hedonic rating of odors [41,42], a function that is associated to the orbitofrontal cortex rather than to the olfactory bulbs [43]. Finally, corticosterone administration during adulthood does not recapitulate strain or ontopathogenic factors. However, this model partly satisfies the etiological validity criterion, as chronic high glucocorticoid levels, such as those observed in Cushing syndrome, renders human subjects vulnerable to depressive episodes [44,45].

Mechanistic validity corresponds to the fact that the organism has been rendered pathological in some aspects. This criterion is satisfied for most models, but not for the bio-assay. Indeed, in all cases, the cognitive and/or biological processes have been rendered pathological by the manipulations that have been performed on the animals. For example, learned helplessness subjects display a cognitive bias similar to that seen in depressed subjects [46,47]. After bulbectomy, the animal displays neurobiological alterations in several distal projection areas of the olfactory bulbs, rendering the alterations close to the ones observed in depressed subjects. After maternal separation, chronic corticosterone or UCMS, hippocampal-related alterations have been observed. Further, the mechanism explaining the therapeutic action for the treatments should be identical as well. For example, if some restoration of functional negative feedback on the HPA underlies the therapeutic action of antidepressant drugs in humans (see [48] for a review), the same should be observed in the animal model, which has indeed been found [49].

All models display ethological validity but at various levels, as the observed alterations concern a more or less wide range of behaviors (recapitulating several symptoms, and not only one) and include more or less crucial symptoms of depression (for example anhedonia is more essential than irritability or anxiety-like behavior). For example, in bioassays such as the forced swim test only one aspect of the behavioral symptomatology is assessed, namely behavioral resignation. In UCMS as well as in the social defeat model, anhedonia has been observed together with other behaviors, such as social avoidance (social defeat) or apathy (UCMS). Measurable changes in biomarkers have been measured in some models, such as altered levels of plasmatic corticosterone or of pro-inflammatory cytokines. It is obvious that chronic alterations in biomarkers require that the animals be subjected to experimental manipulations over long periods of time. For example, no alteration in the regulation of corticosterone release will be observed after forced swimming, while it can be observed after UCMS or targeted mutation.

Finally, as we distinguished two aspects of predictive validity (induction and remission), we have to discuss these two aspects separately. Induction validity is about the similarity of the relationship between the triggering factor and the observable behavioral or biological outcome. Indeed, it could be that the link between a triggering factor and an outcome is similar in the human condition and in the animal model even if the mechanism underlying this relationship is largely unknown: in this case, the model will satisfy the induction validity criterion, but not the mechanistic validity. For example, data concerning the neurobiological alterations displayed by patients with panic disorder is rather sparse: in this case, it is difficult to design an animal model with good mechanistic validity, while it is still possible to achieve induction validity, as it is easy to model the relationship between factors triggering the panic attacks (for example lactate or caffeine administration) and the symptomatology. The reverse can also be observed when some aspects of the pathological mechanism have been modeled, while the relationship between the trigger and the symptom is not reproduced. This is the case for bulbectomy: we have already seen that this model elicits some aspects of the pathological mechanism (and so displays mechanistic validity) but at the same time, because bulbectomy does not cause depression, it does not satisfy induction validity. Concerning remission validity, it focuses on the ability of treatments (both pharmacological and non pharmacological ones) to reverse the pathological features that are observed. As most models or tests have been designed to detect the potential effectiveness of treatments, this criterion is achieved in most but not all models (bioassays, maternal separation, UCMS, corticosterone administration, social defeat, bulbectomy, and so on). First, one has to observe that, in some cases, the characteristics of the treatments are not identical: for example, in the clinic, antidepressants elicit therapeutic effects after chronic administration so when an effect is observed after acute administration in the animal model, this criterion is not achieved. This is the case with bioassays, which in some cases respond after acute or sub-chronic administration of the compound. Further, in the case of targeted mutation, it could be that, as the target of the treatment has been deleted, the model will not answer to pharmacological challenges. For example, knockouts for the noradrenaline transporter may not respond to inhibitors of the noradrenergic transporter [50]. In this case, the null mutant cannot be considered a valid model of depression, but rather as a model of dysfunction of this transporter. As for the induction validity criterion, the remission validity criterion does not overlap with some aspects of mechanisms validity.

Conclusion

What we have proposed is a general framework to assess the validity of animal models of psychiatric disorders, focusing on anxiety disorders and depression. It consists of five general criteria: homological validity, pathogenic validity, mechanistic validity, face validity and predictive validity (the last two being given a rather different meaning than in Willner's proposal). They may be consistent with the procedure to evaluate animal models recently proposed by Van der Staay [10,22]. According to the objectives of a given model, the relevance of these different criteria may have to be hierarchized (see [10] for a discussion of the different targets of modeling). For example, these criteria may not have the same importance if the scope of a model is the search for new therapeutic strategies or if it is to understand the mechanisms explaining the pathology (this is why Van der Staay [22] and Cryan and Sweeney [51] are adamant that models and tests should not be conflated). A step further towards a precise assessment of the validity of these models would be to propose scoring procedures for each of these criteria. This is in part a quite different approach, for it implies, among other things, using mathematical tools, but also paying much more attention to the researcher's various aims when modeling a disease. Moreover, we think that the general framework we propose here could also suit other fields where animal models are used, in psychiatry of course (models of schizophrenia or autism), but also in neurology, and more widely in research into all diseases within the scope of translational medicine. However, they do not apply to models of normal emotions, such as anxiety behavior for example: in this case, it is probable that some criteria will not be relevant, such as pathogenic validity.

Author details

[1]U930, UFR Sciences et Techniques, Parc Grandmont, Rue Monge, Tours, 37200, France. [2]Université François-Rabelais, UFR Médecine, 10 Bd Tonnellé, Tours Cedex, 37032, France.

Authors' contributions

ML is a philosopher of biomedical science and CB is a behavioral neuroscientist. Both authors contributed equally to this paper. CB did the review on classic criteria in animal models of psychiatric disorders, ML reformulated these criteria and this was then applied to examples of models by CB. Both authors read and approved the final manuscript.

Competing interests
The authors declare that they have no competing interests.

References

1. Zerhouni EA: **US biomedical research: basic, translational, and clinical sciences.** *JAMA* 2005, **294**:1352-1358.
2. McArthur RA, Borsini F: **What do *you* mean by "Translational research"? An enquiry through animal and translational models for CNS drug discovery: Psychiatric disorders.** In *Animal and translational models for CNS drug discovery. Vol 1: Psychiatric disorders.* Edited by: McArthur RA, Borsini F. New York: Academic Press; 2008:xvii-xxxviii.
3. Santarelli L, Saxe M, Gross C, Surget A, Battaglia F, Dulawa S, Weisstaub N, Lee J, Duman R, Arancio O, Belzung C, Hen R: **Requirement of hippocampal neurogenesis for the behavioral effects of antidepressants.** *Science* 2003, **301**:805-809.
4. Surget A, Saxe M, Leman S, Ibarguen-Vargas Y, Chalon S, Griebel G, Hen R, Belzung C: **Drug-dependent requirement of hippocampal neurogenesis in a model of depression and of antidepressant reversal.** *Biological Psychiat* 2008, **64**:293-301.
5. Surget A, Tanti A, Leonardo ED, Laugeray A, Rainer Q, Touma C, Palme R, Griebel G, Ibarguen-Vargas Y, Hen R, Belzung C: **Antidepressants recruit new neurons to improve stress response regulation.** *Mol Psychiat* 2011.
6. Snyder JS, Soumier A, Brewer M, Pickel J, Cameron HA: **Adult hippocampal neurogenesis buffers stress responses and depressive behaviour.** *Nature* 2011, **476(7361)**:458-461.
7. Boldrini M, Underwood MD, Hen R, Rosoklija GB, Dwork AJ, John Mann J, Arango V: **Antidepressants increase neural progenitor cells in the human hippocampus.** *Neuropsychopharmacology* 2009, **34(11)**:2376-2389.
8. Lucassen PJ, Stumpel MW, Wang Q, Aronica E: **Decreased numbers of progenitor cells but no response to antidepressant drugs in the hippocampus of elderly depressed patients.** *Neuropharmacology* 2010, **58(6)**:940-949.
9. Geyer MA, Markou A: **Animal models of psychiatric disorders.** In *Psychopharmacology: the fourth generation of progress.* Edited by: Bloom FE, Kupfer DJ. New York: Raven Press; 1995:787-798.
10. Van der Staay FJ, Arndt SS, Nordquist RE: **Evaluation of animal models of neurobehavioral disorders.** *Behav Brain Funct* 2009, **5**:11.
11. Campbell DT, Stanley JC: *Experimental and quasi-experimental designs for research* Chicago: Rand McNally & Cie; 1963.
12. Janssen PAJ: **Screening tests and prediction from animals to man.** In *Animal behavior and drug action. A Ciba Foundation Symposium.* Edited by: Steinberg H, de Reuck AVS, Knight J. London: J.A. Churchill Ltd; 1964:264-268.
13. McKinney WT, Bunney WE: **Animal models of depression.** *Arch Gen Psychiat* 1969, **127**:240-248.
14. Abramson LY, Seligman MEP: **Modeling psychopathology in the laboratory: history and rationale.** In *Psychopathology: Experimental models.* Edited by: Maser JD, Seligman MEP. San Francisco: WH Freeman; 1977:1-26.
15. Willner P: **The validity of animal models of depression.** *Psychopharmacology* 1984, **83**:1-16.
16. Cronbach LJ, Meehl PE: **Construct validity in psychological tests.** *Psycholog Bull* 1955, **52**:281-302.
17. Soubrié P, Simon P: **Les modèles animaux en psychopharmacologie.** *Confrontations psychiatriques* 1989, **30**:113-129.
18. Koob GF, Heinrichs SC, Britton K: **Animal models of anxiety disorders.** In *The American Psychiatric Press Textbook of Psychopharmacology.*. 2 edition. Edited by: Schatzberg AF, Nemeroff CB. Washington DC-London: American Psychiatric Press; 1998:133-144.
19. Sarter M, Bruno JP: **Animal models in Biological psychiatry.** In *Biological Psychiatry. Volume 1.* Edited by: D'Haenen HAH, den Boer JA, Willner P. Chicester: Wiley; 2002:37-44.
20. Robbins TW: **Homology in behavioral pharmacology: an approach to animal models of human cognition.** *Behav Pharmacol* 1998, **9**:509-519.
21. Willner P, Mitchell PJ: **Animal models of depression: A diathesis/Stress approach.** In *Biological Psychiatry. Volume II.* Edited by: D'Haenen H, den Boer JA, Willner P. Chichester, UK: John Wiley 2002:703-726.
22. van der Staay FJ: **Animal models of behavioral dysfunctions: basic concepts and classifications, and an evaluation strategy.** *Brain Res Rev* 2006, **52(1)**:131-159.
23. Keeler JF, Robbins TW: **Translating cognition from animals to humans.** *Biochem Pharmacol* 2011, **81(12)**:1356-1366.
24. Fernando ABP, Robbins TW: **Animal models of neuropsychiatric disorders.** *Ann Rev Clin Psychol* 2011, **7**:39-61.
25. Sartori SB, Landgraf R, Singewald N: **The clinical implications of mouse models of enhanced anxiety.** *Future Neurol* 2011, **6(4)**:531-571.
26. Willner P: **Animal models of depression.** In *Handbook of depression and anxiety. A biological approach.* Edited by: den Boer JA, Ad Sitsen JM. New York-Basel-Hong Kong: Marcel Dekker; 1994:291-316.
27. David DJ, Samuels BA, Rainer Q, Wang JW, Marsteller D, Mendez I, Drew M, Craig DA, Guiard BP, Guilloux JP, Artymyshyn RP, Gardier AM, Gerald C, Antonijevic IA, Leonardo ED, Hen R: **Neurogenesis-dependent and -independent effects of fluoxetine in an animal model of anxiety/depression.** *Neuron* 2009, **62**:479-493.
28. Weiss JM, Kilts CD: **Animals models of depression and schizophrenia.** In *The American Psychiatric Press Textbook of Psychopharmacology.*. 2 edition. Edited by: Schatzberg AF, Nemeroff CB. Washington DC-London: American Psychiatric Press; 1998:89-131.
29. Treit D, Engin E, McEown K: **Animal models of anxiety and anxiolytic drug action.** *Curr Top Behav Neurosci* 2010, **2**:121-160.
30. Krishnan V, Han MH, Graham DL, Berton O, Renthal W, Russo SJ, Laplant Q, Graham A, Lutter M, Lagace DC, Ghose S, Reister R, Tannous P, Green TA, Neve RL, Chakravarty S, Kumar A, Eisch AJ, Self DW, Lee FS, Tamminga CA, Cooper DC, Gershenfeld HK, Nestler EJ: **Molecular adaptations underlying susceptibility and resistance to social defeat in brain reward regions.** *Cell* 2007, **131**:391-404.
31. Schroeder FA, Lin CL, Crusio WE, Akbarian S: **Antidepressant-like effects of the histone deacetylase inhibitor, sodium butyrate, in the mouse.** *Biol Psychiat* 2007, **62**:55-64.
32. Overstreet DH, Friedman E, Mathé AA, Yadid G: **The Flinders Sensitive Line rat: a selectively bred putative animal model of depression.** *Neurosci Biobehav Rev* 2005, **29**:739-759.
33. Pesonen AK, Räikkönen K, Heinonen K, Kajantie E, Forsén T, Eriksson JG: **Depressive symptoms in adults separated from their parents as children: a natural experiment during World War II.** *Am J Epidemiol* 2007, **166(10)**:1126-1133.
34. Noorikhajavi M, Afghah S, Dadkhah A, Holakoyie K, Motamedi SH: **The effect of "parental loss" under 18 on developing "MDD" in adult age.** *Int J Psychiatry Med* 2007, **37(3)**:347-355.
35. Tyrka AR, Wier L, Price LH, Ross NS, Carpenter LL: **Childhood parental loss and adult psychopathology: effects of loss characteristics and contextual factors.** *Int J Psychiatry Med* 2008, **38(3)**:329-344.
36. Tyrka AR, Wier L, Price LH, Ross N, Anderson GM, Wilkinson CW, Carpenter LL: **Childhood parental loss and adult hypothalamic-pituitary-adrenal function.** *Biol Psychiatry* 2008, **63(12)**:1147-1154.
37. Lajud N, Roque A, Cajero M, Gutiérrez-Ospina G, Torner L: **Periodic maternal separation decreases hippocampal neurogenesis without affecting basal corticosterone during the stress hyporesponsive period, but alters HPA axis and coping behavior in adulthood.** *Psychoneuroendocrinology* 2011.
38. Holmes A, Le Guisquet AM, Vogel E, Mollstein RA, Leman S, Belzung C: **Early life genetic, epigenetic and environmental factors shaping emotionality in rodents.** *Neurosci Biobehav Rev* 2005, **29**:1335-1346.
39. Belzung C, Philippot P: **Anxiety from a phylogenetic perspective: is there a qualitative difference between human and animal anxiety?** *Neural Plasticity* 2007, **2007**:59676.
40. Temmel AF, Quint C, Schickinger-Fischer B, Klimek L, Stoller E, Hummel T: **Characteristics of olfactory disorders in relation to major causes of olfactory loss.** *Arch Otolaryngol Head Neck Surg* 2002, **128**:635-641.
41. Atanasova B, Graux J, El Hage W, Hommet C, Camus V, Belzung C: **Olfaction: a potential cognitive marker of psychiatric disorders.** *Neurosci Biobehav Rev* 2008, **32(7)**:1315-1325.
42. Atanasova B, El-Hage W, Chabanet C, Gaillard P, Belzung C, Camus V: **Olfactory anhedonia and negative olfactory alliesthesia in depressed patients.** *Psychiatry Res* 2010, **176(2-3)**:190-196.

43. Anderson AK, Christoff K, Stappen I, Panitz D, Ghahremani DG, Glover G, Gabrieli JD, Sobel N: **Dissociated neural representations of intensity and valence in human olfaction.** *Nat Neurosci* 2003, **6(2)**:196-202.
44. Starkman MN, Schteingart DE, Schork MA: **Depressed mood and other psychiatric manifestations of Cushing's syndrome: relationship to hormone levels.** *Psychosom Med* 1981, **43(1)**:3-18.
45. Langenecker SA, Weisenbach SL, Giordani B, Briceño EM, Guidotti Breting LM, Schallmo MP, Leon HM, Noll DC, Zubieta JK, Schteingart DE, Starkman MN: **Impact of chronic hypercortisolemia on affective processing.** *Neuropharmacology* 2011, **62(1)**:217-225.
46. Disner SG, Beevers CG, Haigh EAP, Beck AT: **Neural mechanisms of the cognitive model of depression.** *Nat Rev Neurosci* 2011, **12**:467-477.
47. Pryce CR, Azzinnari D, Spinelli S, Seifritz E, Tegethoff M, Meinlschmidt G: **Helplessness: A systematic translational review of theory and evidence for its relevance to understanding and treating depression.** *Pharmacol Ther* 2011.
48. Belzung C, Billette de Villemeur E: **The design of new antidepressants: can formal models help? A first attempt using a model of the hippocampal control over the HPA-axis based on a review from the literature.** *Behav Pharmacol* 2010, **21**:677-689.
49. Surget A, Tanti A, Leonardo DE, Laugeray A, Rainer Q, Touma C, Palme R, Griebel G, Ibarguen-Vargas Y, Hen R, Belzung C: **Antidepressants recruit new neurons to improve stress response regulation.** *Mol Psychiat* 2011.
50. Cryan JF, O'Leary OF, Jin SH, Friedland JC, Ouyang M, Hirsch BR, Page ME, Dalvi A, Thomas SA, Lucki I: **Norepinephrine-deficient mice lack responses to antidepressant drugs, including selective serotonin reuptake inhibitors.** *PNAS* 2004, **101**:8186-8191.
51. Cryan JF, Sweeney FF: **The age of anxiety: role of animal models of anxiolytic action in drug discovery.** *Br J Pharmacol* 2011, **164(4)**:1129-1161.

7

Increased anxiety in corticotropin-releasing factor type 2 receptor-null mice requires recent acute stress exposure and is associated with dysregulated serotonergic activity in limbic brain areas

Orna Issler[1], Roderick N Carter[2], Evan D Paul[3], Paul AT Kelly[4], Henry J Olverman[4], Adi Neufeld-Cohen[1], Yael Kuperman[1], Christopher A Lowry[3], Jonathan R Seckl[2], Alon Chen[1] and Pauline M Jamieson[2*]

Abstract

Background: Corticotropin-releasing factor type 2 receptors (CRFR2) are suggested to facilitate successful recovery from stress to maintain mental health. They are abundant in the midbrain raphe nuclei, where they regulate serotonergic neuronal activity and have been demonstrated to mediate behavioural consequences of stress. Here, we describe behavioural and serotonergic responses consistent with maladaptive recovery from stressful challenge in CRFR2-null mice.

Results: CRFR2-null mice showed similar anxiety levels to control mice before and immediately after acute restraint stress, and also after cessation of chronic stress. However, they showed increased anxiety by 24 hours after restraint, whether or not they had been chronically stressed.

Serotonin (5-HT) and 5-hydroxyindoleacetic acid (5-HIAA) contents were quantified and the level of 5-HIAA in the caudal dorsal raphe nucleus (DRN) was increased under basal conditions in CRFR2-null mice, indicating increased 5-HT turnover. Twenty-four hours following restraint, 5-HIAA was decreased only in CRFR2-null mice, suggesting that they had not fully recovered from the challenge. In efferent limbic structures, CRFR2-null mice showed lower levels of basal 5-HT in the lateral septum and subiculum, and again showed a differential response to restraint stress from controls.

Local cerebral glucose utilization (LCMRglu) revealed decreased neuronal activity in the DRN of CRFR2-null mice under basal conditions. Following 5-HT receptor agonist challenge, LCMRglu responses indicated that 5-HT_{1A} receptor responses in the DRN were attenuated in CRFR2-null mice. However, postsynaptic 5-HT receptor responses in forebrain regions were intact.

Conclusions: These results suggest that CRFR2 are required for proper functionality of 5-HT_{1A} receptors in the raphe nuclei, and are key to successful recovery from stress. This disrupted serotonergic function in CRFR2-null mice likely contributes to their stress-sensitive phenotype. The 5-HT content in lateral septum and subiculum was notably altered. These areas are important for anxiety, and are also implicated in reward and the pathophysiology of addiction. The role of CRFR2 in stress-related psychopathologies deserves further consideration.

Keywords: 5-HT_{1A} receptor, Anxiety, Corticotropin-releasing factor type 2 receptor, Raphe nuclei, Serotonin, Stress

* Correspondence: Pauline.Jamieson@ed.ac.uk
[2]Centre for Cardiovascular Science, Queens Medical Research Institute, 47 Little France Crescent, Edinburgh EH16 4TJ, UK
Full list of author information is available at the end of the article

Background

Serotonin (5-HT) is a key neurotransmitter in the control of mood. It is the major target of current antidepressant medications, and often also of treatments for anxiety disorders [1,2]. The principal sources of 5-HT neurons projecting to the forebrain are the midbrain dorsal (DRN) and median (MRN) raphe nuclei [3,4].

Corticotropin-releasing factor (CRF) is a key mediator of the stress response [5-7], and anxiety and affective disorders have been associated with CRF hyperactivity [8]. Corticotropin-releasing factor receptors are abundant in both DRN and MRN [9-11], where they are expressed in serotonergic and non-serotonergic neurons, including regulatory GABAergic neurons [12,13], suggesting the potential for complex interactions between CRF and serotonergic systems. Electrophysiological studies show that exogenous CRF administered to the raphe modulates serotonergic neuronal firing activity [14-16], and therefore CRF receptor-mediated effects on stress-related behaviours may be mediated via 5-HT *in vivo* [17-20].

Type 1 (CRFR1) and type 2 (CRFR2) CRF receptors [21-23] are preferentially activated by CRF or urocortin neuropeptides (Ucn1, Ucn2, Ucn3), respectively [24-28]. The raphe nuclei receive inputs from both CRF and Ucn1 expressing neurons [14,15,29-31], and a potentially important role for the CRF system in controlling 5-HT neurons here is emerging.

CRFR2 is expressed at high levels in the raphe nuclei, while CRFR1 is expressed at lower levels in the raphe nuclei in rats and appears to be absent from this area in mice and human beings [9-11]. Exogenously administered CRFR2 agonists induce c-Fos expression in DRN 5-HT neurons, increase their firing rate, and increase 5-HT release in efferent stress-related nuclei [32-36]. In pharmacological studies, CRFR2 activation in the DRN potentiates immediate fear responses [35], fear conditioning and escape deficits 24 hours later in a model of learned helplessness [37,38], and decreases exploratory behaviours [19] in rodents. Recently, altered anxiety-like behaviour in Ucn-knockout or Ucn-overexpressing mice has been linked to disturbances in serotonergic activity in the neural circuitry controlling anxiety [39-41]. The Ucn1/Ucn2/Ucn3 triple knockout mouse phenotype suggests that CRFR2 and particularly Ucn3 are involved in successful recovery from stress [41]. This interaction with the 5-HT system may provide a major link between the two main arms of the central stress response; the CRF/Ucns peptidergic pathways and the sympathetic monoaminergic system.

5-HT_{1A} receptors (5-HT_{1A}R) are also particularly associated with modulating anxiety [42] and pharmacological stimulation of CRF receptors in the raphe nuclei has been demonstrated to regulate serotonergic neuronal firing here [43,44]. Thus, CRF-containing neuronal projections from the central amygdala (CeA) to the raphe nuclei [45] may modulate activity at postsynaptic 5-HT_{1A}R by directly regulating activity of efferent 5-HT projections or may have wider-ranging effects on 5-HT function via altered raphe 5-HT_{1A}R autoreceptor activity. Conversely, 5-HT_{1A}R activity can influence CRF-induced changes in behaviour; 5-HT_{1A}R-selective agonists can attenuate CRF-induced grooming [46]. We have previously shown that 5-HT_{1A}R responsiveness plays a key role in stress-related behaviours associated with chronic activation of CRFR2 [39] and that interaction is further explored in the studies presented here.

Activation of CRFR2 affects anxiety-like behaviour under stressed conditions [47-49] and CRFR2-null mice have an anxiogenic phenotype [50,51]. This raises the question of what role CRFR2 might play in the pathophysiology of anxiety-related and affective disorders in human beings. To further investigate the mechanisms underlying this, we examined the anxiety phenotype of CRFR2-null mice in detail, and characterized their serotonergic responses to stress.

Methods

Animals

Mice were housed in temperature- and lighting-controlled rooms (lights on, 12 h) with free access to laboratory chow and water. CRFR2-null mice, as previously described [50], and control littermates (C57BL6 × 129) were the adult male offspring of parents heterozygous for the knockout allele. For CRFR2 mRNA studies, adult male wild type C57BL6/J mice (Harlan Laboratories) were used. Mice were group housed, except for the chronic variable mild stress (CVMS) protocols, for which they were singly housed. Principles of laboratory animal care (NIH No. 85-23, 1985) were followed. All procedures were approved by The Weizmann Institute Animal Use and Care Committee or the United Kingdom Animals (Scientific Procedures) Act, 1986.

Behavioural testing

Tests were carried out during the dark phase of the light cycle on adult male mice (2 to 4 months). Mice were habituated in the home cage in a dark room for 2 hours prior to each behavioural test. Separate groups of mice were tested under: (a) basal conditions with no stress applied prior to testing, $n = 12$ for control group, $n = 14$ for CRFR2-null group; (b) immediately following 30 min of acute restraint stress (ARS), $n = 13$, both groups; (c) 24 to 48 hours following ARS, $n = 5$ for control group, $n = 8$ for CRFR2-null group (light/dark transfer test performed at 24 hours post-stress, open-field at 48 hours post-stress); (d) 3 to 4 days following a 4-week CVMS protocol, (light/dark transfer test performed at 3 days post-stress, open-field at 4 days post-stress), $n = 10$ for control group, $n = 11$ for CRFR2-null group. The mice of group d were then retested 3 weeks later, when an ARS was applied and testing was performed at 24 to 48 hours. Figure 1 shows the timeline of the experimental protocols with stress procedures.

Open-field (OF) test

The apparatus and experimental conditions were as previously described [50]. Mice were placed in the centre of the apparatus to initiate a 10-min test session. Visits to, and distance travelled and time spent in the inner zone of the arena were quantified using a video tracking system (VideoMot2; TSE Systems, Bad Hamburg, Germany).

Light/dark transfer test (LDT)

Apparatus and experimental conditions were as previously described [50]. During a 5-min test session, visits to, and distance travelled and time spent in the light compartment were measured.

Stress procedures

Mice were subjected to 30 min ARS in a ventilated 50 ml plastic centrifuge tube. The CVMS regime was modified from Ducottet *et al.* [52]. Mice were singly housed and a variety of mild stressors were applied on an unpredictable schedule, 2 to 3 stressors per day for 4 weeks; these included disruptions to the light-dark cycle, cage shift to one previously inhabited by another male, cage tilt, damp bedding, low-intensity stroboscopic illumination, white noise, restraint stress, short periods of food or water restriction, and housing with no bedding followed by water in the cage. Controls were housed under stress-free conditions.

In the CVMS paradigm, mice were behaviourally tested 48 hours following termination of the last stressor, which was standardized and was 24 hours of constant light for all mice ($n = 10$ or 11). For *in-situ* hybridization and 5-HT transporter (SERT) binding studies, mice ($n = 6$ for control basal group, $n = 8$ for CRFR2-null basal group, $n = 7$ for all stress groups) were killed 12 hours after ARS, or after the last variable stressor, by decapitation within 15 s of disturbing the home cage. The brains were removed, rapidly frozen on dry ice and stored at −80°C until analysis.

Local cerebral glucose utilization (LCMRglu)

Local cerebral glucose utilization (LCMRglu) was determined as described previously [39,53]. Mice ($n = 8$, all groups) were injected (intraperitoneally) with either 10 mg kg^{-1} 8-hydroxy-*N,N*-dipropyl-2-aminotetralin (8-OH-DPAT), 25 mg kg^{-1} 1-(2,5-dimethoxy-4-iodophenyl)-2-aminopropane (DOI) or vehicle (0.1 ml 0.9% NaCl). At 10 min after 8-OH-DPAT, or 20 min after DOI, 5 μCi [^{14}C]-2-deoxyglucose in 0.4 ml 0.9% NaCl was injected intraperitoneally. After 45 min, mice were decapitated and their brains analyzed by quantitative autoradiographic imaging, as described previously [54,55].

Analysis of tissue concentrations of 5-HT and 5-HIAA

Mice ($n = 7$ for unstressed groups, $n = 6$ for ARS groups) were killed by decapitation under basal conditions or 24 hours following ARS. Brains were stored at −80°C until analysis. Areas selected for microdissection were identified by comparison with a standard mouse brain stereotaxic atlas [56]. To ensure accuracy, we used a stereomicroscope to visualize neuroanatomical landmarks for use as reference points in identifying specific nuclei and subdivisions of the DRN. Small diameter microdissection tools (310 to 410 μm diameter) were used to restrict dissections to the subregion of interest. High-pressure liquid chromatography analysis of 5-HT and 5-hydroxyindoleacetic acid (5-HIAA) was performed, as previously described [57].

CRFR2 mRNA qPCR analysis

Quantitative PCR for CRFR2 mRNA expression was carried out as previously reported [40] in brain taken from naïve mice (controls), or 3, 6, 12, 24 or 48 hours after ARS, or, for CVMS mice, one week after the end of the stress protocol ($n = 8$ all groups).

In-situ hybridization (ISH) histochemistry

Coronal brain sections (10 μm) were cut on a cryostat, thaw-mounted onto silanized glass slides, and stored at −80°C until use. *In-situ* hybridization procedures and probes were as previously described [58-60]. Plasmids (generous gifts from Professor M. Holmes and Dr V. Bombail) containing cDNA fragments for glucocorticoid receptor (GR), mineralocorticoid receptor (MR), 5-HT_{1A} R, 5-HT_{2C}R and tryptophan hydroxylase 2 (TPH2) were used to generate ^{35}S-UTP-labelled specific antisense probes to mRNAs. Following ISH, slides were dipped in Kodak Autoradiography Emulsion (Molecular Imaging Systems, New York, USA) and exposed at 4°C for between 24 h and 6 weeks, depending on the probe, developed and counterstained. The hybridization signal for each brain area was determined using computer-assisted grain counting software (Zeiss KS 300 3.0, Carl Zeiss Vision, GmbH). For each animal, silver grains were counted in a fixed circular area over 6 to 10 individual neurons per subregion. The background, counted over areas of white matter, was subtracted. Analysis was carried out blind to treatment group.

5-HT transporter (SERT) binding

Serotonin transporter (SERT) binding was determined on brain sections, cut as above, using (^{3}H)-paroxetine (Perkin Elmer, UK) as previously described [61]. Slides

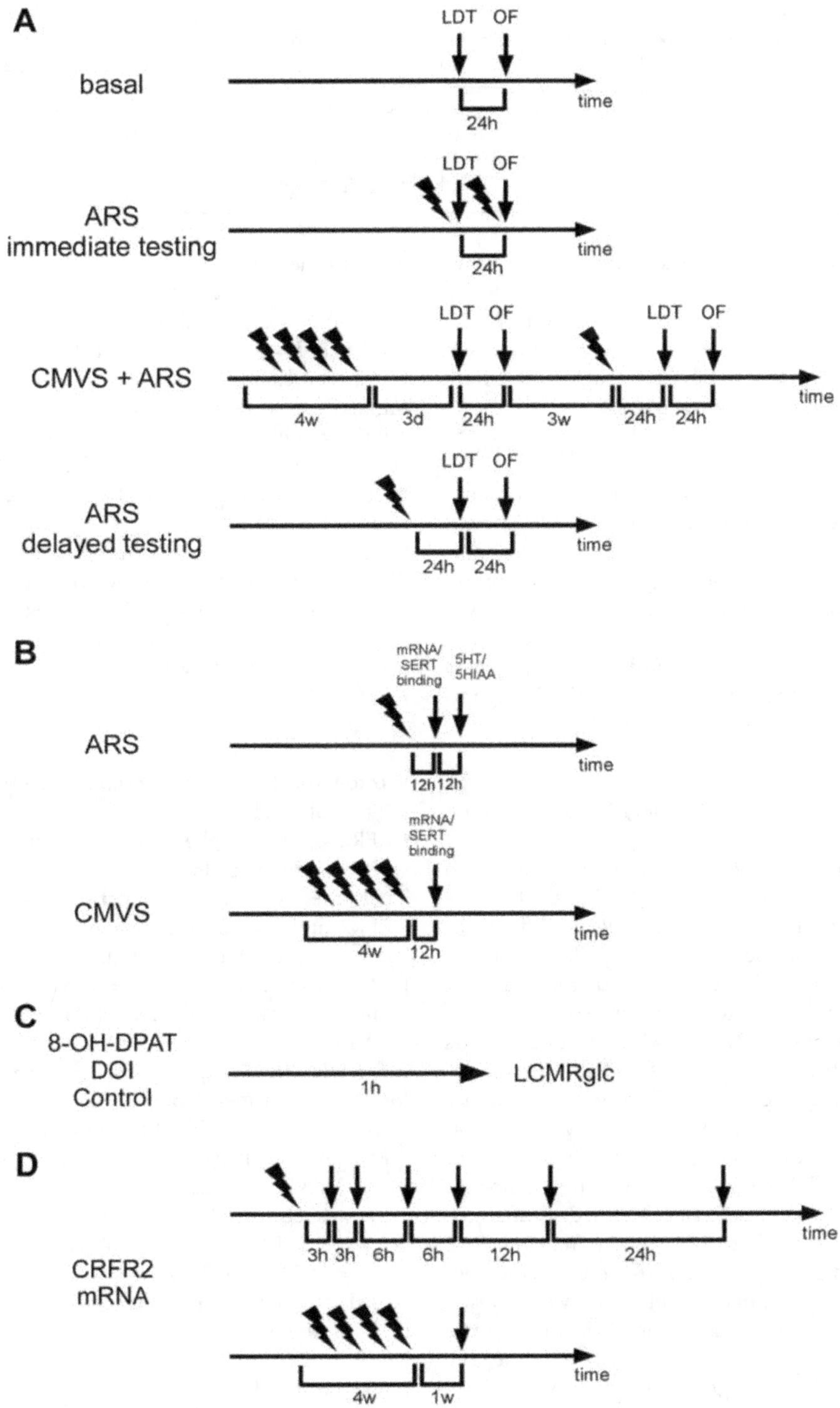

Figure 1 (See legend on next page.)

(See figure on previous page.)
Figure 1 Schematic representation of experimental protocols and timelines. (A) Separate cohorts of CRFR2-null and control mice were tested for anxiety-like behaviour in the light/dark transfer and open-field tests: under basal conditions; immediately following ARS; following CVMS and again 24 to 48 h after an ARS applied 3 weeks after the end of CVMS; 24 to 48 h following ARS. **(B)** CRFR2-null and control mice were exposed to no stress, ARS or CVMS, and mRNA expression of stress-related genes and serotonin transporter (SERT) binding were quantified 12 h after the end of stress. 5-HT/5HIAA content in brain nuclei were quantified in unstressed mice and 24 h after ARS. **(C)** LCMRglu was measured in CRFR2-null and control mice one hour after administration of saline or 5-HTR agonist. **(D)** CRFR2 mRNA levels in brain were quantified over a 48-h time course following ARS or 7 days after CVMS in control mice. , ARS; , CVMS; d, days; w, weeks.

were then exposed to (^{3}H)-sensitive film (Amersham Hyperfilm MP, GE Healthcare, UK) at −80°C for 6 weeks. Analysis of autoradiographs was performed by measuring the signal over the area of interest with densitometry software (MCID Basic 7.0, Imaging Research, Inc.). The background was subtracted.

Statistical analyses

Statistical analyses employed the two-tailed Student's *t* test or two-way analysis of variance (ANOVA) with post-hoc analysis using Fisher's protected least significant difference test as appropriate, with the exception of time course of CRFR2 expression, where one-way ANOVA with Dunnett's post-hoc analysis was used. Data are presented as mean ± standard error of the mean (SEM). Differences were considered statistically significant at $P < 0.05$.

Results

CRFR2-null mice show increased anxiety 24 to 48 h after acute restraint stress (ARS)

Under basal conditions, where mice were not exposed to stress (other than that caused by the test itself), CRFR2-null mice and littermate controls showed no differences in anxiety-related behaviour in two well-validated behavioural tests, the LDT (Figure 2) and the OF test (Figure 3), compared with littermate controls.

Because this finding contrasted with previous reports [50,51], we hypothesized that stressful challenge was required to reveal the role of CRFR2 in anxiety. Another group of mice was tested immediately following 30 min ARS. Again, no effect of genotype on anxiety-like behaviour was observed (Figures 2 and 3). A further cohort of mice exposed to CVMS was tested 3 to 4 days after the end of the protocol, to allow for recovery from the final acute stressor, and again no differences were observed between control and CRFR2 mice in either behavioural test.

However, 3 weeks later, these same CVMS mice were exposed to a single 30-min ARS, and 24 to 48 h later the CRFR2-null mice showed significantly increased indices of anxiety compared with controls, with fewer visits to ($t = 3.022$, $P = 0.007$, $n = 10$ or 11), shorter distance travelled in ($t = 2.360$, $P = 0.029$, $n = 10$ or 11), and a trend to less time spent in the light chamber in the LDT ($t = 2.062$, $P = 0.053$, $n = 10$ or 11) (Figure 2), and fewer visits to the centre of ($t = 2.271$, $P = 0.036$, $n = 10$ or 11) and less time spent in ($t = 2.231$, $P = 0.039$, $n = 10$ or 11) the centre and a trend to less time spent in the OF test ($t = 1.825$, $P = 0.085$, $n = 10$ or 11) (Figure 3).

We then examined whether this delayed effect of ARS on anxiety was dependent on prior CVMS by subjecting a further cohort of mice to ARS alone, and observed the same increased anxiety-like behaviour 24 to 48 hours post-stress (Figures 2 and 3). In the LDT, CRFR2-null mice spent less time ($t = 2.650$, $P = 0.023$, $n = 5$ to 8) and travelled a shorter distance ($t = 2.833$, $P = 0.016$, $n = 5$ to 8) in the light chamber. In the OF test, CRFR2-null mice spent less time in ($t = 2.675$, $P = 0.022$, $n = 5$ to 8) and made fewer visits to the centre ($t = 3.604$, $P = 0.004$, $n = 10$ to 11), and travelled a shorter distance ($t = 5.078$, $P = 0.0004$, $n = 10$ to 11).

Serotonergic function is altered in the raphe nuclei of CRFR2-null mice

CRFR2 in the raphe nuclei modulate 5-HT activity, with consequences for stress-related behaviours [32-38]. Therefore serotonergic functions were examined in CRFR2-null and control mice. Neuronal metabolic activity, as measured by LCMRglu, was lower in both the DRN ($t = 2.626$, $P = 0.048$, $n = 8$ for 8-OH-DPAT experiment, $t = 2.804$, $P = 0.036$, $n = 8$ for DOI experiment) and median raphe nucleus (MRN) ($t = 2.472$, $P = 0.049$, $n = 8$ for 8-OH-DPAT experiment, $t = 2.785$, $P = 0.038$, $n = 8$ for DOI experiment) of CRFR2-null mice as compared with controls under basal conditions (Figure 4).

Following challenge with the 5-HT_{1A}R-specific agonist 8-OH-DPAT, a main effect of treatment (ANOVA: $F_{(1,28)} = 4.558$, $P = 0.044$), and an interaction between genotype and treatment was observed in DRN (ANOVA: $F_{(1,28)} = 5.953$, $P = 0.021$) (Figure 4). Post-hoc analysis revealed that controls responded with decreased LCMRglu in both the DRN ($t = 3.235$, $P = 0.0124$, $n = 8$) and the MRN ($t = 2.520$, $P = 0.047$, $n = 8$) as expected, whereas the raphe nuclei of CRFR2-null mice were unresponsive to 5-HT_{1A}R agonist. Following 5-HT_2R-specific agonist DOI challenge, only a main effect of genotype was seen in both the DRN (ANOVA: $F_{(1,28)} = 5.224$, $P = 0.030$) and the MRN (ANOVA: $F_{(1,28)} = 5.333$, $P = 0.029$). The pattern of responses was, however, the same as for 8-OH-DPAT.

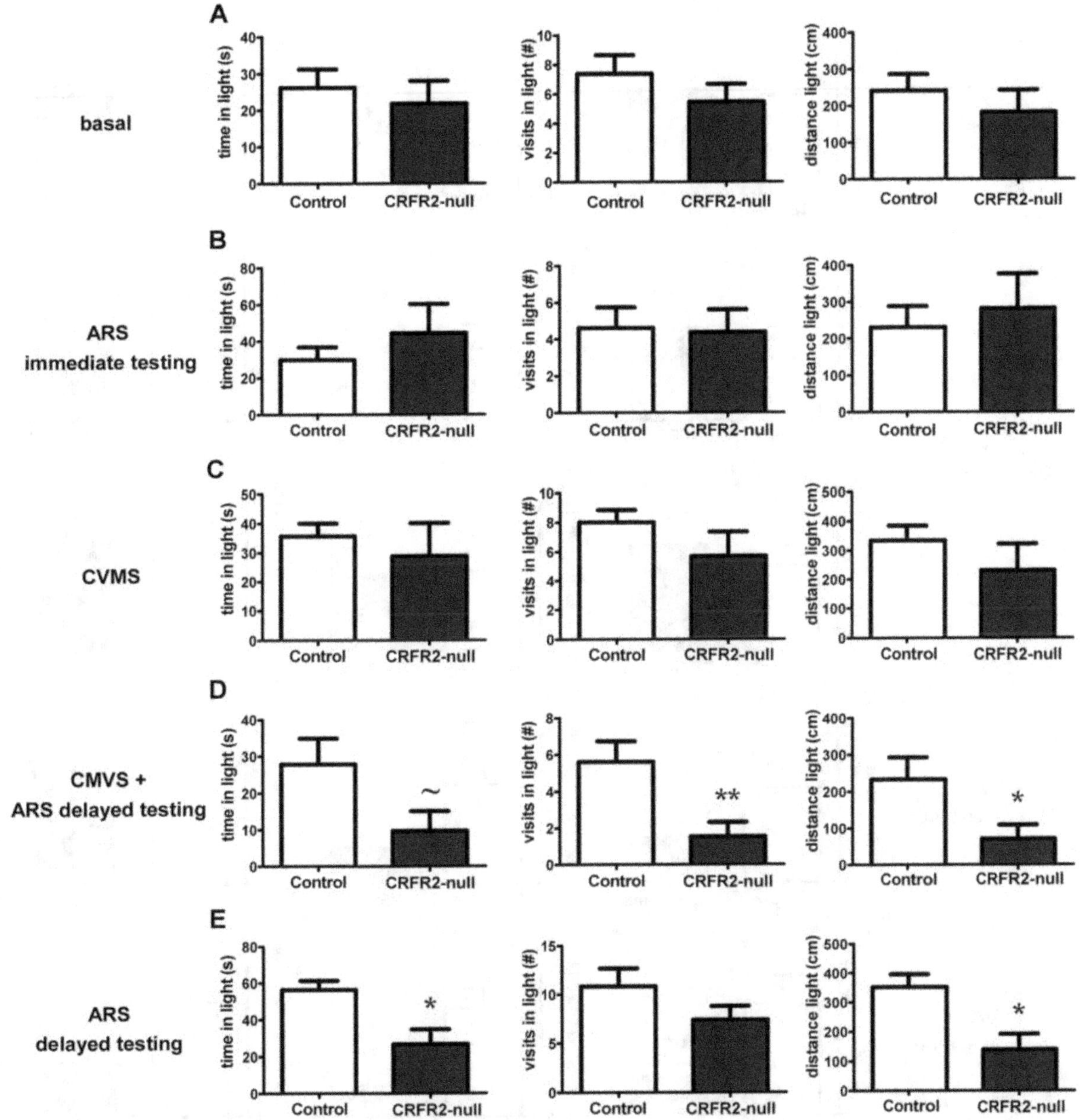

Figure 2 CRFR2-null mice exhibit increased anxiety-like behaviour 24 hours after ARS in the LDT. Under basal conditions **(A)**, immediately following ARS **(B)**, or after CVMS **(C)**, no differences were observed in behaviour between CRFR2-null mice and controls. However, when CVMS mice **(D)** or naïve mice **(E)** were exposed to ARS and tested 24 to 48 hours later, CRFR2-null mice showed increased anxiety-like behaviour compared with control mice. Data expressed as mean ± SEM. $N = 10$ to 14 for **A-D**, $N = 5$ to 8 for **E**. *$P < 0.05$, **$P < 0.01$, ~ $P = 0.53$, compared with control.

Studies to date have largely concentrated on the role of the DRN in respect to behaviour and anxiety. Therefore, we measured 5-HT and 5-HIAA within subregions of the DRN (Figure 4). Within the caudal DRN, there was a main effect of genotype on 5-HIAA (ANOVA: $F_{(1,22)} = 7.094$, $P = 0.014$) and a genotype X ARS interaction on 5-HIAA:5-HT ratio (ANOVA: $F_{(1,22)} = 6.153$, $P = 0.021$). Post-hoc analysis revealed an increase in 5-HIAA ($t = 3.472$, $P = 0.002$, $n = 7$) and 5-HIAA:5-HT ratio ($t = 3.242$, $P = 0.004$, $n = 7$) in CRFR2-mice under basal conditions, indicating increased serotonin turnover here. 24 hours following ARS, both the caudal ($t = 2.759$, $P = 0.011$, $n = 6$ or 7) and the dorsal

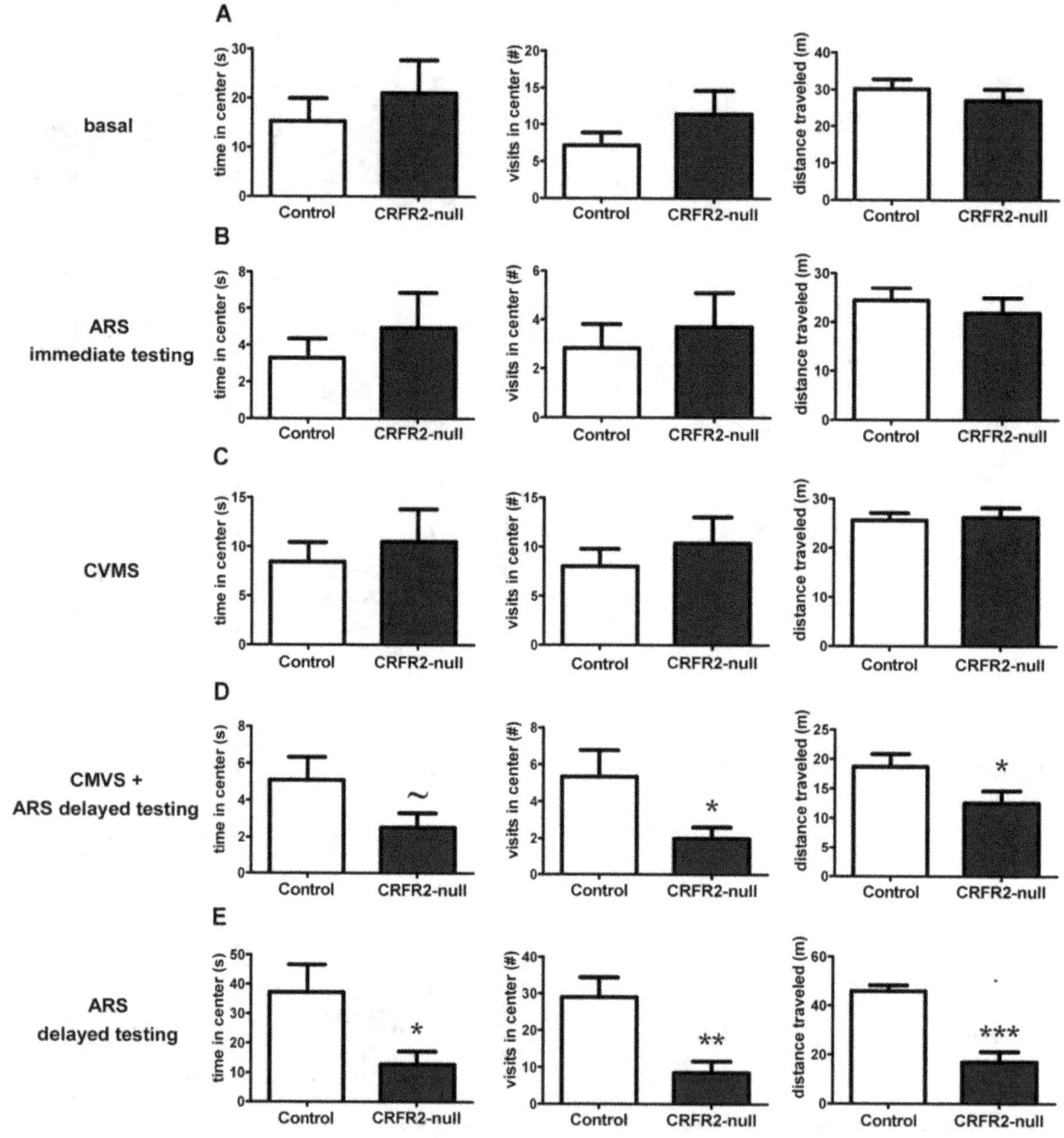

Figure 3 CRFR2-null mice exhibit increased anxiety-like behaviour 48 hours after ARS in the OF test. Under basal conditions **(A)**, immediately following ARS **(B)**, or after CVMS **(C)**, no differences were observed in behaviour between CRFR2-null mice and controls. However, when CVMS mice **(D)** or naïve mice **(E)** were exposed to ARS and tested 24 to 48 h later, CRFR2-null mice showed increased anxiety-like behaviour compared with control mice. Data expressed as mean ± SEM. $N = 10$ to 14 for **A-D**, $N = 5$ to 8 for **E**. $^{*}P < 0.05$, $^{**}P < 0.01$, $^{***}P < 0.001$, $^{\sim}P = 0.085$, compared with control.

($t = 4.087$, $P = 0.0005$, $n = 6$ or 7) DRN showed decreases in 5-HIAA:5-HT ratio in CRFR2-null mice, with an associated decrease in 5-HIAA in the caudal DRN of CRFR2-null mice ($t = 2.554$, $P = 0.018$, $n = 6$ or 7), whereas controls showed no effect of ARS on these parameters.

5-HT responses to stress and 5-HTR agonists are altered in efferent brain regions of CRFR2-null mice

Following challenge with the 5-HT_{1A}R-specific agonist 8-OH-DPAT, there was a main effect of treatment throughout the forebrain (ANOVA: $F_{(1,28)} = 4.196$ for

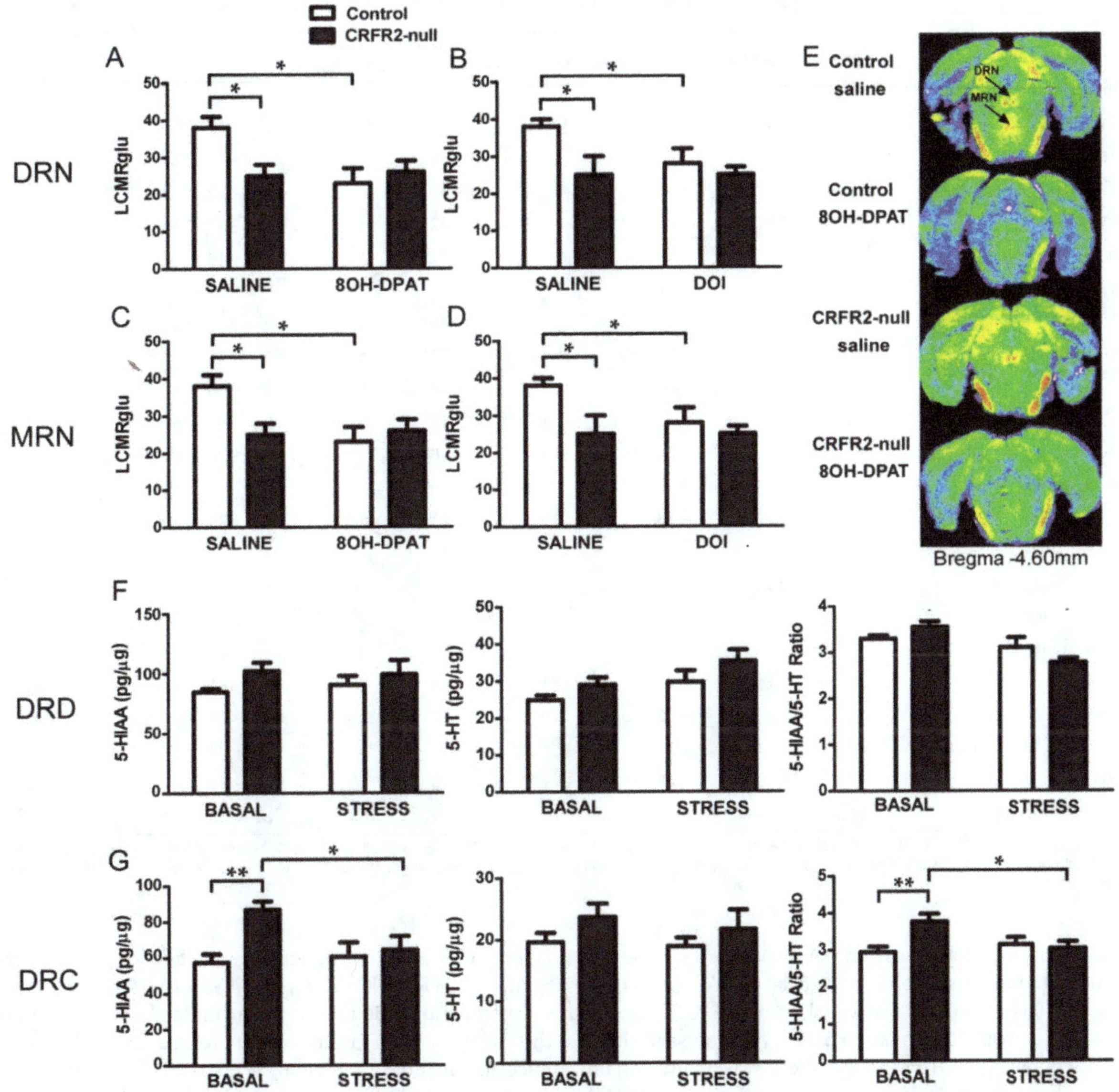

Figure 4 Serotonergic function is altered in the raphe nuclei of CRFR2-null mice. (A-E) LCMRglu in the dorsal raphe nucleus (DRN) and median raphe nucleus (MRN) is lower in CRFR2-null mice than controls under basal conditions. **(A,C)** 8-OH-DPAT or **(B,D)** DOI administration decreased LCMRglu in the **(A,B)** DRN or **(C,D)** MRN only in control mice. **(E)** Colour-coded autoradiograms from coronal brain sections at the level of the midbrain raphe. 'Warm' colours represent high levels of [^{14}C]-2-deoxyglucose accumulation while 'cold' colours represent low tracer accumulation. Images were selected from animals with matched plasma tracer and glucose concentrations. 5-HIAA and 5-HT content of the **(F)** dorsal and **(G)** caudal subdivisions of the DRN showed that the 5-HIAA:5-HT ratio was higher in CRFR2-null mice under basal conditions in the dorsal DRN (DRD) and was lowered by ARS only in CRFR2-null mice in both DRD and caudal DRN (DRC). Data expressed as mean ± SEM. $N = 8$ for LCMRglu, ANOVA critical $F_{(1,28)}$ value = 4.196 for $P \leq 0.05$, 7.636 for $P \leq 0.01$, 13.500 for $P \leq 0.001$. $N = 6$ or 7 for 5-HIAA and 5-HT content, ANOVA critical $F_{(1,22)}$ values = 4.301 for $P \leq 0.05$, 7.945 for $P \leq 0.01$, 14.380 for $P \leq 0.001$. $^*P < 0.05$, $^{**}P < 0.01$ in post-hoc analysis.

$P = 0.05$) (Table 1) with a genotype × 8-OH-DPAT interaction observed in some extrapyramidal and limbic structures. Post-hoc analysis revealed that while controls had decreased LCMRglu in response to 8-OH-DPAT in extrapyramidal regions as expected, CRFR2-null mice showed no response. These areas receive projections from the DRN but lack their own 5-HT$_{1A}$R, indicating that this reflects attenuated DRN response to 5-HT$_{1A}$R agonist.

In limbic areas, both genotypes decreased LCMRglu significantly (Table 1), but the genotype × 8-OH-DPAT

Table 1 LCMRglu in efferent brain regions of control and CRFR2-null mice in response to 5-HT$_{1A}$R or 5-HT$_2$R agonist

	Control			CRFR2-null			Control			CRFR2-null		
	Saline	8-OH-DPAT	%	Saline	8-OH-DPAT	%	Saline	DOI	%	Saline	DOI	%
Neocortex												
Frontal	46 ± 3	33 ± 3*	**−28**	47 ± 3	42 ± 3*	**−21**[a]	47 ± 3	38 ± 2*	**−19**	45 ± 2	30 ± 2*	**−33**[a, b]
Anterior cingulate	48 ± 3	35 ± 2*	**−27**	49 ± 2	39 ± 4*	**−35**[a]	50 ± 3	40 ± 2*	**−15**	51 ± 3	34 ± 2*	**−33**[a]
Prefrontal	47 ± 3	35 ± 3*	**−26**	47 ± 3	42 ± 2	**−6**[a]	50 ± 3	39 ± 3*	**−22**	50 ± 3	30 ± 2*	**−40**[a]
Somatosensory	55 ± 2	33 ± 4*	**−40**	51 ± 4	45 ± 3*	**−22**[a]	56 ± 2	53 ± 3	**−5**	55 ± 4	44 ± 3*	**−20**[a]
Parietal	53 ± 2	35 ± 2*	**−34**	50 ± 4	43 ± 3	**−21**[a]	55 ± 2	45 ± 1*	**−18**	54 ± 3	37 ± 2*	**−31**[a, b]
Hippocampus												
Subiculum	40 ± 3	26 ± 3*	**−35**	45 ± 3	23 ± 3*	**−49**[a]	42 ± 2	43 ± 3	**2**	43 ± 3	33 ± 3*	**−23**
Dentate gyrus	26 ± 3	16 ± 3*	**−38**	30 ± 2	15 ± 3*	**−50**[a]	28 ± 3	18 ± 2*	**−36**	27 ± 3	16 ± 2*	**−14**[a]
CA1	37 ± 3	22 ± 4*	**−41**	38 ± 3	16 ± 2*	**−58**[a]	36 ± 3	26 ± 3*	**−28**	37 ± 2	26 ± 2*	**−30**[a]
CA2	35 ± 3	20 ± 3*	**−43**	36 ± 3	19 ± 2*	**−47**[a]	35 ± 3	34 ± 3	**−3**	36 ± 3	29 ± 2*	**−19**
CA3	38 ± 2	20 ± 2*	**−47**	41 ± 2	17 ± 2*	**−58**[a]	36 ± 2	28 ± 3	**−22**	36 ± 2	22 ± 3*	**−39**[a]
Extrapyramidal areas												
Medial striatum	43 ± 3	33 ± 2*	**−23**	42 ± 3	39 ± 3	**−7**[a]	45 ± 3	34 ± 2*	**−24**	46 ± 3	29 ± 2*	**−37**[a]
Lateral striatum	46 ± 3	29 ± 3*	**−37**	44 ± 3	41 ± 3	**−7**[c]	46 ± 4	30 ± 3*	**−35**	48 ± 4	31 ± 3*	**−35**[a]
Globus pallidus	33 ± 2	20 ± 2	**−39**	32 ± 2	33 ± 2	**−3**[a, b, c]	32 ± 2	30 ± 2	**−6**	35 ± 2	23 ± 3*	**−34**[a, c]
Substantia nigra	30 ± 3	20 ± 1*	**−27**	27 ± 3	25 ± 4	**−7**	28 ± 4	30 ± 2	**7**	28 ± 2	18 ± 4	**−36**
Limbic areas												
Medial septal nucleus	41 ± 3	30 ± 2*	**−27**	39 ± 3	22 ± 2*	**−44**[a]	45 ± 2	31 ± 2*	**−31**	48 ± 3	30 ± 2*	**−38**[a]
Lateral septal nucleus	38 ± 3	27 ± 3*	**−29**	40 ± 2	18 ± 2*	**−55**[a, c]	37 ± 3	28 ± 3	**−24**	40 ± 4	27 ± 3*	**−33**[a]
Bed nucleus of the stria terminalis	27 ± 4	18 ± 2*	**−33**	31 ± 2	16 ± 3*	**−48**[a]	30 ± 4	20 ± 2	**−33**	30 ± 2	18 ± 3*	**−40**[a]
Basolateral amygdala	36 ± 3	26 ± 3*	**−28**	36 ± 2	15 ± 2*	**−58**[a, b, c]	38 ± 2	27 ± 4	**−29**	38 ± 2	24 ± 4*	**−37**[a]
Central amygdala	26 ± 2	20 ± 2*	**−23**	25 ± 3	15 ± 2*	**−40**[a]	25 ± 2	17 ± 2	**−32**	24 ± 3	15 ± 2*	**−38**[a]

Local cerebral glucose utilization (LCMRglu), shown as mean ± SEM and percentage change in LCMRglu in 8-OH-DPAT or DOI compared with saline-treated mice. $n = 8$. [a]Main effect of drug; [b]main effect of genotype, [c]genotype X drug interaction in 2-way ANOVA, where critical $F_{(1,28)}$ value was 4.20 for $P \le 0.05$. *$P < 0.05$ vs saline in post-hoc analysis.

interaction in lateral septum (ANOVA: $F_{(1,28)} = 4.654$, $P = 0.040$) and basolateral amygdala (BLA) (ANOVA: $F_{(1,28)} = 4.654$, $P = 0.040$) revealed that the CRFR2-null mice had a greater response to 5-HT$_{1A}$R agonist in these areas. Following DOI challenge, there was again a main effect of treatment throughout the forebrain (ANOVA: $F_{(1,28)} = 4.196$ for $P = 0.05$) (Table 1). Post-hoc analysis revealed that many brain regions showed a significant response to DOI in CRFR2-null mice but not controls (Table 1), suggesting greater postsynaptic 5-HT$_2$R responsiveness throughout the forebrain in CRFR2-null mice.

We then analyzed 5-HT and 5-HIAA content in the components of an anxiety-related amygdala-subiculum-septal circuit (Figure 5). There was a main effect of ARS on 5-HT content in the intermediate part of the lateral septum (LSI) (ANOVA: $F_{(1,22)} = 15.41$, $P = 0.0008$) and of genotype on the 5-HIAA:5-HT ratio (ANOVA: $F_{(1,22)} = 19.460$, $P = 0.0002$). There was also a genotype × ARS interaction in subiculum on both 5-HT (ANOVA: $F_{(1,22)} = 5.196$, $P = 0.033$) and 5-HIAA:5-HT ratio (ANOVA: $F_{(1,22)} = 10.87$, $P = 0.004$), and a main effect of genotype on 5-HIAA:5-HT (ANOVA: $F_{(1,22)} = 4.585$, $P = 0.045$).

Post-hoc analysis revealed that under basal conditions the 5-HIAA:5-HT ratio was increased in CRFR2-null mice (subiculum; $t = 3.846$, $P = 0.001$, $n = 6$: LSI; $t = 4.657$, $P < 0.0001$, $n = 7$). However, in contrast with the DRN, this was due to lower 5-HT (subiculum; $t = 2.474$, $P = 0.022$, $n = 6$-7: LSI; $t = 2.759$, $P < 0.012$, $n = 7$) with unchanged 5-HIAA. In response to ARS, 24 h later there was an increase in 5-HT in the LSI of CRFR2-null mice ($t = 3.878$, $P = 0.0009$, $n = 6$ or 7) and a decrease in the 5-HIAA:5-HT ratio ($t = 2.516$, $P = 0.020$, $n = 6$ or 7). The genotype x ARS interaction in the subiculum was such that 5-HIAA:5-HT was increased by ARS in controls ($t = 2.569$, $P = 0.018$, $n = 6$ or 7), but decreased in CRFR2-null mice ($t = 2.094$, $P = 0.049$, $n = 6$ or 7). In the CeA, there was a main effect of ARS (ANOVA: $F_{(1,22)} = 17.71$, $P = 0.004$) to increase 5-HT content in both genotypes ($t = 2.838$, $P = 0.010$, $n = 6$ or 7 for controls; $t = 3.113$, $P = 0.005$ for CRFR2-null mice, $n = 6$ or 7). 5-HT

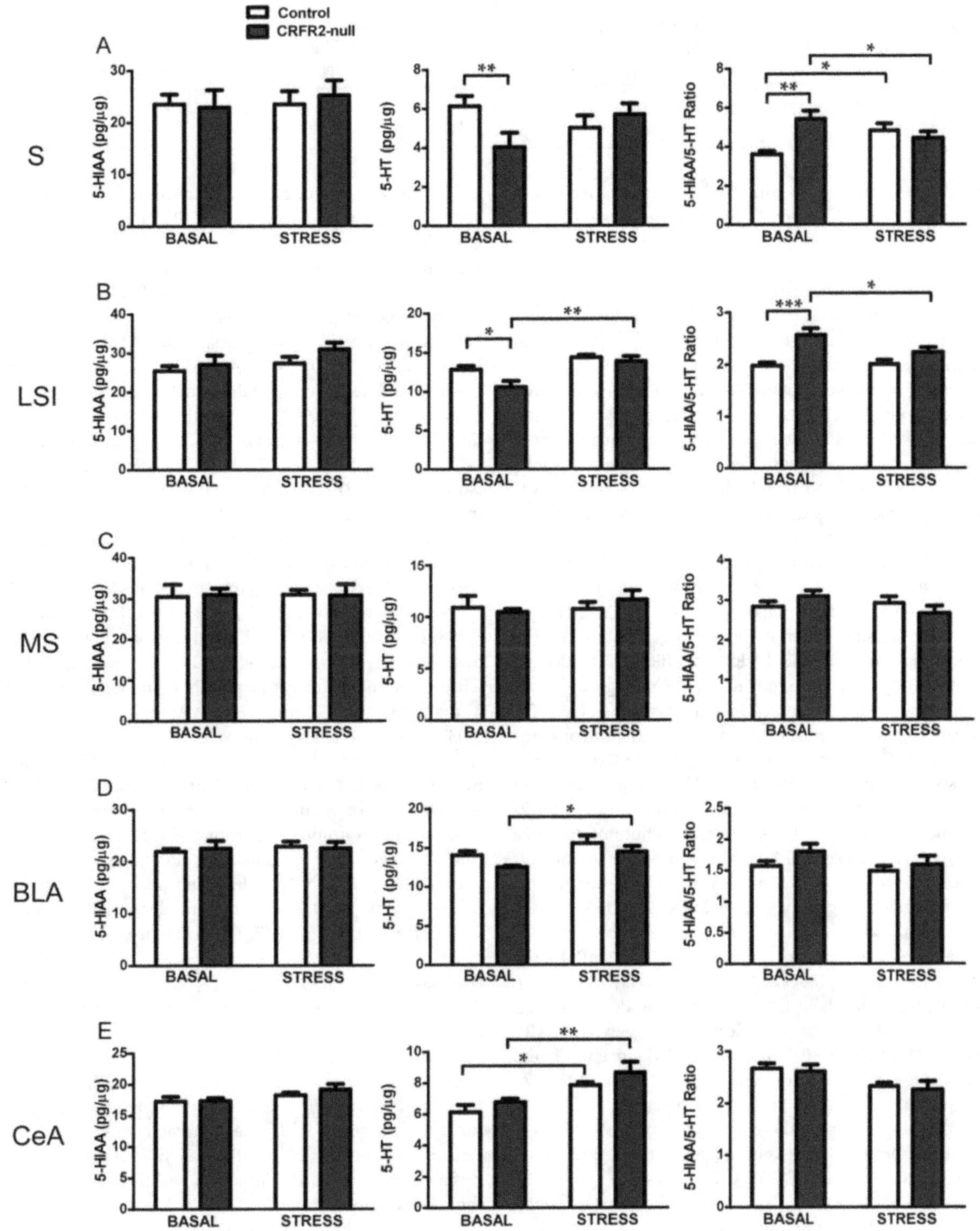

Figure 5 (See legend on next page.)

(See figure on previous page.)

Figure 5 5-HT responses to stress are altered in efferent brain regions of CRFR2-null mice. 5-HIAA and 5-HT levels as well as 5-HIAA/5-HT ratios are shown in the **(A)** subiculum (S), **(B)** intermediate part of the lateral septum (LSI), **(C)** medial septum (MS), **(D)** basolateral amygdala (BLA) and **(E)** central amygdala (CeA). CRFR2-null mice showed differences in basal levels of 5-HT and or 5-HIAA:5-HT ratio in the S and LSI, and a differential response to stress in the LSI and BLA. Data expressed as mean ± SEM. $N = 8$ for LCMRglu, ANOVA critical $F_{(1,28)}$ value = 4.196 for $P \leq 0.05$, 7.636 for $P \leq 0.01$, 13.500 for $P \leq 0.001$. $N = 6$ or 7 for 5-HIAA and 5-HT content, ANOVA critical $F_{(1,22)}$ values = 4.301 for $P \leq 0.05$, 7.945 for $P \leq 0.01$, 14.380 for $P \leq 0.001$. * $P < 0.05$, ** $P < 0.01$, *** $P < 0.001$ in post-hoc analysis.

levels also increased in the BLA ($t = 2.168$, $P = 0.041$, $n = 6$ or 7) of CRFR2-null mice in response to ARS (Figure 5).

Serotonergic and corticosteroid receptor gene expression are altered in response to stress in CRFR2-null mice

To investigate which factors potentially involved in the processes of adaptation to acute stress might be differentially regulated in CRFR2-null mice as compared with controls, SERT protein levels (ligand binding) and mRNA levels of serotonergic genes and corticosteroid receptors (ISH) were quantified in apposite brain nuclei following ARS or end of CVMS. A time of 12 h post-stress was chosen as appropriate, as altered expression of these factors at this time has previously been observed by many investigators. Full results are in Additional file 1; only key significant differences are presented here.

In agreement with responses to 8-OH-DPAT, 5-$HT_{1A}R$ mRNA expression did not differ with genotype in the hippocampus or amygdala (Additional file 1). No effect of genotype or stress was seen in the DRN (Figure 6), but a genotype x stress interaction (ANOVA: $F_{(2,36)} = 3.328$, $P = 0.048$) whereby decreased expression in control compared with CRFR2-null mice ($t = 2.181$, $P = 0.036$, $n = 7$) was seen in the MRN following CVMS, and there were trends for ARS to reduce 5-$HT_{1A}R$ expression in CRFR2-null mice ($t = 1.702$, $P = 0.098$, $n = 6$ or 7) but not controls, and for CVMS to reduce 5-$HT_{1A}R$ expression in controls alone ($t = 2.020$, $P = 0.052$, $n = 6$ or 7). There was no appreciable effect of genotype on 5-$HT_{2C}R$ mRNA expression (Additional file 1).

There was a main genotype effect on TPH2 mRNA expression in MRN (ANOVA: $F_{(2,36)} = 5.311$, $P = 0.027$), with increased levels in CRFR2-null mice. Post-hoc analysis detected this as significant only between ARS groups ($t = 2.080$, $P = 0.045$, $n = 6$ or 7) (Figure 6). There was a main effect of stress on TPH2 in DRN (ANOVA: $F_{(2,36)} = 3.684$, $P = 0.036$) across genotypes.

In the hippocampus, there was a main effect of stress on SERT protein expression (CA1 ANOVA: $F_{(2,36)} = 4.106$, $P = 0.027$; CA2 ANOVA: $F_{(2,36)} = 4.387$, $P = 0.020$; subiculum ANOVA: $F_{(2,36)} = 8.474$, $P = 0.001$), owing to increased expression after the end of CVMS, only reaching statistical significance in CRFR2-null mice (CA1 $t = 2.151$, $P = 0.038$, $n = 7$ or 8; CA2 $t = 2.139$, $P = 0.026$, $n = 7$ or 8; subiculum $t = 3.490$, $P = 0.0013$, $n = 7$ or 8) and not in controls (Figure 6). There were no effects of genotype or stress on SERT expression in the amygdala (Additional file 1).

Expression of GR mRNA showed differential effects between brain regions and genotypes (Figure 6). In the dorsal hippocampus, there was a trend towards higher GR expression in CRFR2-null mice (CA1 ANOVA: $F_{(2,36)} = 3.976$, $P = 0.054$; CA2 ANOVA: $F_{(2,36)} = 4.008$, $P = 0.067$). There was a main effect of stress (ANOVA: $F_{(2,36)} = 7.312$, $\underline{P} = 0.002$) with both ARS and CVMS reducing expression in CA1 of CRFR2-null mice (ARS $t = 2.420$, $P = 0.021$, $n = 7$ or 8; CVMS $t = 2.962$, $P = 0.005$, $n = 7$ or 8), but only CVMS had a significant effect in controls ($t = 2.962$, $P = 0.043$, $n = 6$ or 7). In CA2, only CVMS had an effect to reduce GR expression, and this was only significant in CRFR2-null mice ($t = 2.725$, $P = 0.010$, $n = 7$ or 8). In the paraventricular nucleus (PVN) there was a main effect of genotype (ANOVA: $F_{(2,36)} = 6.788$, $P = 0.003$) with CRFR2-null mice having lower GR mRNA expression, although this was not significant within treatment groups in post-hoc analysis. There was a main effect of stress (ANOVA: $F_{(2,36)} = 4.974$, $P = 0.032$); post-hoc analysis showed increased GR following CVMS, but only reaching significance in CRFR2-null mice ($t = 2.341$, $P = 0.025$, $n = 7$ or 8). Expression of MR mRNA was not regulated by stress or genotype in any brain region examined (Additional file 1). Finally, CRFR2 mRNA levels, as quantified by qPCR, were increased over a time period of 3 to 48 hours post-ARS (ANOVA: $F_{(5,42)} = 3.750$, $P = 0.007$) but were decreased following CVMS ($t = 2.164$, $P = 0.047$, $n = 8$) (Figure 6).

Discussion

This study extends the evidence regarding the importance of CRFR2 in mediating the processes towards successful behavioural recovery in the period following stress, and moreover demonstrates that CRFR2 is engaged in the control of serotonergic function during the same time frame. It further characterizes the stress-sensitive phenotype of CRFR2-null mice [50,51,62] and reveals fundamental disturbances within components of their serotonergic system.

In contrast with original reports of increased basal levels of anxiety [50,51], in our hands, similar to the findings of Coste *et al.* [62], CRFR2-null mice do not show increased anxiety-like behaviour compared to

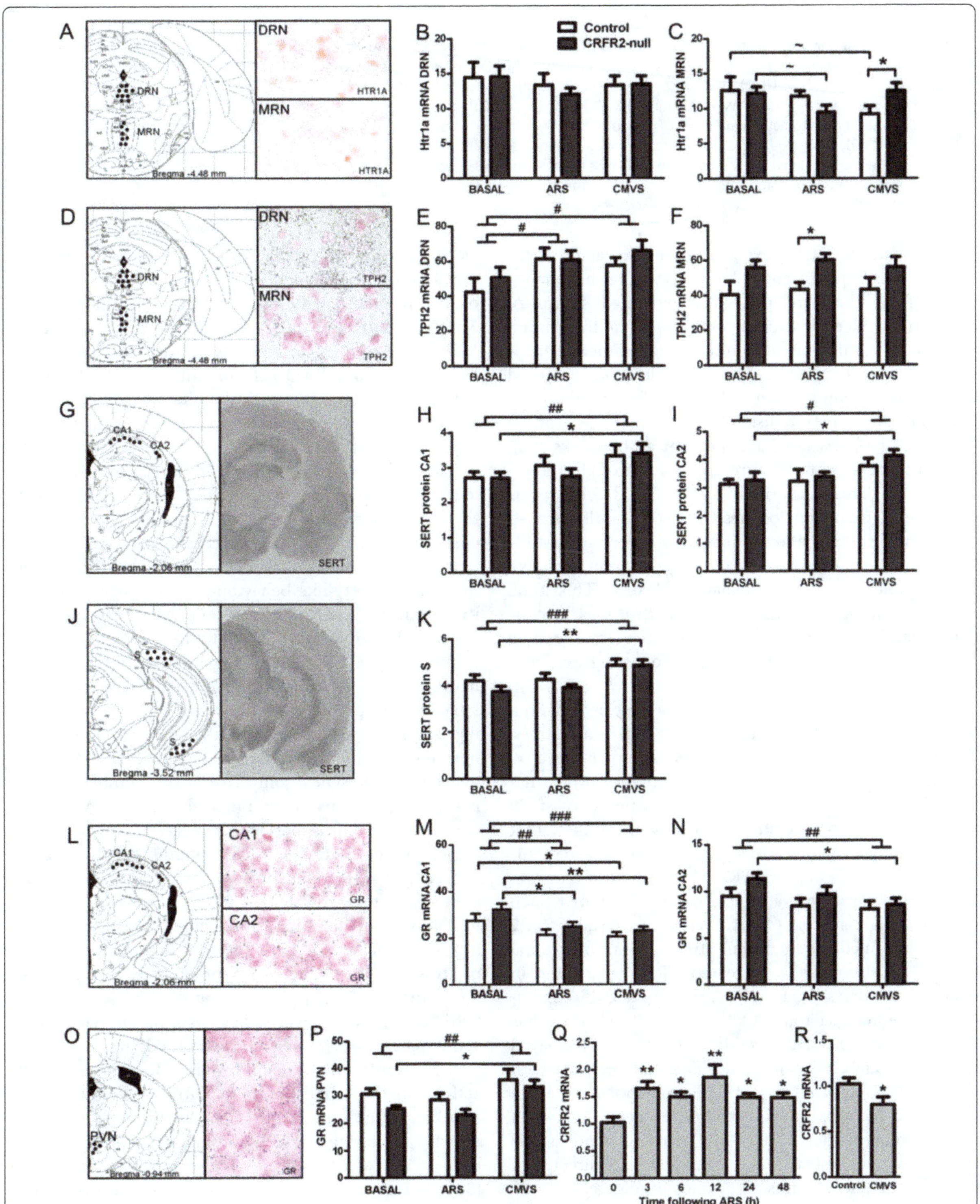

Figure 6 (See legend on next page.)

(See figure on previous page.)
Figure 6 Serotonergic and corticosteroid receptor expression are regulated differentially in response to stress in CRFR2-null mice. (A) mRNA expression of 5-HT$_{1A}$R in the **(B)** dorsal raphe nucleus (DRN) and **(C)** median raphe nucleus (MRN); **(D)** tryptophan hydroxylase 2 (TPH2) mRNA in **(E)** DRN and **(F)** MRN; **(G)** serotonin transporter (SERT) protein expression in **(H)** hippocampal CA1, **(I)** CA2 and **(J,K)** subiculum (S); **(L)** glucocorticoid receptor (GR) mRNA expression in **(M)** CA1, **(N)** CA2 and **(O,P)** the paraventricular nucleus (PVN). Data presented as mean ± SEM for mRNA levels or densitometry signal (SERT). $N = 6$ to 8. ANOVA critical $F_{(2,36)}$ value = 3.259 for $P \leq 0.05$, 5.248 for $P \leq 0.01$, 8.420 for $P \leq 0.001$. $^{\#}P < 0.05$, $^{\#\#}P < 0.01$, $^{\#\#\#}P < 0.001$ for effect of stress across genotypes. $^{*}P < 0.05$, $^{**}P < 0.01$, $^{***}P < 0.001$ ~$P < 0.10$ in post-hoc analysis. ARS increased CRFR2 mRNA expression in whole brain of mice at all times points up to 48 h post-stress **(Q)**, whereas CVMS decreased CRFR2 expression 7 days after the end of the CVMS protocol **(R)**. Data presented as mean ± SEM. $N = 8$. ANOVA critical $F_{(5,42)}$ value = 2.438 for $P \leq 0.05$, 3.488 for $P \leq 0.01$. $^{*}P < 0.05$, $^{**}P < 0.01$ as compared with 0 hours in post-hoc analysis or with control group.

controls until 24 h after exposure to a prior acute stressor. This discrepancy could be due to differing phenotypes of the three independently generated strains of CRFR2-null mice, or factors such as age or husbandry. However, the mice in this study are the same strain as reported with increased anxiety by Bale *et al.* [50] and an anxious phenotype was described for both group- [50] and singly [51] housed CRFR2-null mice from 9 [40] to 24 [50] weeks of age, but not at 16 weeks [62], meaning that these factors are unlikely to explain the inconsistency. This study indicates the need for a prior stress for increased anxiogenesis in CRFR2-null mice, so an alternative explanation is that mice in previous studies might have been inadvertently previously stressed, for example, by a prior behavioural test. This time course of the behavioural effects of ARS led us to conclude that CRFR2 has a key role in the processes leading to behavioural recovery in the hours following exposure to a stressor.

While CRFR2-null mice in our study appear to be in a maladaptive state at 24 hours following an acute stress, CRFR2-null mice exposed to CVMS are not more anxious than controls. It could be interpreted from this that CRFR2-null mice have the ability to cope successfully with this more chronic stress, but it is more likely that both CRFR2-null mice and controls are affected adversely by CVMS, while CRFR2-null mice show an exaggerated response to a single acute stressor. Such stressors might release CRF sufficient to recruit CRFR2 [20], which mediate successful stress coping in normal mice [63]. Alternatively, increased CRFR1 signalling in response to stress might occur; increased CRF expression in the amygdala and PVN of CRFR2-null mice has been reported [50]. However, the time frame of delayed anxiogenesis in CRFR2-null mice does not correlate with the expected rapid release of CRF in response to acute stress and its subsequent negative feedback. The time interval required for CRFR2-null mice to acquire this anxiety trait suggests that the processes are indirect, and the serotonergic system is an obvious candidate.

Exogenous CRF administered to the DRN inhibits firing of 5-HT neurons via CRFR1 [15,18], while Ucns or higher levels of CRF increase firing via CRFR2 [32-36]. The raphe nuclei receive inputs from both CRF and Ucn1 neurons [14,15,29], which may therefore regulate serotonergic raphe function physiologically. In support of this hypothesis, CRFR2-null mice show altered 5-HT/5-HIAA content in the DRN, LSI, subiculum, CeA and BLA 24 h after ARS, whereas control mice showed a clear change only in 5-HT content of the CeA. Recent studies of mice with genetically altered Ucn levels have shown that 5-HT function is dysregulated in these models [39-41] and that CRFR2-null mice show greater sensitivity to elevation of 5-HT levels by pharmacological means, an observation suggested to be linked to their stress-sensitive phenotype [64]. Notably, mice deficient in all three Ucns do indeed show a similar phenotype [41] to our observations in CRFR2-null mice, with increased anxiety-like behaviour and dysregulated activity within 5-HT circuits 24 h following ARS, again evidencing the importance of CRFR2 here.

Interestingly, CRFR2-null mice show decreased basal neuronal metabolic activity in the raphe nuclei. This is typically interpreted as evidence of decreased 5-HT firing activity levels, as while both 5-HT and GABAergic neurons are important functionally here, GABAergic neurons are present at only 10% of the number of 5-HT neurons [65]. This is an unusual finding under basal conditions in our experience and could be due to increased raphe 5-HT$_{1A}$R inhibitory autoreceptor activity, altered 5-HT$_{1A}$R modulation of raphe GABAergic interneurons that express both CRFR2 and 5-HT$_{1A}$R, or by inhibition from forebrain postsynaptic receptors including 5-HT$_{1A}$R and 5-HT$_2$R [66-69]. Increased sensitivity of structures throughout the forebrain to 5-HT$_2$R agonists and to 5-HT$_{1A}$R in some limbic structures in CRFR2-null mice suggests that postsynaptic receptor responsiveness is increased, and thus the latter mechanism may be significant. A shift towards unopposed CRFR1 activity in the raphe nuclei of CRFR2-null mice could also be a significant factor in mediating these effects or directly inhibiting 5-HT neuronal activity. Uncontrollable stress, which activates DRN serotonergic neurons [38], is associated with a functional desensitization of 5-HT$_{1A}$R [70]. We observed no significant differences in 5-HTR expression in the DRN of CRFR2-null mice and so it is likely that these effects are also mediated by decreased internalization and desensitization of receptors

[71], providing a mechanism for potentially very dynamic responses to stress. Detailed electrophysiological studies would be required to resolve the mechanism further.

In contrast with forebrain structures, the lack of LCMRglu response in the raphe nuclei to 5-HTR agonists in CRFR2-null mice suggests tonic inhibition of neuronal activity here may be close to maximal under basal conditions. The response to 5-HT_{1A}R agonist in extrapyramidal brain areas receiving projections from the DRN [72,73] but lacking their own 5-HT_{1A}R [74,75] was also attenuated. Thus CRFR2 appear to be required for maintaining normal basal neuronal activity in the raphe nuclei and, in particular, for the balance of 5-HT_{1A}R function here.

CRFR2 are present in both the DRN and the MRN [11,13]. However, studies of stress biology have largely concentrated on the DRN, and so to relate this altered raphe function to the CRFR2-null behavioural phenotype, we examined 5-HT responses to stress in the DRN and associated anxiety-related nuclei. Concentrations of 5-HIAA and the 5-HIAA:5-HT ratio were elevated in CRFR2-null mice under baseline conditions within the caudal subregion of the DRN (DRC), and these effects approached significance in the adjacent dorsal subregion (DRD). The DRD and DRC mediate CRF receptor responses and are considered to be anxiety-related subregions of the DRN based on anatomical and functional criteria [76,77]. For example, they are activated by anxiogenic drugs [78], CRF-related peptides *in vivo* [33,79] and *in vitro* [80], inescapable shock [70], noise stress [80], social defeat [81], the avoidance task on the elevated T-maze [82], acoustic startle [83] and anxiety due to prior experience of intimate partner violence [84]. In support of the specificity of these anxiety-related effects on DRD/DRC serotonergic systems, in none of these studies were serotonergic neurons in the adjacent ventrolateral part of the DRN activated. Elevation of 5-HIAA and 5-HIAA:5-HT ratios in the DRC could be due to an organizational difference in 5-HT systems as a consequence of CRFR2-null phenotype, or to differential activity that develops later in life. In either case, DRC neurons appear to have altered baseline activity in adult CRFR2 null mice, which may reflect a vulnerability to increased anxiety states.

Despite lower 5-HT content in efferent stress-related nuclei under unstressed conditions in CRFR2-null mice, stress had a greater effect on their 5-HT content at 24 h, in keeping with their stress-sensitive phenotype. This was particularly evident in LSI, which receives significant 5-HT projections from the caudal DRN [85,86], in the subiculum and, to a lesser extent, in the CeA. The subiculum is a key structure in inhibiting the hypothalamic-pituitary-adrenal axis (HPAA) during termination of the stress response [87] and so altered function here might relate to the higher responsiveness of the HPAA in CRFR2-null mice following acute stress [50,62].

Not all anxiety-related nuclei examined showed such changes. We found no differences in the LCMRglu of the bed nucleus of the stria terminalis (BNST) between control and CRFR2-null mice at either baseline or in response to 8-OH-DPAT or DOI challenge. This was unexpected, given the pivotal role of the BNST in the control of anxiety states [88]. However, the serotonergic dysregulation in CRFR2-null mice may be downstream of the BNST which projects strongly to the DRD/DRC region [89], where CRFR2 are abundant [12,13]. Overexpression of CRF in the BNST induces a decrease in CRFR2 binding selectively in the DRD/DRC [90] and so it may be that the observed effects in CRFR2-null mice are primarily mediated here.

5-HT firing activity is generally increased by stress [20] and negative feedback to the DRN ultimately restores balance [66-69,71], as evidenced by essentially unchanged 5-HT and 5-HIAA levels in control mice at 24 h following ARS. It has been previously reported that CRFR2-null mice show greater sensitivity to 5-HT modulation of stress-induced behaviours [64]. The pattern of increased responses in CRFR2-null mice to both 5-HT_{1A}R and 5-HT_2R receptor agonists in areas expressing postsynaptic receptors is in keeping with this finding. The LSI and BLA are key components of the limbic stress circuitry that were more responsive to 5-HT_{1A}R agonist in CRFR2-null mice. This might therefore relate to their stress-sensitive phenotype and indicate a role for these structures in stress recovery.

The MRN has been implicated in mediating a delayed coping response following fear behaviour induced by CRF in the DRN [35,91]. A delayed increase in 5-HT in the mPFC mediated by CRFR2 in MRN is associated with cessation of intra-DRN CRF-induced freezing behaviour [91] and is therefore proposed to mediate stress resilience effects [92]. In CRFR2-null mice, the CRFR2-mediated surges in 5-HT neuronal firing from DRN and MRN cannot occur, and unopposed CRFR1-mediated inhibition in DRN might further contribute to this [15,18]. The normal 5-HT response in mPFC occurs one to two hours after intra-DRN CRFR2 receptor activation [35,91], and we infer that the maladaptive state in CRFR2-mice develops after the peak of this CRFR2-induced increase in mPFC 5-HT and by 24 h after the stress. Thus, we propose that this delayed activity in efferent 5-HT neurons, which is critical for successful adaptation to acute stress, is disrupted in CRFR2-null mice. The consequences for CRFR2-null mice beyond 24 h are unknown, but unlike controls, 5-HT levels at this time point are increased from basal levels in several limbic nuclei, indicating that homeostasis has not been restored It is feasible that a lack of negative feedback within the 5-HT system due to the failure of CRFR2-mediated 5-HT activity might contribute to this.

Therefore, we propose that a rapid and highly regulated increase in CRFR2 signalling in response to acute stress, the resultant increase in efferent 5-HT activity and subsequent negative feedback to restore homeostasis are important for a normal and successful coping response. The delayed increase in 5-HT in mPMC is of key importance. Without this orchestrated response, CRFR2-null mice do not respond to stress appropriately, and there is prolonged anxiety that might account for their well-recognized anxiety phenotype. This proposed model is presented in Figure 7. There is significant evidence for a role for the MRN in stress recovery [91,92], and this model is consistent with our observation that LCMRglu is lower under basal conditions in the MRN of CRFR2-null mice while the robust elevation of TPH2 mRNA in CRFR2-null MRN might be a compensatory response to a lack of CRFR2 activation here. More detailed analysis of the dynamics of CRF and 5-HT processes in this time frame and beyond in appropriate subregions of the raphe nuclei, and consideration of the roles of other mediators of the stress response in CRFR2-null mice, are required to substantiate this further.

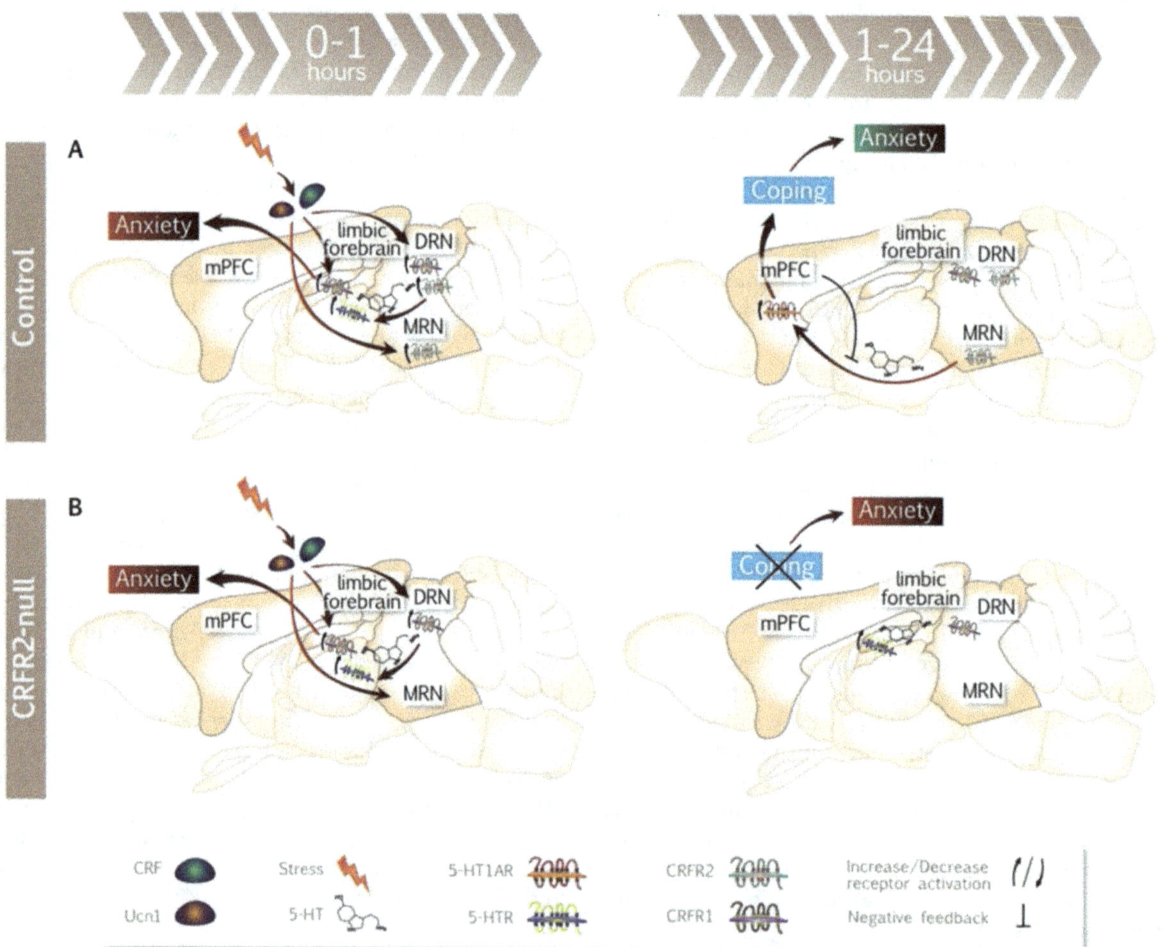

Figure 7 Proposed model for development of prolonged anxiety following acute stress in CRFR2-null mice. Following acute stress in control mice **(A)** CRF acting at CRFR1 in the limbic forebrain produces immediate anxiety. High levels of CRF and potentially Ucn1 activate CRFR1 and more abundant CRFR2 in the DRN with a net effect to promote early firing of efferent 5-HT neurons to limbic nuclei. Activation of CRFR2 in the MRN promotes delayed 5-HT release in the mPFC at 1 to 2 h, which acts at 5-HT1AR to mediate successful coping and anxiolysis by 24 h. Negative feedback in the 5-HT system restores homeostasis by 24 h. **(B)** In CRFR2-null mice, the CRFR2-mediated increase in 5-HT firing cannot occur and unopposed CRFR1 activity might inhibit 5-HT neuronal firing in limbic nuclei even further. Absence of negative feedback within the 5-HT system contributes to the increased 5-HT levels observed in limbic areas at 24 h. The temporal dynamics of the 5-HT system following acute stress are dysregulated and homeostasis has not been restored. Crucially, the delayed 5-HT activity in mPFC is disrupted and successful coping has not occurred, resulting in prolonged anxiety.

Owing to the number of mediators involved in stress responses and the complex interactions among them, other factors in addition to the serotonergic system are likely to be modified in CRFR2-null mice in the hours following stress exposure, which might have implications for the longer term. Indeed Ucn1 expression in the Edinger-Westphal nucleus and CRF in CeA (but not the PVN) are increased in CRFR2 mice [50], which may be a developmental compensatory change that is also responsible at least in part for their phenotype. Expression of CRFR1 is, however, unaltered. We found that changes in serotonergic and corticosteroid receptor gene expression in response to stress were generally greater in CRFR2-null mice, again in keeping with their stress-sensitive behavioural phenotype. CRFR2-null mice have normal basal HPAA activity, but higher responsiveness following acute stress [50,62]. Hence, changes such as the observed greater stress-induced increases in hippocampal SERT levels in CRFR2-null mice may be mediated by glucocorticoids [93,94], adding potentially further complexity to the relationship between CRFR2 and 5-HT function. Stress also downregulated hippocampal GR mRNA to a greater degree in CRFR2-null mice, potentially reflecting this expected HPAA hyperactivation. CRFR2-null mice also had lower basal GR expression in the PVN, possibly reflecting chronically higher HPAA tone, and CVMS unexpectedly increased this. Discordant regulation of GR expression in the hippocampus and PVN has been reported previously [95,96], with upregulation of GR by stress suggested to maintain glucocorticoid signalling to limit HPAA responses during prolonged stress. 5-HT also regulates GR expression, and this may be mediated through TPH2 activity, in order to regulate HPAA activity [97]. Both TPH2 and 5-HT_{1A}R mRNAs in MRN were differentially expressed in CRFR2-null mice. TPH2 mRNA levels in MRN were higher in CRFR2-null mice, and there may be altered afferent control of DRN activity from here [98], suggesting that the MRN should be more carefully considered in future studies of CRFR2 function.

Given this proposed role of CRFR2, we might expect expression to be regulated by stress exposure. We found expression to increase, reaching a maximum at 3 to 12 h post-ARS and subsequently declining, an effect similar to that seen for CRFR1 when acutely exposed to ligand [99], while chronic stress decreased CRFR2 mRNA expression in this and a previous study [100]. Others have observed lower CRFR2 expression in adult rats subjected to maternal deprivation or in genetically stress-sensitive rodent strains [101,102], suggesting that CRFR2 downregulation has the potential to be permanent in anxious or stress-sensitive animals. The interesting exceptions are where CRFR2 is increased by chronically elevated levels of CRF [103] or corticosterone [104], or in a model of maladaptive post-traumatic stress disorder-like behaviour [105]. We hypothesize that while increased CRFR2 activity is required for successful recovery from stress and subsequent downregulation is a normal adaptive response associated with healthy coping, that ongoing hyperactivity of CRFR2 might be associated with a maladaptive stress response. The role of CRFR2 in mediating learned helplessness in response to uncontrollable stress has implicated CRFR2 activity in the development of maladaptive behavioural responses [38,79]. However equally, CRFR2 upregulation might be an appropriate secondary adaptation to a chronic stress. This issue requires further investigation, to assess whether CRFR2 is a potential target in stress-related psychiatric disorders.

In this study, 5-HT function in the lateral septum and subiculum, sites linked with anxiety as well as the neural circuitry of reward and addiction [106-108], was particularly altered. Dysregulated serotonergic function has long been linked to stress-related psychopathologies [109,110] and direct effects of Ucns on CRFR2 in LSI have been observed in rodent models of these disorders; hence, CRFR2 may play an important role in these processes [111-113].

Conclusions

While the role of CRFR2 in stress recovery was proposed some time ago [63,114], this study provides new information regarding the mechanisms by which this may be mediated and highlights the importance in the immediate post-stress period. This has implications for the pathophysiology of psychiatric conditions associated with acute stress exposure, such as post-traumatic stress disorder, reactive depression and relapse to substance abuse. As evidence continues to emerge that CRFR2 may mediate its effects on stress primarily through 5-HT, the potential for involvement in further mood disorders and ultimately for therapeutic targeting is clear.

Additional file

Additional file 1: Serotonergic and corticosteroid gene expression in control and CRFR2-null mice in response to ARS or CVMS.

Abbreviations

5-HT: serotonin; 5-HTR: 5-HT receptor; 5-HIAA: 5-hydroxyindoleacetic acid; 8-OH-DPAT: 8-hydroxy-*N*,*N*-dipropyl-2-aminotetralin; ANOVA: analysis of variance; ARS: acute restraint stress; BLA: basolateral amygdala; BNST: bed nucleus of the stria terminalis; CeA: central amygdala; CVMS: chronic variable mild stress; CRF: corticotropin-releasing factor; CRFR1: corticotropin-releasing factor type 1 receptors; CRFR2: corticotropin-releasing factor type 2 receptors; DOI: 1-(2,5-dimethoxy-4-iodophenyl)-2-aminopropane; DRC: dorsal raphe nucleus, caudal part; DRD: dorsal raphe nucleus, dorsal part; DRN: dorsal raphe nucleus; GR: glucocorticoid receptor; HPAA: hypothalamic-pituitary-adrenal axis; ISH: *in-situ* hybridization histochemistry; LCMRglu: local cerebral glucose utilization; LDT: light/dark transfer test; LSI: intermediate part of the lateral septum; MR: mineralocorticoid receptor; MRN: median raphe nucleus; MS: medial septum; OF: open-field; PVN: paraventricular nucleus of the hypothalamus; qPCR: quantitative polymerase chain reaction; S: subiculum; SEM: standard error of the mean; SERT: serotonin transporter; TPH2: tryptophan hydroxylase 2; Ucn: urocortin.

Competing interests
The authors declare that they have no competing interests.

Authors' contributions
PMJ acquired funding, designed the study, performed experiments, analyzed and interpreted data and wrote the manuscript. OI designed and performed experiments, analyzed and interpreted data and prepared figures. RNC, EDP, AN-C and YK performed experiments and analyzed data. PATK and HJO designed and performed experiments and analyzed and interpreted data. CAL acquired related funding, designed experiments and analyzed and interpreted data. JRS and AC acquired related funding and participated in study design and data interpretation. All authors provided comments and suggestions during manuscript preparation. All authors read and approved the final manuscript.

Acknowledgements
We are grateful to our funding sources, including Wellcome Trust (grant 083192/Z/07/Z; PMJ, JRS, AC), the European Research Council (FP7 grant 260463; AC), the National Institute of Mental Health (NIH Award MH086539; CAL), the Israel Science Foundation (AC) and the Legacy Heritage Biomedical Science Partnership (AC). The content is solely the responsibility of the authors and does not necessarily represent the official views of the National Institute of Mental Health or the National Institutes of Health.

Author details
[1]Department of Neurobiology, Weizmann Institute of Science, Rehovot 76100, Israel. [2]Centre for Cardiovascular Science, Queens Medical Research Institute, 47 Little France Crescent, Edinburgh EH16 4TJ, UK. [3]Department of Integrative Physiology and Center for Neuroscience, University of Colorado Boulder, Boulder, CO 80309, USA. [4]Centre for Cognitive and Neural Systems, University of Edinburgh, 1 George Square, Edinburgh EH8 9JZ, UK.

References
1. Reid S, Barbui C: **Long term treatment of depression with selective serotonin reuptake inhibitors and newer antidepressants.** *BMJ* 2010, **340**:c1468.
2. Bandelow B, Zohar J, Hollander E, Kasper S, Möller HJ, WFSBP Task Force on Treatment Guidelines for Anxiety, Obsessive-Compulsive and Post-Traumatic Stress Disorders, Zohar J, Hollander E, Kasper S, Möller HJ, Bandelow B, Allgulander C, Ayuso-Gutierrez J, Baldwin DS, Buenvicius R, Cassano G, Fineberg N, Gabriels L, Hindmarch I, Kaiya H, Klein DF, Lader M, Lecrubier Y, Lépine JP, Liebowitz MR, Lopez-Ibor JJ, Marazziti D, Miguel EC, Oh KS, Preter M, *et al*: **World Federation of Societies of Biological Psychiatry (WFSBP) guidelines for the pharmacological treatment of anxiety, obsessive-compulsive and post-traumatic stress disorders - first revision.** *World J Biol Psychiatry* 2008, **9**:248–312.
3. Steinbusch HW: **Distribution of serotonin-immunoreactivity in the central nervous system of the rat-cell bodies and terminals.** *Neuroscience* 1981, **6**:557–618.
4. Steinbusch HW, Verhofstad AA, Joosten HW: **Localization of serotonin in the central nervous system by immunohistochemistry: description of a specific and sensitive technique and some applications.** *Neuroscience* 1978, **3**:811–819.
5. Vale W, Spiess J, Rivier C, Rivier J: **Characterization of a 41 residue ovine hypothalamic peptide that stimulates the secretion of corticotropin and β-endorphin.** *Science* 1981, **213**:1394–1397.
6. Müller MB, Zimmermann S, Sillaber I, Hagemeyer TP, Deussing JM, Timpl P, Kormann MS, Droste SK, Kühn R, Reul JM, Holsboer F, Wurst W: **Limbic corticotropin-releasing hormone receptor 1 mediates anxiety-related behavior and hormonal adaptation to stress.** *Nat Neurosci* 2003, **6**:1100–1107.
7. Vale W, Rivier C, Brown MR, Spiess J, Koob G, Swanson L, Bilezikjian L, Bloom F, Rivier J: **Chemical and biological characterization of corticotropin releasing factor.** *Recent Prog Horm Res* 1983, **39**:245–270.
8. Lloyd RB, Nemeroff CB: **The role of corticotropin-releasing hormone in the pathophysiology of depression: therapeutic implications.** *Curr Top Med Chem* 2011, **11**:609–617.
9. Sanchez MM, Young LJ, Plotsky PM, Insel TR: **Autoradiographic and *in situ* hybridization localization of corticotropin-releasing factor 1 and 2 receptors in nonhuman primate brain.** *J Comp Neurol* 1999, **408**:365–377.
10. Chalmers DT, Lovenberg TW, De Souza EB: **Localization of novel corticotropin-releasing factor receptor (CRF2) mRNA expression to specific subcortical nuclei in rat brain: comparison with CRF1 receptor mRNA expression.** *J Neurosci* 1995, **15**:6340–6350.
11. Van Pett K, Viau V, Bittencourt JC, Chan RKW, Li H-Y, Arias C, Prins GS, Perrin M, Vale W, Sawchenko PE: **Distribution of mRNAs encoding CRF receptors in brain and pituitary of rat and mouse.** *J Comp Neurol* 2000, **428**:191–212.
12. Lukkes JL, Staub DR, Dietrich A, Truitt W, Neufeld-Cohen A, Chen A, Johnson PL, Shekhar A, Lowry CA: **Topographical distribution of corticotropin-releasing factor type 2 receptor-like immunoreactivity in the rat dorsal raphe nucleus: co-localization with tryptophan hydroxylase.** *Neuroscience* 2011, **183**:47–63.
13. Day HE, Greenwood BN, Hammack SE, Watkins LR, Fleshner M, Maier SF, Campeau S: **Differential expression of 5HT-1A, α_{1b} adrenergic, CRF-R1, and CRF-R2 receptor mRNA in serotonergic, γ-aminobutyric acidergic, and catecholaminergic cells of the rat dorsal raphe nucleus.** *J Comp Neurol* 2004, **474**:364–378.
14. Lowry CA, Rodda JE, Lightman SL, Ingram CD: **Corticotropin-releasing factor increases *in vitro* firing rates of serotonergic neurons in the rat dorsal raphe nucleus: evidence for activation of a topographically organized mesolimbocortical serotonergic system.** *J Neurosci* 2000, **20**:7728–7736.
15. Kirby LG, Rice KC, Valentino RJ: **Effects of corticotropin-releasing factor on neuronal activity in the serotonergic dorsal raphe nucleus.** *Neuropsychopharmacology* 2000, **22**:148–162.
16. Waselus M, Nazzaro C, Valentino RJ, Van Bockstaele EJ: **Stress-induced redistribution of corticotropin-releasing factor receptor subtypes in the dorsal raphe nucleus.** *Biol Psychiatry* 2009, **66**:76–83.
17. Lukkes J, Vuong S, Scholl J, Oliver H, Forster G: **Corticotropin-releasing factor receptor antagonism within the dorsal raphe nucleus reduces social anxiety-like behavior after early-life social isolation.** *J Neurosci* 2009, **29**:9955–9960.
18. Valentino RJ, Lucki I, Van Bockstaele E: **Corticotropin-releasing factor in the dorsal raphe nucleus: linking stress coping and addiction.** *Brain Res* 2010, **1314**:29–37.
19. Clark MS, McDevitt RA, Hoplight BJ, Neumaier JF: **Chronic low dose ovine corticotropin releasing factor or urocortin II into the rostral dorsal raphe alters exploratory behavior and serotonergic gene expression in specific subregions of the dorsal raphe.** *Neuroscience* 2007, **146**:1888–1905.
20. Linthorst ACE: **Stress, corticotropin-releasing factor and serotonergic neurotransmission.** In *Handbook of Stress and the Brain. Volume 1.* 1st edition. Edited by Steckler T, Kalin NH, Reul JMHM. Amsterdam: Elsevier; 2005:503–524.
21. Lovenberg TW, Liaw CW, Grigoriadis DE, Clevenger W, Chalmers DT, De Souza EB, Oltersdorf T: **Cloning and characterization of a functionally distinct corticotropin-releasing factor receptor subtype from rat brain.** *Proc Natl Acad Sci U S A* 1995, **92**:836–840.
22. Perrin MH, Donaldson C, Chen R, Blount A, Berggren T, Bilezikjian L, Sawchenko P, Vale WW: **Identification of a second corticotropin-releasing factor receptor gene and characterization of a cDNA expressed in heart.** *Proc Natl Acad Sci U S A* 1995, **92**:2969–2973.
23. Chen R, Lewis KA, Perrin MH, Vale WW: **Expression cloning of a human corticotropin releasing factor (CRF) receptor.** *Proc Natl Acad Sci USA* 1993, **90**:8967–8971.
24. Fekete EM, Zorrilla EP: **Physiology, pharmacology, and therapeutic relevance of urocortins in mammals: ancient CRF paralogs.** *Front Neuroendocrinol* 2007, **28**:1–27.
25. Lewis K, Li C, Perrin MH, Blount A, Kunitake K, Donaldson C, Vaughan J, Reyes TM, Gulyas J, Fischer W, Bilezikjian L, Rivier J, Sawchenko PE, Vale WW: **Identification of Urocortin III, an additional member of the corticotropin-releasing factor (CRF) family with high affinity for the CRF2 receptor.** *Proc Natl Acad Sci U S A* 2001, **98**:7570–7575.
26. Reyes TM, Lewis K, Perrin MH, Kunitake KS, Vaughan J, Arias CA, Hogenesch JB, Gulyas J, Rivier J, Vale WW, Sawchenko PE: **Urocortin II: a member of the corticotropin-releasing factor (CRF) neuropeptide family that is**

selectively bound by type 2 CRF receptors. *Proc Natl Acad Sci USA* 2001, **98:**2843–2848.

27. Vaughan JM, Donaldson C, Bittencourt J, Perrin MH, Lewis K, Sutton S, Chan R, Turnbull A, Lovejoy D, Rivier C, Sawchenko PE, Vale W: **Urocortin, a mammalian neuropeptide related to fish urotensin I and to corticotropin-releasing factor.** *Nature* 1995, **378:**287–292.
28. Hsu SY, Hsueh AJ: **Human stresscopin and stresscopin-related peptide are selective ligands for the type 2 corticotropin-releasing hormone receptor.** *Nat Med* 2001, **7:**605–611.
29. Bittencourt JC, Vaughan J, Arias C, Rissman RA, Vale WW, Sawchenko PE: **Urocortin expression in rat brain: evidence against a pervasive relationship of urocortin-containing projections with targets bearing type 2 CRF receptors.** *J Comp Neurol* 1999, **415:**285–312.
30. Kozicz T, Yanaihara H, Arimura A: **Distribution of urocortin-like immunoreactivity in the central nervous system of the rat.** *J Comp Neurol* 1998, **391:**1–10.
31. Weitemier AZ, Ryabinin AE: **Lesions of the Edinger-Westphal nucleus alter food and water consumption.** *Behav Neurosci* 2005, **119:**1235–1243.
32. Pernar L, Curtis AL, Vale WW, Rivier JE, Valentino RJ: **Selective activation of corticotropin-releasing factor-2 receptors on neurochemically identified neurons in the rat dorsal raphe nucleus reveals dual actions.** *J Neurosci* 2004, **24:**1305–1311.
33. Staub DR, Evans AK, Lowry CA: **Evidence supporting a role for corticotropin-releasing factor type 2 (CRF2) receptors in the regulation of subpopulations of serotonergic neurons.** *Brain Res* 2006, **1070:**77–89.
34. Amat J, Tamblyn JP, Paul ED, Bland ST, Amat P, Foster AC, Watkins LR, Maier SF: **Microinjection of urocortin 2 into the dorsal raphe nucleus activates serotonergic neurons and increases extracellular serotonin in the basolateral amygdala.** *Neuroscience* 2004, **129:**509–519.
35. Forster GL, Pringle RB, Mouw NJ, Vuong SM, Watt MJ, Burke AR, Lowry CA, Summers CH, Renner KJ: **Corticotropin-releasing factor in the dorsal raphe nucleus increases medial prefrontal cortical serotonin via type 2 receptors and median raphe nucleus activity.** *Eur J Neurosci* 2008, **28:**299–310.
36. Lukkes JL, Forster GL, Renner KJ, Summers CH: **Corticotropin-releasing factor 1 and 2 receptors in the dorsal raphe differentially affect serotonin release in the nucleus accumbens.** *Eur J Pharmacol* 2008, **578:**185–193.
37. Hammack SE, Pepin JL, DesMarteau JS, Watkins LR, Maier SF: **Low doses of corticotropin-releasing hormone injected into the dorsal raphe nucleus block the behavioral consequences of uncontrollable stress.** *Behav Brain Res* 2003, **147:**55–64.
38. Hammack SE, Schmid MJ, LoPresti ML, Der-Avakian A, Pellymounter MA, Foster AC, Watkins LR, Maier SF: **Corticotropin releasing hormone type 2 receptors in the dorsal raphe nucleus mediate the behavioral consequences of uncontrollable stress.** *J Neurosci* 2003, **23:**1019–1025.
39. Neufeld-Cohen A, Kelly PA, Paul ED, Carter RN, Skinner E, Olverman HJ, Vaughan JM, Issler O, Kuperman Y, Lowry CA, Vale WW, Seckl JR, Chen A, Jamieson PM: **Chronic activation of corticotropin-releasing factor type 2 receptors reveals a key role for 5-HT1A receptor responsiveness in mediating behavioral and serotonergic responses to stressful challenge.** *Biol Psychiatry* 2012, **72:**437–447.
40. Neufeld-Cohen A, Evans AK, Getselter D, Spyroglou A, Hill A, Gil S, Tsoory M, Beuschlein F, Lowry CA, Vale W, Chen A: **Urocortin-1 and -2 double-deficient mice show robust anxiolytic phenotype and modified serotonergic activity in anxiety circuits.** *Mol Psychiatry* 2010, **15:**426–441. 339.
41. Neufeld-Cohen A, Tsoory MM, Evans AK, Getselter D, Gil S, Lowry CA, Vale WW, Chen A: **A triple urocortin knockout mouse model reveals an essential role for urocortins in stress recovery.** *Proc Natl Acad Sci USA* 2010, **107:**19020–19025.
42. Akimova E, Lanzenberger R, Kasper S: **The serotonin-1A receptor in anxiety disorders.** *Biol Psychiatry* 2009, **66:**627–635.
43. Price ML, Curtis AL, Kirby LG, Valentino RJ, Lucki I: **Effects of corticotropin-releasing factor on brain serotonergic activity.** *Neuropsychopharmacology* 1998, **18:**492–502.
44. Waselus M, Valentino RJ, Van Bockstaele EJ: **Collateralized dorsal raphe nucleus projections: a mechanism for the integration of diverse functions during stress.** *J Chem Neuroanat* 2011, **41:**266–280.
45. Gray TS: **Amygdaloid CRF pathways. Role in autonomic, neuroendocrine, and behavioral responses to stress.** *Ann NY Acad Sci* 1993, **697:**53–60.
46. Lazosky AJ, Britton DR: **Effects of 5-HT-1A receptor agonists on CRF-induced behavior.** *Psychopharmacology (Berl)* 1991, **104:**132–136.
47. Todorovic C, Radulovic J, Jahn O, Radulovic M, Sherrin T, Hippel C, Spiess J: **Differential activation of CRF receptor subtypes removes stress-induced memory deficit and anxiety.** *Eur J Neurosci* 2007, **25:**3385–3397.
48. Bakshi VP, Smith-Roe S, Newman SM, Grigoriadis DE, Kalin NH: **Reduction of stress-induced behavior by antagonism of corticotropin-releasing hormone 2 (CRH2) receptors in lateral septum or CRH1 receptors in amygdala.** *J Neurosci* 2002, **22:**2926–2935.
49. Kuperman Y, Issler O, Regev L, Musseri I, Navon I, Neufeld-Cohen A, Gil S, Chen A: **Perifornical urocortin-3 mediates the link between stress-induced anxiety and energy homeostasis.** *Proc Natl Acad Sci USA* 2010, **107:**8393–8398.
50. Bale TL, Contarino A, Smith GW, Chan R, Gold LH, Sawchenko PE, Koob GF, Vale WW, Lee K-F: **Mice deficient for corticotropin-releasing hormone receptor-2 display anxiety-like behaviour and are hypersensitive to stress.** *Nat Gen* 2000, **24:**410–414.
51. Kishimoto T, Radulovic J, Radulovic M, Lin CR, Schrick C, Hooshmand F, Hermanson O, Rosenfeld MG, Spiess J: **Deletion of Crhr2 reveals an anxiolytic role for corticotropin-releasing hormone receptor-2.** *Nat Genet* 2000, **24:**415–419.
52. Ducottet C, Griebel G, Belzung C: **Effects of the selective nonpeptide corticotropin-releasing factor receptor 1 antagonist antalarmin in the chronic mild stress model of depression in mice.** *Prog Neuropsychopharmacol Biol Psych* 2003, **27:**625–631.
53. Dawson N, Ferrington L, Olverman HJ, Kelly PA: **Novel analysis for improved validity in semi-quantitative 2-deoxyglucose autoradiographic imaging.** *J Neurosci Methods* 2008, **175:**25–35.
54. Dawson N, Ferrington L, Lesch KP, Kelly PA: **Cerebral metabolic responses to 5-HT2A/C receptor activation in mice with genetically modified serotonin transporter (SERT) expression.** *Eur Neuropsychopharmacol* 2011, **21:**117–128.
55. Dawson N, Ferrington L, Olverman HJ, Harmar AJ, Kelly PA: **Sex influences the effect of a lifelong increase in serotonin transporter function on cerebral metabolism.** *J Neurosci Res* 2009, **87:**2375–2385.
56. Paxinos G, Franklin KBJ: *The Mouse Brain in Stereotaxic Coordinates.* 2nd edition. San Diego: Academic Press; 2001.
57. Evans AK, Reinders N, Ashford KA, Christie IN, Wakerley JB, Lowry CA: **Evidence for serotonin synthesis-dependent regulation of *in vitro* neuronal firing rates in the midbrain raphe complex.** *Eur J Pharmacol* 2008, **590:**136–149.
58. Harris HJ, Kotelevtsev Y, Mullins JJ, Seckl JR, Holmes MC: **Intracellular regeneration of glucocorticoids by 11β-hydroxysteroid dehydrogenase (11β-HSD)-1 plays a key role in regulation of the hypothalamic-pituitary-adrenal axis: analysis of 11β-HSD-1-deficient mice.** *Endocrinology* 2001, **142:**114–120.
59. Seckl JR, Dickson KL, Fink G: **Central 5,7-dihydroxytryptamine lesions decrease hippocampal glucocorticoid and mineralocorticoid receptor messenger ribonucleic acid expression.** *J Neuroendocrinol* 1990, **2:**911–916.
60. Holmes MC, French KL, Seckl JR: **Modulation of serotonin and corticosteroid receptor gene expression in the rat hippocampus with circadian rhythm and stress.** *Brain Res Mol Brain Res* 1995, **28:**186–192.
61. De Souza EB, Kuyatt BL: **Autoradiographic localization of 3H-paroxetine-labeled serotonin uptake sites in rat brain.** *Synapse* 1987, **1:**488–496.
62. Coste SC, Kesterson RA, Heldwein KA, Stevens SL, Heard AD, Hollis JH, Murray SE, Hill JK, Pantely GA, Hohimer AR, Hatton DC, Phillips TJ, Finn DA, Low MJ, Rittenberg MB, Stenzel P, Stenzel-Poore MP: **Abnormal adaptations to stress and impaired cardiovascular function in mice lacking corticotropin-releasing hormone receptor-2.** *Nat Genet* 2000, **24:**403–409.
63. Reul JM, Holsboer F: **Corticotropin-releasing factor receptors 1 and 2 in anxiety and depression.** *Curr Opin Pharmacol* 2002, **2:**23–33.
64. McEuen JG, Semsar KA, Lim MA, Bale TL: **Influence of sex and corticotropin-releasing factor pathways as determinants in serotonin sensitivity.** *Endocrinology* 2009, **150:**3709–3716.
65. Stamp JA, Semba K: **Extent of colocalization of serotonin and GABA in the neurons of the rat raphe nuclei.** *Brain Res* 1995, **677:**39–49.
66. Sharp T, Boothman L, Raley J, Queree P: **Important messages in the 'post': recent discoveries in 5-HT neurone feedback control.** *Trends Pharmacol Sci* 2007, **28:**629–636.
67. Boothman L, Raley J, Denk F, Hirani E, Sharp T: ***In vivo* evidence that 5-HT (2C) receptors inhibit 5-HT neuronal activity via a GABAergic mechanism.** *Br J Pharmacol* 2006, **149:**861–869.
68. Boothman LJ, Sharp T: **A role for midbrain raphe gamma aminobutyric acid neurons in 5-hydroxytryptamine feedback control.** *Neuroreport* 2005, **16:**891–896.

69. Celada P, Puig MV, Casanovas JM, Guillazo G, Artigas F: **Control of dorsal raphe serotonergic neurons by the medial prefrontal cortex: involvement of serotonin-1A, GABA(A), and glutamate receptors.** *J Neurosci* 2001, **21**:9917–9929.
70. Rozeske RR, Evans AK, Frank MG, Watkins LR, Lowry CA, Maier SF: **Uncontrollable, but not controllable, stress desensitizes 5-HT1A receptors in the dorsal raphe nucleus.** *J Neurosci* 2011, **31**:14107–14115.
71. Flugge G: **Regulation of monoamine receptors in the brain: dynamic changes during stress.** *Int Rev Cytol* 2000, **195**:145–213.
72. McQuade R, Sharp T: **Functional mapping of dorsal and median raphe 5-hydroxytryptamine pathways in forebrain of the rat using microdialysis.** *J Neurochem* 1997, **69**:791–796.
73. Vertes RP: **A PHA-L analysis of ascending projections of the dorsal raphe nucleus in the rat.** *J Comp Neurol* 1991, **313**:643–668.
74. Laporte AM, Lima L, Gozlan H, Hamon M: **Selective *in vivo* labelling of brain 5-HT1A receptors by [^{3}H]WAY 100635 in the mouse.** *Eur J Pharmacol* 1994, **271**:505–514.
75. Verge D, Daval G, Marcinkiewicz M, Patey A, el Mestikawy S, Gozlan H, Hamon M: **Quantitative autoradiography of multiple 5-HT1 receptor subtypes in the brain of control or 5,7-dihydroxytryptamine-treated rats.** *J Neurosci* 1986, **6**:3474–3482.
76. Lowry CA, Hale MW, Evans AK, Heerkens J, Staub DR, Gasser PJ, Shekhar A: **Serotonergic systems, anxiety, and affective disorder: focus on the dorsomedial part of the dorsal raphe nucleus.** *Ann NY Acad Sci* 2008, **1148**:86–94.
77. Lowry CA, Johnson PL, Hay-Schmidt A, Mikkelsen J, Shekhar A: **Modulation of anxiety circuits by serotonergic systems.** *Stress* 2005, **8**:233–246.
78. Abrams JK, Johnson PL, Hay-Schmidt A, Mikkelsen JD, Shekhar A, Lowry CA: **Serotonergic systems associated with arousal and vigilance behaviors following administration of anxiogenic drugs.** *Neuroscience* 2005, **133**:983–997.
79. Staub DR, Spiga F, Lowry CA: **Urocortin 2 increases c-Fos expression in topographically organized subpopulations of serotonergic neurons in the rat dorsal raphe nucleus.** *Brain Res* 2005, **1044**:176–189.
80. Evans AK, Heerkens JL, Lowry CA: **Acoustic stimulation *in vivo* and corticotropin-releasing factor *in vitro* increase tryptophan hydroxylase activity in the rat caudal dorsal raphe nucleus.** *Neurosci Lett* 2009, **455**:36–41.
81. Gardner KL, Thrivikraman KV, Lightman SL, Plotsky PM, Lowry CA: **Early life experience alters behavior during social defeat: focus on serotonergic systems.** *Neuroscience* 2005, **136**:181–191.
82. Spiacci A Jr, Coimbra NC, Zangrossi H Jr: **Differential involvement of dorsal raphe subnuclei in the regulation of anxiety- and panic-related defensive behaviors.** *Neuroscience* 2012, **227**:350–360.
83. Meloni EG, Reedy CL, Cohen BM, Carlezon WA Jr: **Activation of raphe efferents to the medial prefrontal cortex by corticotropin-releasing factor: correlation with anxiety-like behavior.** *Biol Psychiatry* 2008, **63**:832–839.
84. Cordero MI, Poirier GL, Marquez C, Veenit V, Fontana X, Salehi B, Ansermet F, Sandi C: **Evidence for biological roots in the transgenerational transmission of intimate partner violence.** *Transl Psychiatry* 2012, **2**:e106.
85. Waselus M, Galvez JP, Valentino RJ, Van Bockstaele EJ: **Differential projections of dorsal raphe nucleus neurons to the lateral septum and striatum.** *J Chem Neuroanat* 2006, **31**:233–242.
86. Kohler C, Chan-Palay V, Steinbusch H: **The distribution and origin of serotonin-containing fibers in the septal area: a combined immunohistochemical and fluorescent retrograde tracing study in the rat.** *J Comp Neurol* 1982, **209**:91–111.
87. O'Mara S: **Controlling hippocampal output: the central role of subiculum in hippocampal information processing.** *Behav Brain Res* 2006, **174**:304–312.
88. Walker DL, Toufexis DJ, Davis M: **Role of the bed nucleus of the stria terminalis versus the amygdala in fear, stress, and anxiety.** *Eur J Pharmacol* 2003, **463**:199–216.
89. Peyron C, Petit JM, Rampon C, Jouvet M, Luppi PH: **Forebrain afferents to the rat dorsal raphe nucleus demonstrated by retrograde and anterograde tracing methods.** *Neuroscience* 1998, **82**:443–468.
90. Sink KS, Walker DL, Freeman SM, Flandreau EI, Ressler KJ, Davis M: **Effects of continuously enhanced corticotropin releasing factor expression within the bed nucleus of the stria terminalis on conditioned and unconditioned anxiety.** *Mol Psychiatry* 2013, **18**:308–319.
91. Forster GL, Feng N, Watt MJ, Korzan WJ, Mouw NJ, Summers CH, Renner KJ: **Corticotropin-releasing factor in the dorsal raphe elicits temporally distinct serotonergic responses in the limbic system in relation to fear behavior.** *Neuroscience* 2006, **141**:1047–1055.
92. Paul ED, Lowry CA: **Functional topography of serotonergic systems supports the Deakin/Graeff hypothesis of anxiety and affective disorders.** *J Psychopharmacol* 2013, **27**:1090–1106.
93. Racca S, Spaccamiglio A, Esculapio P, Abbadessa G, Cangemi L, DiCarlo F, Portaleone P: **Effects of swim stress and α-MSH acute pre-treatment on brain 5-HT transporter and corticosterone receptor.** *Pharmacol Biochem Behav* 2005, **81**:894–900.
94. Zhang J, Fan Y, Li Y, Zhu H, Wang L, Zhu MY: **Chronic social defeat up-regulates expression of the serotonin transporter in rat dorsal raphe nucleus and projection regions in a glucocorticoid-dependent manner.** *J Neurochem* 2012, **123**:1054–1068.
95. Gomez F, Lahmame A, de Kloet ER, Armario A: **Hypothalamic-pituitary-adrenal response to chronic stress in five inbred rat strains: differential responses are mainly located at the adrenocortical level.** *Neuroendocrinology* 1996, **63**:327–337.
96. Neal CR Jr, VanderBeek BL, Vazquez DM, Watson SJ Jr: **Dexamethasone exposure during the neonatal period alters ORL1 mRNA expression in the hypothalamic paraventricular nucleus and hippocampus of the adult rat.** *Brain Res Dev Brain Res* 2003, **146**:15–24.
97. Chen GL, Miller GM: **Advances in tryptophan hydroxylase-2 gene expression regulation: new insights into serotonin-stress interaction and clinical implications.** *Am J Med Genet* 2012, **159B**:152–171.
98. Vertes RP, Fortin WJ, Crane AM: **Projections of the median raphe nucleus in the rat.** *J Comp Neurol* 1999, **407**:555–582.
99. Brunson KL, Grigoriadis DE, Lorang MT, Baram TZ: **Corticotropin-releasing hormone (CRH) downregulates the function of its receptor (CRF1) and induces CRF1 expression in hippocampal and cortical regions of the immature rat brain.** *Exp Neurol* 2002, **176**:75–86.
100. Chen A, Perrin M, Brar B, Li C, Jamieson P, Digruccio M, Lewis K, Vale W: **Mouse corticotropin-releasing factor receptor type 2α gene: isolation, distribution, pharmacological characterization and regulation by stress and glucocorticoids.** *Mol Endocrinol* 2005, **19**:441–458.
101. Bravo JA, Dinan TG, Cryan JF: **Alterations in the central CRF system of two different rat models of comorbid depression and functional gastrointestinal disorders.** *Int J Neuropsychopharmacol* 2011, **14**:666–683.
102. Eghbal-Ahmadi M, Hatalski CG, Avishai-Eliner S, Baram TZ: **Corticotropin releasing factor receptor type II (CRF2) messenger ribonucleic acid levels in the hypothalamic ventromedial nucleus of the infant rat are reduced by maternal deprivation.** *Endocrinology* 1997, **138**:5048–5051.
103. Korosi A, Veening JG, Kozicz T, Henckens M, Dederen J, Groenink L, van der Gugten J, Olivier B, Roubos EW: **Distribution and expression of CRF receptor 1 and 2 mRNAs in the CRF over-expressing mouse brain.** *Brain Res* 2006, **1072**:46–54.
104. Hashimoto K, Nishiyama M, Tanaka Y, Noguchi T, Asaba K, Hossein PN, Nishioka T, Makino S: **Urocortins and corticotropin releasing factor type 2 receptors in the hypothalamus and the cardiovascular system.** *Peptides* 2004, **25**:1711–1721.
105. Lebow M, Neufeld-Cohen A, Kuperman Y, Tsoory M, Gil S, Chen A: **Susceptibility to PTSD-like behavior is mediated by corticotropin-releasing factor receptor type 2 levels in the bed nucleus of the stria terminalis.** *J Neurosci* 2012, **32**:6906–6916.
106. Belujon P, Grace AA: **Hippocampus, amygdala, and stress: interacting systems that affect susceptibility to addiction.** *Ann NY Acad Sci* 2011, **1216**:114–121.
107. Martin-Fardon R, Ciccocioppo R, Aujla H, Weiss F: **The dorsal subiculum mediates the acquisition of conditioned reinstatement of cocaine-seeking.** *Neuropsychopharmacology* 2008, **33**:1827–1834.
108. Sartor GC, Aston-Jones GS: **A septal-hypothalamic pathway drives orexin neurons, which is necessary for conditioned cocaine preference.** *J Neurosci* 2012, **32**:4623–4631.
109. Mann JJ: **Role of the serotonergic system in the pathogenesis of major depression and suicidal behavior.** *Neuropsychopharmacology* 1999, **21**:99S–105S.
110. Kirby LG, Zeeb FD, Winstanley CA: **Contributions of serotonin in addiction vulnerability.** *Neuropharmacology* 2011, **61**:421–432.
111. Ryabinin AE, Yoneyama N, Tanchuck MA, Mark GP, Finn DA: **Urocortin 1 microinjection into the mouse lateral septum regulates the acquisition and expression of alcohol consumption.** *Neuroscience* 2008, **151**:780–790.
112. Liu J, Yu B, Orozco-Cabal L, Grigoriadis DE, Rivier J, Vale WW, Shinnick-Gallagher P, Gallagher JP: **Chronic cocaine administration switches**

corticotropin-releasing factor2 receptor-mediated depression to facilitation of glutamatergic transmission in the lateral septum. *J Neurosci* 2005, **25**:577–583.

113. Henry B, Vale W, Markou A: **The effect of lateral septum corticotropin-releasing factor receptor 2 activation on anxiety is modulated by stress.** *J Neurosci* 2006, **26**:9142–9152.
114. Bale TL, Vale WW: **CRF and CRF receptors: role in stress responsivity and other behaviors.** *Annu Rev Pharmacol Toxicol* 2004, **44**:525–557.

8

The relationship between Hippocampal asymmetry and working memory processing in combat-related PTSD – a monozygotic twin study

Timothy Hall[1†], Cherrie Galletly[1,2,7*†], C Richard Clark[3†], Melinda Veltmeyer[4,8†], Linda J Metzger[†], Mark W Gilbertson[4†], Scott P Orr[5†], Roger K Pitman[5†] and Alexander McFarlane[6†]

Abstract

Background: PTSD is associated with reduction in hippocampal volume and abnormalities in hippocampal function. Hippocampal asymmetry has received less attention, but potentially could indicate lateralised differences in vulnerability to trauma. The P300 event-related potential component reflects the immediate processing of significant environmental stimuli and has generators in several brain regions including the hippocampus. P300 amplitude is generally reduced in people with PTSD.

Methods: Our study examined hippocampal volume asymmetry and the relationship between hippocampal asymmetry and P300 amplitude in male monozygotic twins discordant for Vietnam combat exposure. Lateralised hippocampal volume and P300 data were obtained from 70 male participants, of whom 12 had PTSD. We were able to compare (1) combat veterans with current PTSD; (2) their non-combat-exposed co-twins; (3) combat veterans without current PTSD and (4) their non-combat-exposed co-twins.

Results: There were no significant differences between groups in hippocampal asymmetry. There were no group differences in performance of an auditory oddball target detection task or in P300 amplitude. There was a significant positive correlation between P300 amplitude and the magnitude of hippocampal asymmetry in participants with PTSD.

Conclusions: These findings suggest that greater hippocampal asymmetry in PTSD is associated with a need to allocate more attentional resources when processing significant environmental stimuli.

Background

Post Traumatic Stress Disorder (PTSD) is characterised by recurrent and intrusive memories, avoidance, and hyperarousal. PTSD is also associated with impairment in attention, and some studies have shown deficits in learning and memory [1] It has been suggested that disturbed processing of new environmental information in PTSD is due to continuous background re-processing of traumatic events, resulting in modifications of neural circuits [2,3]. The resources required to maintain these autonomous loops may therefore not be available for general attention and memory function. The capacity of working memory has been shown to be directly related to the severity of intrusive memories [4], providing empirical support for this theory.

The hippocampus (HC), located within the ventral medial temporal lobe, is central to the encoding and reconstruction of episodic memories [5]. The hippocampus is part of a large extended network involving the learning of material available within working memory. Plasticity in the physical connections between the HC and the neocortex is crucial for integrating multi-modal sensory information and modifying memory dynamics over time [6]. In addition the HC has a significant role in executive processing systems [7,8]. The HC also contributes to regulation of the hypothalamic-pituitary-adrenocortical system, which is crucial in both acute and chronic responses to stress [9].

* Correspondence: cherrie.galletly@adelaide.edu.au
†Equal contributors
[1]Discipline of Psychiatry, School of Medicine, University of Adelaide, Adelaide, Australia
[2]Ramsay Health Care (SA) Mental Health Services, Adelaide, South Australia
Full list of author information is available at the end of the article

The hippocampus, located within the ventral medial temporal lobe, has long been known to be central to explicit long-term recognition memory. Olsen et al. (2012) [10], reviewed recent research showing that the hippocampus is also involved in short-delay recognition and perception. Olsen et al. (2012) [10] concluded that the hippocampus rapidly and continuously forms associations between disparate environmental inputs, including comparing current perceptual input with internal representations. The hippocampus is therefore part of a large extended network involving the recognition and learning of material available within working memory. This network incorporates multiple brain regions, including the prefrontal cortex. Failure in a significant part of this extended network will compromise the functioning of the network as a whole. The hippocampus also contributes to regulation of the hypothalamic-pituitary-adrenocortical system, which is crucial in both acute and chronic responses to stress [9].

Psychological trauma has been found to have damaging effects on the HC [11-14], and animal studies have shown that stress induces changes in hippocampal morphology and function [15,16]. In normal subjects the volume of the right hippocampus is larger than the left hippocampus [17,18]. Numerous studies have shown that hippocampal volume (HCV) is smaller in people with PTSD compared to controls [19-21]. A recent meta-analysis of 39 studies reporting hippocampal volume in PTSD [22] found that people with PTSD and trauma-exposed people without PTSD had smaller left, right and total hippocampal volumes than people never exposed to trauma. This suggests that trauma has an impact on the hippocampus bilaterally. In addition, people with PTSD had smaller volumes of the right, but not the left, hippocampus compared to people who had been exposed to trauma but did not have PTSD. The reduction in right hippocampal volume in PTSD reported by Woon et al. [22] is consistent with an MRI study showing reduced neuronal density in the right medial temporal cortex in people with PTSD, compared to trauma-exposed people without PTSD [23]. These findings suggest that the right hippocampus is differentially reduced in volume in people who develop PTSD.

Disruption of the normal pattern of hippocampal asymmetry has been found in people with schizophrenia [24,25] and in young people meeting criteria for an at-risk mental state for psychosis [26]. Studies in mild cognitive impairment and dementia suggest that there may be changes in hippocampal asymmetry as memory deteriorates [27]. Taken together, these findings demonstrate that abnormal hippocampal asymmetry is found in people subject to pathological processes that affect brain function and manifest as disorders affecting mental state and cognitive function.

Our participants consisted of male Vietnam combat veterans with and without PTSD, and their non-combat exposed monozygotic twins. The contributions of familial vulnerability and trauma exposure to biological abnormalities in this study population have been investigated by Pitman and colleagues [28]. Gilbertson et al. [29] demonstrated that total hippocampal volumes were about 10% smaller in men with severe PTSD, compared to men who did not have PTSD. Consistent with this finding, there was a significant correlation between total hippocampal volume and PTSD symptom severity in the PTSD group. However, these investigators also found that there was no difference in hippocampal volume between participants with severe PTSD, and their combat-unexposed identical twins, suggesting that smaller hippocampal volume might be a biological risk factor, rather than a consequence of trauma exposure and the pathophysiological processes associated with PTSD.

In the present study, we investigated the relationship between hippocampal asymmetry and the capacity to process information about the immediate environment in a sample of identical twins discordant for Vietnam combat exposure. We utilised the amplitude of the event related potential (ERP) P300 component as a measure of the controlled allocation of attentional resources to an anticipated stimulus. The P300 reflects processing of information about a significant stimulus, including context updating, context disclosure, event-categorisation and memory updating [30,31]. The P300 is most commonly elicited by asking participants to identify target tones in an auditory oddball task. The P300 has generators in a number of brain regions, including the temporo-parietal cortex, the cingulate cortex, the thalamus and the inferior and middle frontal cortex [32]. There are two separate generators in the hippocampus, located in the anterior subiculum and the posterior hippocampal body [33].

Numerous studies [34-39] including a meta-analysis by Karl et al. [40] have indicated that the amplitude of the P300 at midline electrodes in relation to trauma-neutral target tones is generally reduced in patients with PTSD. In a study involving the same monozygotic twin population as the present study, Metzger et al. [41] found smaller P300 amplitude in non-medicated, non-smoking twins with PTSD, compared to their combat-unexposed co-twins. In the full sample, there was no difference in reaction time or P300 amplitude between any of the groups (combat veterans with and without PTSD, and their combat-unexposed co-twins respectively). A recent study [42] found that P300 current source density was significantly reduced in people with PTSD in the inferior frontal gyrus, insula, and anterior cingulate.

The aim of the present study was to investigate the relationship between P300 amplitude and hippocampal asymmetry in the twin sample described above. As noted above, it has been established that hippocampal volume has a role in predisposing to PTSD, and there may be further changes related to both trauma exposure and to the development of PTSD. The amplitude of the P300 to trauma-neutral stimuli is generally reduced in PTSD, indicating that the information processing abnormalities characteristic of PTSD are reflected in changes in the P300. In addition, hippocampal generators contribute to P300 amplitude.

Given that both reduced P300 amplitude and greater hippocampal asymmetry (with relatively great volume reduction of the right hippocampus) are likely to reflect pathological changes related to PTSD, we hypothesised that there would be a negative correlation between P300 amplitude to trauma-neutral target tones and the magnitude of hippocampal asymmetry in people with combat-related PTSD (such that smaller P300 amplitude would be found in participants with greater hippocampal asymmetry).

Methods

Participants

Participant recruitment, informed consent, and data collection procedures have been described in previous publications [29,43]. Participants completed the 18-item Combat Severity Scale [44], employed in Vietnam Era Twin Registry research and previously validated against combat related medals, which yielded a measure of the severity of their combat exposure; and the Mississippi Scale for Combat-Related PTSD [45], a 35-item instrument for quantifying PTSD and related symptoms. The presence of PTSD in participants was determined by The Clinician-Administered PTSD Scale (CAPS): Current and Lifetime Diagnosis Version [46,47]. All subjects with PTSD included in this study had CAPS scores greater than 65 indicating severe PTSD. In addition, a Structured Clinical Interview for DSM-IV [48] was used to screen for the presence of Axis 1 mental disorders.

Sixty-four male subjects, comprising 32 monozygotic twin pairs where one twin had experienced combat in Vietnam while the other had not, participated in the present study. The mean age of the twin pairs in which the combat-exposed member had PTSD was 53.1 years (SD = 3.3) and the mean age of twin pairs in which the combat-exposed member did not have PTSD was 51.8 years (SD = 2.3) (F(1,76) = 3.8, p = .050). The mean years of education was 13.5 (SD = 2.6) for combat-exposed subjects with PTSD, 14.3 (SD = 2.8) for their non-combat exposed co-twins, 14.7 (SD = 2.4) for combat-exposed subjects without PTSD, and 14.7 (SD = 2.6) for their non-combat exposed co-twins (NS). Combat-exposed subjects with PTSD had higher combat severity scores (Mean = 7.9, SD = 1.9) than combat-exposed subjects without PTSD (Mean = 3.5, SD = 2.6) and this difference was significant (F(1,76) = 67.4, p < .001). The participants have been described in more detail by Gilbertson et al. [29].

Oddball paradigm

Participants were seated upright in a sound-attenuated room. E-A-RTONE (Aearo Company, Santa Barbara, California, USA) earphones were used to present tones binaurally. A five dB descending and ascending staircase method was used to gauge the hearing threshold for a 1,000 Hz test-tone in each participant. All participants completed an auditory target detection task involving 285 tone-stimulus presentations. Three distinctly pitched tones were used: a target (2,000 Hz), a common (1,000 Hz) and infrequent distractor (500 Hz). The entire sequence included 40 target, 40 distracter and 205 common tones with a random inter-stimulus interval varying between 1,950 and 2,050 ms. The task was to identify the high pitched tones as quickly and accurately as possible, by pressing a button with the dominant hand. The presentation sequence was pseudo-randomised to prevent the consecutive occurrence of two infrequent tones. Tones were generated by STIM software (Neuro Scan Inc, Herndon, Virginia, USA) and tone amplitude was verified using an Abbeon AB-85 sound meter (Abbeon, Indianapolis, Indiana, USA).

EEG measurement

EEG activity was recorded from parietal sites (Pz, P3, and P4) [49], using tin electrodes embedded in a nylon cap (Electro-Cap International, Eaton, UK). EEG was grounded from the forehead and referenced to linked ear lobes. Electrooculogram (EOG) activity was recorded at the outer canthus and infraorbitally to the left eye. Trials with excessive eye-movement artefact (EOG range ±85 μV) were excluded from the averaging process.

EEG impedances were approximately equal and kept below 5 k Ohms. Signals were amplified using Coulbourn High Gain Bioamplifiers (Coulbourn, Allentown, Pennsylvania, USA), band-pass filtered (0.1-150 Hz) and digitally sampled at 1,000 Hz, with a resultant signal sensitivity of .049 μV/bit. The EEG epoch extended from 100 ms pre-stimulus to 900 ms post-stimulus, and was averaged at each site according to stimulus type. It was digitally bandpass filtered between .1 and 14 Hz (12 dB/Oct). Peak measures for P300 were determined from each subject's averaged waveforms for each stimulus type, using a Neuro Scan interactive scoring program. P300 was defined as the most positive peak between 300–500 ms post-stimulus onset.

MRI

A 1.5 Tesla MRI scanner (General Electric Signa System, Milwaukee, Wisconsin, USA) was used to perform a whole-brain scan. Automated step algorithms were used to calculate whole brain volume. Subsequently, hippocampal volume was determined by a person blind to the individual's group characteristics, using a manual tracing procedure [50]. Although hippocampal volume was the focus of the present study, left and right amygdala volumes, and total brain volume, were also measured to provide control data [29]. The reliability of the volume measures was confirmed by a second 'blind' rater as previously described [29].

Statistical analysis

Participants were classified into four groups designated by PTSD diagnosis and combat exposure: (1) combat veterans with current PTSD and (2) their non-combat-exposed co-twins; (3) combat veterans without current PTSD and (4) their non-combat-exposed co-twins. An absolute magnitude HCV asymmetry (HCVA) measure was created for each participant according to the formula: | (right HCV − left HCV)/(right HCV + left HCV) |.

Hippocampal volumes and P300 amplitudes at all electrode sites were screened for outliers more than three standard deviations from the mean. Square root or logarithmic transformations were used as required to correct violations of homogeneity and the Greenhouse-Geisser epsilon correction was used for violations of sphericity. A one-way Analysis of Variance (ANOVA) was used to compare accuracy of target detection between groups, and a repeated measure ANOVA was used to compare P3 amplitude across the three electrodes.

One-way ANOVA was used to compare the total hippocampal volume, and the volumes of the left and right hippocampus, between the four groups. A one-way ANOVA was also performed to compare the asymmetry measures across groups. As EEG scalp potentials are not independent, a principal components analysis was performed across the P300 amplitude data to quantify the number of independent dimensions accounting for 95% of the data variance. A Pearson product–moment correlation coefficient was used to investigate the relationship between the magnitude of asymmetry and P300 amplitude at the three parietal sites (Pz, P3 and P4) in all four diagnosis and exposure groups separately. Finally, separate correlations were performed to evaluate whether significant correlations could be accounted for either 'right side greater than left' (R > L) or 'left side greater than right' (L > R) hippocampal volume changes. The Pearson product–moment correlation coefficient was also used to investigate the relationships between HC volume and HC asymmetry, total CAPS scores, and scores on individual CAPS dimensions.

Results

HC asymmetry

Hippocampal volumes are presented in Table 1. There was a significant main effect for diagnosis for right hippocampal volume ($F(1,66) = 9.63$, $p = .003$) and total hippocampal volume ($F(1,66) = 8.73$, $p = .004$). The mean volume of the left hippocampus was also smaller in the PTSD group but this difference did not reach significance ($F(1,66) = 3.35$, $p = 0.07$). We found that seven subjects with PTSD had a reversal of normal asymmetry with a larger left than right hippocampus, and five had a normal asymmetry with a larger right hippocampus. However, when one-way ANOVAs were performed to investigate between group differences in absolute asymmetry, no significant differences were found between any of the four diagnosis/exposure groups. There was no significant difference between groups in the volumes of the left or right amygdala or in total brain volume.

Correlations between HC asymmetry and P300 amplitude

There was no significant difference between the four groups in performance of the target detection task or in P3 amplitude. A principal components analysis of the P300 data across the three electrodes demonstrated that two components accounted for >97% of the total variance, so a Bonferroni corrected p value of $\leq .025$ was taken as significant.

We found positive correlations between hippocampal volume asymmetry and P300 amplitude in participants with PTSD at sites Pz ($r = .69$, $n = 12$, $p \leq .025$) and P3 ($r = .64$, $n = 12$, $p \leq .025$), with higher magnitudes of hippocampal volume asymmetry associated with larger P300 values (Table 2). Neither of the two non-combat exposed co-twin groups, nor the non-PTSD combat-exposed group demonstrated significant correlations between these two variables. The inclusion or exclusion of outliers did not significantly affect the results.

Comparing those with normal HC asymmetry and those with abnormal HC asymmetry, there was no significant difference in P300 amplitude at any electrode, and no group difference in asymmetry of amplitude at the individual electrodes.

HC asymmetry and symptom measures

In the PTSD group, there was no difference in CAPS scores between those with normal vs abnormal HC asymmetry. There was a negative correlation between total HC volume and re-experiencing symptoms (($r = -.56$, $n = 13$, $p \leq .043$), and between left HC volume and re-experiencing symptoms (($r = -.71$, $n = 13$, $p \leq .006$).

Table 1 Mean (SD) Hippocampal volumes in monozygotic twins with PTSD, their trauma-unexposed twins, and in trauma-exposed and trauma-unexposed monozygotic twins without PTSD

	PTSD (n = 24)		Non-PTSD (n = 46)	
	Trauma exposed (n = 12)	Trauma unexposed (n = 12)	Trauma exposed (n = 23)	Trauma unexposed (n = 23)
Right HC volume (ml)	3.32 (0.59)	3.26 (0.39)	3.76 (0.54)	3.61 (0.48)
Left HC volume (ml)	3.34 (0.46)	3.49 (0.57)	3.65 (0.50)	3.63 (0.45)
Total HC volume (ml)	6.66 (0.83)	6.75 (0.90)	7.41 (0.93)	7.25 (0.69)

Discussion

Based on the results of their meta-analysis, Woon et al. [22] conclude that there may be a differential sensitivity to the effects of trauma, with the right hippocampus being more vulnerable than the left hippocampus. It should be noted however that the subjects from the present study were included in this meta-analysis, contributing about 3% of the PTSD subjects and 11% of the non-PTSD subjects. Our findings were consistent with the findings of this meta-analysis in that the PTSD group had a reversal of normal asymmetry; on average the left hippocampus was slightly larger than the right hippocampus. However their co-twins, and the trauma-unexposed subjects, similarly had slightly larger mean left than right hippocampal volumes. These differences were small and none of these comparisons reached significance. Our results do not support previous findings that the right HC is more sensitive to the effects of trauma than the left HC [22]. In our data, the mean volume of the right HC in trauma-exposed co-twins, both with and without PTSD, was larger than the mean right HC volume of the non-trauma exposed co-twins.

Our results did not support the hypothesis that there would be a negative correlation between P300 amplitude and hippocampal asymmetry. We expected that greater asymmetry, taken to indicate greater pathology, would correlate with a smaller allocation of attentional resources to the working memory task. Instead, we found that although there was no significant asymmetry difference between the four groups, there were significant positive correlations between hippocampal asymmetry and P300 amplitude to target tones in participants with PTSD, at midline (Pz) and left (P3) parietal sites.

The lack of correlation between hippocampal asymmetry and P300 amplitude in the monozygotic co-twins of the PTSD participants, and in the other two groups (including participants with combat exposure) suggests that the correlations are associated with PTSD itself, rather than being genetically determined or related to combat exposure. It has previously been suggested [51] that the presence of such correlations in subjects with psychiatric illness, but not in normal subjects, may reflect disease-associated pathology. This conclusion might be strengthened if there was a correlation between P300 amplitude or the magnitude of hippocampal asymmetry, and symptom severity. Bae et al. (2011) [42] have demonstrated associations between P300 current source density (CSD) in regions in the frontal, parietal and temporal cortices, and various PTSD symptoms including re-experiencing and increased arousal (positively correlated with P300 CSD) and avoidance and numbing (negatively correlated with P300 CSD). Investigation of the associations between hippocampal volume asymmetry, P300 amplitude, and symptom severity, was beyond the scope of the present study. However, further research is required looking at the links between brain structure, brain function, and measures of disease severity. In addition, we did not have information about handedness, although co-twins would be expected to be matched for handedness. The proportion of people with mixed or right hemisphere dominance in the general population is small so it is unlikely that the presence of such subjects would have affected the overall conclusions.

Whilst most ERP studies of subjects with PTSD have found P300 amplitude reduction, an increase in P300

Table 2 Bivariate correlations: Hippocampal asymmetry v P300 amplitude

	Pearson correlation	Sig. (2-tailed)
	Asymmetry magnitude	
1: PTSD/Exposed Group N = 12		
Pz P300	0.69	0.01**
P3 P300	0.64	0.03**
P4 P300	0.33	0.29
2: Non-PTSD/Non-Exposed Group (co-twins of Group 1) N = 12		
Pz P300	−0.13	0.70
P3 P300	0.34	0.28
P4 P300	0.41	0.18
3: Non-PTSD/Exposed Group N = 23		
Pz P300	0.12	0.63
P3 P300	0.00	0.98
P4 P300	−0.10	0.67
4: Non-PTSD/Non-Exposed Group (co-twins of Group 3) N = 23		
Pz P300	−0.21	0.37
P3 P300	0.01	0.97
P4 P300	0.02	0.95

**$p \leq .025$

amplitude to trauma-neutral stimuli has been reported in a population of nurses who developed PTSD following exposure to wounded combatants in Vietnam [52]. P300 amplitude has been shown to be increased to trauma-relevant stimuli in people with PTSD, indicating an increase in allocation of attention resources towards elements in the environment that may be immediately threatening [43].

It is possible that the larger P300 in our subjects with greater hippocampal asymmetry might reflect a greater allocation of attention, in an effort to overcome difficulties performing the task. Amman et al. [53] report that in multiple sclerosis, a disease that is associated with neuropsychological impairment, patients showed stronger fMRI activation change in the right parahippocampal cortex and in the middle and medial frontal regions during the performance of simple tasks involving attention and working memory, compared to normal controls. There was a linear increase in activation with increasing task complexity, until the task load became excessive. Similarly, Fabiani and Friedman [54] found increased P300 amplitude was associated with poorer performance on the Wisconsin Card Sorting Test.

Our results might therefore indicate that the subjects with PTSD needed to give greater attention to the task in order to achieve normal results. Both auditory and visual stimulus processing in working memory are associated with hippocampal activation [55], and the hippocampus is involved in the processing mechanisms that determine attentional allocation and P300 amplitude [56]. A large asymmetry of hippocampal structures may necessitate a change in the neurophysiology of non-traumatic stimulus encoding, reflected in the enlarged P300 components.

Working memory capability has been shown to be decreased in those individuals who experience intrusive memories, indicating that a proportion of finite working memory resources is required during re-experiencing of traumatic memories, leaving fewer resources available for updating online content [57]. Nadel et al. [5] have shown that the hippocampus is intimately related to the processing and retrieval of spatial and episodic memories, long after they have been established, supporting the role of the hippocampus in the re-experiencing of intrusive memories. Our PTSD subjects may therefore have less capacity to process non-trauma related stimuli, because of the ongoing processing of intrusive trauma-related material. As noted above, this could result in a greater allocation of effort, to overcome these difficulties. Our results are consistent with the proposition that the increased allocation of attention was maximal in those with greatest hippocampal pathology, reflected in greater hippocampal asymmetry. In PTSD, the availability of hippocampal neurons required for encoding the stimuli in the oddball task may act as a rate-limiting step in non-trauma related information processing. In addition, the correlation between smaller HC volume and re-experiencing symptoms could suggest that HC damage is associated with an inability to process and eventually recover from traumatic memories.

Whilst this study focussed on hippocampal pathology, following on from previous research demonstrating hippocampal abnormalities associated both with trauma, and with PTSD, there is also evidence of volume reductions in other brain regions in PTSD. Araki et al. (2004) [58] investigated the relationship between lower P300 amplitude and anterior cingulate grey matter volume in people who developed PTSD as a result of the Tokyo subway sarin attack. The numbers were quite small (8 subjects with PTSD and 13 subjects without PTSD who had been exposed to the sarin attack). There was a trend-level correlation ($p = 0.077$) between P300 amplitude at Pz and left anterior cingulate grey matter volume. Further research into brain structure and function in PTSD should therefore extend to other brain regions beyond the hippocampus.

Conclusions

In conclusion, the hippocampus is clearly sensitive to the effects of trauma, with changes in both structure and function. Further, smaller hippocampal volume appears to be associated with vulnerability to developing PTSD when the person is exposed to trauma. Hippocampal volumes and hippocampal asymmetry have therefore been taken as reflecting both genetically determined vulnerability and trauma-related damage to the hippocampus. Our monozygotic twin sample enables us to control for genetic factors, so hippocampal volume differences are therefore related to trauma exposure, in some cases with the addition of the pathological processes associated with PTSD. The oddball P300 event related potential reflects the allocation of attentional resources during working memory processing, and hippocampal structures make a substantial contribution to P300 amplitude. Previous research has shown that the P300 is sensitive to the effects of PTSD [38]. Our results show that, in people with PTSD only, there is a positive correlation between hippocampal asymmetry and allocation of attentional resources. This could be because a proportion of finite processing capacity is being utilised by the constant re-experiencing of traumatic memories, leaving limited resources for non-trauma related cognitive tasks.

Competing interests

The authors declare that they have no competing interests.

Authors' contributions

TH undertook the analyses of hippocampal asymmetry and ERP measures. CG, CRC and AM were responsible for the planning and supervision of this work. LM, MV, CRC, AM, RP and SO undertook the initial ERP analyses. MG, RP and SO undertook the measurement of hippocampal volume. TH, CG, CRC and AM wrote the first drafts of the manuscript. All authors read and approved the final manuscript

Acknowledgements
The authors would like to acknowledge NHMRC program grant number 300403 held by R. Bryant, A.McFarlane, D. Silove, R. Clark and M. Creamer. We would also like to acknowledge the untimely death of our colleague and fellow contributor to this work, Linda Metzger.

Author details
[1]Discipline of Psychiatry, School of Medicine, University of Adelaide, Adelaide, Australia. [2]Ramsay Health Care (SA) Mental Health Services, Adelaide, South Australia. [3]Cognitive Neuroscience Laboratory and School of Psychology, Flinders University of South Australia, Adelaide, Australia. [4]Veterans Affairs Medical Centre Research Service, Manchester, New Hampshire, England. [5]Massachusetts General Hospital and Harvard Medical School, Boston, USA. [6]The Centre of Military and Veterans' Health, Adelaide, Australia. [7]Northern Mental Health, Adelaide Metro Mental Health Directorate, Adelaide, South Australia. [8]Harvard Medical School, Boston, USA.

References

1. Qureshi SU, Long ME, Bradshaw MR, Pyne JM, Magruder KM, Kimbrell T, Hudson TJ, Jawaid A, Schulz PE, Kunik ME: **Does PTSD impair cognition beyond the effect of trauma?** *J Neuropsychiatry Clin Neuroscience* 2011, **23**:16–28.
2. McFarlane AC, Yehuda R, Clark CR: **Biologic models of traumatic memories and post-traumatic stress disorder: The role of neural networks.** In *The Psychiatric Clinics of North America: Recent Advances in the Study of Biological Alterations in Post-Traumatic Stress Disorder 25*. Edited by Yehuda R. Philadelphia: WB Saunders; 2002:253–270.
3. Clark CR, McFarlane AC, Morris P, Weber DL, Sonkkilla C, Shaw M, Tochon-Danguy HJ, Egan GF: **Cerebral function in posttraumatic stress disorder during verbal working memory updating: A positron emission tomography study.** *Biol Psychiatry* 2003, **53**:474–481.
4. Brewin CR, Smart L: **Working memory capacity and suppression of intrusive thoughts.** *J Behav Ther Exp Psychiatry* 2005, **36**:61–68.
5. Nadel L, Samsonovich A, Ryan L, Moscovitch M: **Multiple trace theory of human memory: computational, neuroimaging, and neuropsychological results.** *Hippocampus* 2000, **10**:352–368.
6. Nadel L, Moscovitch M: **Hippocampal contributions to cortical plasticity.** *Neuropharmacology* 1998, **37**:431–439.
7. Corkin S: **Beware of frontal lobe deficits in hippocampal clothing.** *Trends Cogn Sci* 2001, **5**:321.323.
8. Antonova E, Sharma T, Morris R, Kumari V: **The relationship between brain structure and neurocognition in schizophrenia: a selective review.** *Schizophr Res* 2004, **70**:117–145.
9. Buchanan TW, Kern S, Allen JS, Tranel D, Kirschbaum C: **Circadian regulation of cortisol after hippocampal damage in humans.** *Biol Psychiatry* 2004, **56**:651–656.
10. Olsen RK, Moses SN, Riggs L, Ryan JD: **The hippocampus supports multiple cognitive processes through relational building and comparison.** *Front Hum Neurosci* 2012, **6**:146–159.
11. Bremner JD, Vythilingam M, Vermetten E, Southwick SM, McGlashan T, Nazeer A, Khan S, Vaccarino LV, Soufer R, Garg PK, Ng CK, Staib LH, Duncan JS, Charney DS: **MRI and PET study of deficits in hippocampal structure and function in women with childhood sexual abuse and posttraumatic stress disorder.** *Am J Psychiatry* 2003, **160**:924–932.
12. Shin LM, Shin PS, Heckers S, Krangel TS, Macklin ML, Orr SP, Lasko NB, Segal E, Makris N, Richert K, Levering J, Schacter DL, Alpert NM, Fischman AJ, Pitman RK, Rauch SL: **Hippocampal function in posttraumatic stress disorder.** *Hippocampus* 2004, **14**:292–300.
13. Geuze E, Vermetten E, Bremner JD: **MR-based in vivo hippocampal volumetrics: 2. Findings in neuropsychiatric disorders.** *Mol Psychiatry* 2005, **10**:160–184.
14. Nemeroff C, Bremner J, Foa E, Mayberg H, North C, Stein M: **Posttraumatic stress disorder: a state-of-the-science review.** *J Psychiatr Res* 2006, **40**:1–21.
15. Lee T, Jarome T, Li SJ, Kim JJ, Helmstetter FJ: **Chronic stress selectively reduces hippocampal volume in rats: a longitudinal magnetic resonance imaging study.** *Neuroreport* 2009, **25**:1554–1558.
16. Takei S, Morinobu S, Yamamoto S, Fuchikami M, Matsumoto T, Yamawaki S: **Enhanced hippocampal BDNF/TrkB signalling in response to fear conditioning in an animal model of posttraumatic stress disorder.** *J Psychiatr Res* 2011, **45**:460–468.
17. Pedraza O, Bowers D, Gilmore R: **Asymmetry of the hippocampus and amygdala in MRI volumetric measurements of normal adults.** *J Int Neuropsychol Soc* 2004, **10**:664–678.
18. Watson C, Andermann F, Gloor P, Jones-Gotman M, Peters T, Evans A, Olivier A, Melanson D, Leroux G: **Anatomic basis of amygdaloid and hippocampal volume measurement by magnetic resonance imaging.** *Neurology* 1992, **42**:1743–1750.
19. Villarreal G, King CY: **Brain imaging in posttraumatic stress disorder.** *Semin Clin Neuropsychiatry* 2001, **6**:131–145.
20. Kitayama N, Vaccarino V, Kutner M, Weiss P, Bremner J: **Magnetic resonance imaging (MRI) measurement of hippocampal volume in posttraumatic stress disorder: a meta analysis.** *J Affect Disord* 2005, **88**:79–86.
21. Smith M: **Bilateral hippocampal volume reduction in adults with post-traumatic stress disorder: a meta-analysis of structural MRI studies.** *Hippocampus* 2005, **15**:798–807.
22. Woon FL, Sood S, Hedges DW: **Hippocampal volume deficits associated with exposure to psychological trauma and posttraumatic stress disorder in adults: A meta-analysis.** *Prog Neuropsychopharmacol Biol Psychiatry* 2010, **34**:1181–1188.
23. Freeman TW, Cardwell D, Karson CN, Komoroski RA: **In vivo proton magnetic resonance spectroscopy of the medial temporal lobes of subjects with combat-related posttraumatic stress disorder.** *Magn Reson Med* 1998, **40**:66–71.
24. Kim SH, Lee JM, Kim HP, Jang DP, Shin YW, Ha TH, Kim JJ, Kim IY, Kwon JS, Kim SI: **Asymmetry analysis of deformable hippocampal model using the principal component in schizophrenia.** *Hum Brain Mapp* 2005, **25**:361–369.
25. Qiu A, Wang L, Younes L, Harms MP, Ratnanather JT, Miller MI, Csernansky JG: **Neuroanatomical asymmetry patterns in individuals with schizophrenia and their non-psychotic siblings.** *Neuroimage* 2009, **47**:1221–1229.
26. Buehlmann E, Berger GE, Aston J, Cschwandtner U, Pflueger MO, Borgwardt SJ, Radue E, Riecher-Rössler A: **Hippocampus abnormalities in at risk mental states for psychosis? A cross-sectional high resolution region of interest magnetic resonance imaging study.** *J Psychiatr Res* 2010, **44**:447–453.
27. Shi F, Liu B, Zhou Y, Yu C, Jiang T: **Hippocampal volume and asymmetry in mild cognitive impairment and Alzheimer's disease: Meta-analyses of MRI studies.** *Hippocampus* 2009, **19**:1055–1064.
28. Pitman RK, Gilbertson MW, Gurvits TV, May FS, Lasko NB, Metzger LJ, Shenton ME, Yehuda R, Orr SP: **Clarifying the origin of biological abnormalities in PTSD through the study of identical twins discordant for combat exposure.** *Ann N Y Acad Sci* 2006, **1071**:242–254.
29. Gilbertson MW, Shenton ME, Ciszewski A, Kasai K, Lasko NB, Orr SP, Pitman RK: **Smaller hippocampal volume predicts pathologic vulnerability to psychological trauma.** *Nat Neurosci* 2002, **5**:1242–1247.
30. Nulsen CE, Fox AM, Hammond GR: **Processes contributing to forward and backward: an ERP investigation.** *Neuroreport* 2010, **21**:298–302.
31. Polich J: **Updating P300: an integrative theory of P3a and P3b.** *Clin Neurophysiol* 2007, **118**:2128–2148.
32. Kiehl KA, Laurens KR, Duty TL, Forster BB, Liddle PF: **Neural sources involved in auditory target detection and novelty processing: an event related fMRI study.** *Psychophysiology* 2001, **38**:133–142.
33. Ludowig E, Bien CG, Elger CE, Rosburg T: **Two P300 generators in the hippocampal formation.** *Hippocampus* 2010, **20**:186–195.
34. Weber DL, Clark CR, McFarlane AC, Morris P, Egan G: **Abnormal stimulus evaluation in post-traumatic stress disorder.** *Biol Psychiatry* 1993, **34**:311–320.
35. Metzger LJ, Orr SP, Lasko NB, Pitman RK: **Auditory event-related potentials to tone stimuli in combat-related posttraumatic stress disorder.** *Biol Psychiatry* 1997, **42**:1006–1015.
36. Metzger LJ, Orr SP, Lasko NB, Berry NJ, Pitman RK: **Evidence for diminished P3 amplitudes in PTSD.** *Ann N Y Acad Sci* 1997, **821**:499–503.
37. Felmingham KL, Bryant RA, Kendall C, Gordon E: **Event-related potential dysfunction in posttraumatic stress disorder: the role of numbing.** *Psychiatr Res* 2002, **109**:171–179.

38. Galletly C, Clark CR, McFarlane AC, Weber DL: **Working memory in posttraumatic stress disorder – an event-related potential study.** *J Trauma Stress* 2001, **14:**295–309.
39. Veltmeyer M, Clark C, McFarlane A, Felmingham K, Bryant R, Gordon E: **Integrative assessment of brain and cognitive function in post-traumatic stress disorder.** *J Integr Neurosci* 2005, **4:**145–159.
40. Karl A, Malta L, Maercker A: **Meta-analytic review of event related potential studies in post-traumatic stress disorder.** *Biol Psychol* 2006, **71:**123–147.
41. Metzger LJ, Clark CR, McFarlane AC, Veltmeyer M, Lasko NB, Paige SR, Orr SP, Pitman RK: **Event-related potential components to auditory target stimuli in monozygotic twins discordant for combat exposure: Association with PTSD.** *Psychophysiology* 2009, **46:**172–178.
42. Bae KY, Kim DW, Im CH, Lee SH: **Source imaging of P300 auditory evoked potentials and clinical correlations in patients with posttraumatic stress disorder.** *Prog Neuropsychopharmacol Biol Psychiatry* 2011, **35:**1908–1917.
43. Orr SP, Metzger LJ, Lasko NB, Macklin ML, Hu FB, Shalev AY, Pitman RK: **Physiologic responses to sudden, loud tones in monozygotic twins discordant for combat exposure.** *Arch Gen Psychiatry* 2003, **60:**283–288.
44. Janes GR, Goldberg J, Eisen SA, True WR: **Reliability and validity of a combat exposure index for Vietnam era veterans.** *J Clin Psychol* 1991, **47:**80–86.
45. Keane TM, Caddell JM, Taylor KL: **Mississippi scale for combat-related posttraumatic stress disorder: three studies in reliability and validity.** *J Consult Clin Psychol* 1988, **56:**85–90.
46. Blake DD, Weathers FW, Nagy LM, Kaloupek DG, Gusman FD, Charney DS, Keane TM: **The development of a clinician-administered PTSD scale.** *J Trauma Stress* 1995, **8:**75–90.
47. Weathers FW, Keane TM, Davidson JR: **Clinician-administered PTSD scale: a review of the first ten years of research.** *Depress Anxiety* 2001, **13:**132–156.
48. First M, Spitzer R, Gibbon M, Williams J: *Structured Clinical Interview for Axis I DSM-IV Disorders.* Biometrics Research Department: New York; 1994.
49. Jasper HH: **The ten-twenty electrode system of the International Federation.** *Electroencephalogr Clin Neurophysiol* 1958, **10:**371–375.
50. Shenton ME, Kilkinis R, Jolesz FA, Pollak SD, LeMay M, Wible CG, Hokama H, Martin J, Metcalf D, Coleman M: **Abnormalities of the left temporal lobe and thought disorder in schizophrenia. A quantitative magnetic resonance imaging study.** *N Engl J Med* 1992, **327:**604–612.
51. Bertolino A, Breier A, Callicott JH, Adler C, Mattay VS, Shapiro M, Frank JA, Pickar D, Weinberger DR: **The relationship between dorsolateral prefrontal neuronal *N*-acetylaspartate and evoked release of striatal dopamine in schizophrenia.** *Neuropsychopharmacology* 2000, **22:**125–132.
52. Metzger LJ, Carson MA, Paulus LA, Lasko NB, Paige SR, Pitman RK, Orr SP: **Event-related potentials to auditory stimuli in female Vietnam nurse veterans with posttraumatic stress disorder.** *Psychophysiology* 2002, **39:**49–63.
53. Amann M, Dössegger LS, Penner IK, Hirsch JG, Raselli C, Calabrese P, Weier K, Radü EW, Kappos L, Gass A: **Altered functional adaptation to attention and working memory tasks with increasing complexity in relapsing-remitting multiple sclerosis patients.** *Hum Brain Mapp*, in press.
54. Fabiani M, Friedman D: **Changes in brain activity patterns in aging: the novelty oddball.** *Psychophysiology* 1995, **32:**579–594.
55. Crottaz-Herbette S, Lau KM, Glover GH, Menon V: **Hippocampal involvement in detection of deviant auditory and visual stimuli.** *Hippocampus* 2005, **15:**132–139.
56. Kato T, Erhard P, Takayama Y, Strupp J, Le TH, Ogawa S, Ugurbil K: **Human hippocampal long-term sustained response during word memory processing.** *Neuroreport* 1998, **9:**1041–1047.
57. Brewin CR, Beaton A: **Thought suppression, intelligence, and working memory capacity.** *Behav Res Ther* 2002, **40:**923–930.
58. Araki T, Kasai K, Yamasue H, Kato N, Kudo N, Ohtani T, Nakagome, Kirihara K, Yamada H, Abe O, Iwanami A: **Association between lower P30 amplitude and smaller anterior cingulate cortex volume in patients with posttraumatic stress disorder: a study of victims of Tokyo subway sarin attack.** *Neuroimage* 2005, **25:**43–50.

9

Daily stress reactivity and serotonin transporter gene (5-HTTLPR) variation: internalizing responses to everyday stress as a possible transdiagnostic phenotype

Christopher C Conway[1*], George M Slavich[2,3] and Constance Hammen[1,3]

Abstract

Background: Recent studies examining the interaction between the 5-HTTLPR locus in the serotonin transporter gene and life stress in predicting depression have yielded equivocal results, leading some researchers to question whether 5-HTTLPR variation indeed regulates depressive responses to stress. Two possible sources of inconsistent data in this literature are imprecise stress assessment methodologies and a restricted focus on depression phenotypes as the outcome of interest, as opposed to transdiagnostic emotional symptoms such as internalizing and externalizing dimensions. The present study aimed to address these critical limitations in prior research by examining how 5-HTTLPR acts in concert with idiographically assessed daily life stress to predict transdiagnostic emotional outcomes.

Results: One hundred and four healthy young adults genotyped for 5-HTTLPR reported on their life stress exposure and internalizing and externalizing experiences for 14 consecutive days. As hypothesized, daily stress levels were associated with severity of internalizing symptoms, but only for 5-HTTLPR S allele carriers. Additional analyses revealed that these interactive effects of 5-HTTLPR and daily life stress on internalizing symptoms extended to both the distress and fear subdomains of internalizing symptoms.

Conclusions: Considered together, these results support the validity of the 5-HTTLPR stress sensitivity hypothesis and suggest for the first time that variation at 5-HTTLPR moderates the effects of daily life stress on broadband symptom profiles.

Keywords: Anxiety, Depression, Daily diary, Gene-environment interaction, Intermediate phenotype, Life events, RDoC, Serotonin transporter gene, Young adulthood

Background

The most widely studied topic in gene-environment interaction (G × E) research over the past decade has been the interplay between a polymorphism in the promoter region of the serotonin transporter gene and life stress in predicting risk for depression. A number of studies have either partly or fully replicated the finding that short (S) allele carriers at 5-HTTLPR are more susceptible to depression in the face of stress than long (L) allele homozygotes [1]. Yet, null results have also been reported; indeed, one recent meta-analysis did not find convincing evidence for the 5-HTTLPR G × E phenomenon [2].

The manner in which life stress is assessed has likely contributed to inconsistent findings across G × E studies. One meta-analytic review that evaluated methodological influences on the magnitude of 5-HTTLPR G × E concluded that the 5-HTTLPR genotype moderates the effects of stress on depression, but only when investigator-based procedures (for example, interview measures, inspection of objective records) are used for stress assessment [3]. Additionally, when exposed to standardized emotional or stressful cues in laboratory settings, S allele carriers consistently exhibit potentiated limbic system activation, cortisol responses, and attentional biases to threat-related

* Correspondence: conwayc@ucla.edu
[1]Department of Psychology, University of California, Los Angeles, Box 951563, Los Angeles, CA 90095-1563, USA
Full list of author information is available at the end of the article

stimuli compared to L allele homozygotes [4-6]. Together, these observations suggest that the methods researchers use to assess properties of the environment play a critical role in tests of the 5-HTTLPR stress sensitivity hypothesis [7].

Another pressing and unanswered question is whether 5-HTTLPR is relevant just for depression or, alternatively, for a broader range of stress-linked psychopathology. Whereas initial evidence suggested that 5-HTTLPR genotype, in concert with stress, does not influence anxiety [8], other studies have since implicated the S allele in risk for diverse anxiety and depressive symptoms [7]. Further, the S allele's association with basic neural, endocrine, and cognitive phenotypes that are linked to a broad array of disorders provides indirect evidence for its involvement in multiple psychopathologies [9].

The goal of the present study was to advance this research by examining the relation of 5-HTTLPR variation to a novel social-environmental context: everyday stressful life events. Using a daily diary methodology, we were able to make an idiographic assessment of fluctuations in stress exposure by determining a person's average stress levels with repeated measurements; evaluate whether the putative stress-sensitizing effects of 5-HTTLPR extend to day-to-day emotional symptoms; and substantially reduce the interval between stress occurrence and report of symptomatic reactions. Based on prior research, we hypothesized that 5-HTTLPR S allele carriers would exhibit stronger internalizing responses to daily life stress than L allele homozygotes.

We also investigated the specificity of 5-HTTLPR-mediated individual differences in stress reactivity by assessing transdiagnostic emotional phenotypes. Drawing on latent variable research on the meta-structure of mental disorders [10], we collected daily reports of fear (underlying panic and the phobias), distress (unipolar depression and generalized anxiety), and externalizing (disinhibited behavior and substance misuse) phenotypes. These transdiagnostic dimensions are theorized to capture homogeneous clinical traits that are more amenable to genetic analysis than categorical psychiatric diagnoses [11]. Given existing evidence of an association between the S allele and heightened emotional reactivity, we hypothesized that S allele carriers would exhibit stronger fear, distress, and externalizing reactions to everyday stressors than L allele homozygotes.

Methods

Participants

Participants were 104 undergraduate students enrolled in an introductory psychology course. The sample included 76 women (73.1%) and 28 men (26.9%), with a mean age of 19.64 years (*standard deviation* = 4.61). Forty-seven participants (45.2%) self-identified as Caucasian, 45 (43.3%) as Latino/a, 5 (4.8%) as biracial, 3 (2.9%) as Asian, 1 (1.0%) as Native American, and 3 (3.0%) as 'other.'

Procedures

At a baseline interview, participants completed the Young Adult Self Report questionnaire (YASR; [12]) to assess trait levels of internalizing and externalizing symptoms (see below). They also supplied a saliva sample for genotyping procedures. Participants were then provided instructions for the daily online diary. Diary data were collected on the day of the baseline assessment and the following 13 consecutive days during the middle of the fall and winter academic quarters. The 14-day study period was selected so that the number of weekdays (versus weekend days) would be constant across all participants. Participants were asked to complete the diary as late at night as was convenient for them (from 8pm to 2am); diaries could only be submitted if all questionnaire items were completed. Study procedures were approved by the institutional review board of the University of California, Los Angeles, and all participants provided written informed consent prior to participating in the study.

Measures

Daily stressful life events

Daily stressors were assessed with a 16-item inventory composed of items adapted from instruments designed to elicit self-reports of stressful life events relevant to student life (for example, [13,14]). These items queried daily stressors occurring in several life domains, including interpersonal, achievement, financial and health events. Example events included 'A friendship ended,' 'Failed to achieve an important school-related goal,' 'Did not have enough money to do something or buy something,' and 'Was sick or had a medical issue' (see Appendix for complete list). Prior research has shown that life events from this inventory are associated with internalizing symptoms both on a daily basis and over several months [14,15]. Participants indicated whether each event occurred over the course of the current day and, if so, how many times it occurred. The total count of stressors was used in analyses to represent daily stress exposure.

Baseline internalizing and externalizing symptoms

The YASR consists of 119 items that assess internalizing and externalizing symptoms, as well as other problem behavior dimensions, including somatic complaints and attention problems. Achenbach [12] provided data to support the internal consistency, test-retest reliability, and criterion validity of the YASR internalizing and externalizing scales. In the present sample, Cronbach's alpha values for the internalizing and externalizing scales were 0.87 and 0.72, respectively.

Daily symptoms

Fear, distress, and externalizing symptoms have not been assessed in previous daily process research. Assessment measures for the present study were created by selecting items from existing instruments that have been constructed to distinguish between these symptom domains in between-subjects research. For example, items that had the largest factor loadings on the YASR externalizing subscale, and that were also relevant to college students, were selected to index daily externalizing behavior. Internalizing items were selected from the Inventory of Depression and Anxiety Symptoms [16], which includes scales that are psychometrically derived to distinguish the fear and distress domains. Inventory of Depression and Anxiety Symptoms items that were judged to be most applicable to the college student population were chosen for inclusion on the daily fear and distress scales.

Daily internalizing symptoms

Five items were chosen to represent the fear domain (for example, 'I felt self-conscious knowing that others were watching me') and six items were chosen to represent the distress domain (for example, 'I felt inadequate') (see Appendix for complete list). Participants were prompted to respond on a five-point Likert-type scale according to 'How much you have felt or experienced things this way today?' Responses to distress and fear symptom items were summed to represent the total level of daily internalizing symptoms.

Daily externalizing symptoms

The same prompt and response format were used to assess daily severity of externalizing symptoms. Nine items (for example, 'I was mean to others') were adapted from the YASR to assess the externalizing domain (see Appendix for complete list).

Genotyping

Saliva samples were collected under researcher observation for DNA analyses using Oragene saliva collection kits (DNA Genotek, Inc, Ottawa, ON, Canada). Genotyping was performed at the University of California, Los Angeles, Genotyping and Sequencing Core. Polymerase chain reaction (PCR) primers were labeled with fluorescent dye, and PCR was performed on Applied Biosystems dual block PCR thermal cyclers (Foster City, CA, USA). Microsatellite genotypes were run on an Applied Biosystems 3730 capillary DNA sequencer and analyzed using the Applied Biosystems GeneMapper software version 4.0. The 5-HTTLPR polymorphism was assayed on an Applied Biosystems GeneMapper 7900HT Fast Real-Time PCR System and analyzed using the Sequence Detection Systems software version 2.3. Each run included two positive control samples (individual 2 in CEPH family 1347; Coriell Institute). Genotype frequencies were LL = 34, SL = 42, SS = 28, and they were in Hardy-Weinberg equilibrium for the entire sample, as well as for Caucasian and Latino subgroups ($\chi^2(2)$ <2, P >0.10. In accord with prior research [17], the rs25531 locus was assayed using the protocol described by Wray *et al.* [18] and eight L_G alleles were reclassified as S alleles.

Data analyses

Data analyses were conducted within a hierarchical linear modeling (HLM) framework. HLM is ideal for diary studies because observations at multiple time-points are nested within individuals, resulting in dependencies among residuals. G × E hypotheses were investigated using the following HLM functions:

$$\text{INT}_t = \pi_0 + \pi_1(\text{STRESS}_t) + \pi_2(\text{INT}_{t-1}) + e_t$$

$$\pi_{0j} = \beta_{00} + \beta_{01}(\text{GENDER}_j) + \beta_{02}(\text{GENO1}_j) + \beta_{03}(\text{GENO2}_j) + u_{0j}$$

$$\pi_{1j} = \beta_{10} + \beta_{11}(\text{GENDER}_j) + \beta_{12}(\text{GENO1}_j) + \beta_{13}(\text{GENO2}_j) + u_{1j}$$

$$\pi_{2j} = \beta_{20} + u_{2j}$$

where INT_t represents internalizing symptoms on Day t, INT_{t-1} represents internalizing symptoms on Day t-1, STRESS_t represents the count of stressors on Day t, GENO1_j represents the contrast between SS and LL genotypes, and GENO2_j represents the contrast between SL and LL genotypes. Gender was controlled by including it as a between-subjects predictor of the overall intercept (π_0) on Level 2.

All Level 1 variables were person-mean centered, such that STRESS_t indicates the difference between the number of stressors occurring on Day t for a given participant and this participant's mean number of daily stressors across all 14 days. Gender and the genotype contrasts were entered uncentered into Level 2 equations.

The cross-level interactions between the 5-HTTLPR contrasts and daily stress were of primary interest in G × E analyses. A likelihood ratio test was performed to evaluate the significance of the simultaneous addition of genotype contrasts into the π_1 equation. In a secondary analysis, product terms composed of genotype and gender, and genotype and ethnicity, were added at Level 2 to examine the consistency of G × E effects across these demographic factors.

We expected to observe main effects of daily life stress on same-day symptoms, but not next-day symptoms, given that lagged effects are rarely detected in daily process studies involving non-clinical populations [19]. Nevertheless, we tested for lagged main effects and G × E on an exploratory basis. It is possible that genetically vulnerable individuals experience a more enduring emotional impact of stressful events, although this was not observed in one previous study of 5-HTTLPR stress reactivity and anxious mood [15]. Along these lines, we used effect size estimates from a prior study of 5-HTTLPR and daily stress reactivity (Table 2 in [15]) to compute *post hoc* power. Following Hox's [20] equations, and setting alpha to the conventional 0.05 level, we found the present study to have *post hoc* power of 0.74, suggesting sufficient statistical power to detect significant results if they exist.

Data were checked preliminarily for outliers and non-normality. Four participants were considered as possible univariate outliers on the internalizing dimension and four on the externalizing dimension (one case was a possible outlier on both), defined as symptom scores that were greater than two standard deviations from the mean (all were above the mean) across all 14 measurements. The pattern and significance of results were unchanged when these cases were removed, and analyses presented below therefore include all cases. Given positive skew across all four outcome variables, significance testing was based on robust standard errors (also known as Huber/White estimators), which do not depend on the normality of errors assumption [20].

Results

Descriptive statistics

The average scores on the YASR internalizing and externalizing scales at baseline were 15.76 (*standard deviation* = 7.56) and 7.90 (*standard deviation* = 4.62), respectively. According to Achenbach's [12] guidelines, 18 participants (17.3%) were in the borderline clinical or clinical range for internalizing, and 4 participants (3.8%) were in the borderline clinical or clinical range for externalizing. The Pearson correlation between internalizing and externalizing scales was 0.29 ($P<0.01$).

Descriptive statistics for the daily variables are presented in Table 1. Averaged across 14 days, all daily symptom scales demonstrated high levels of internal consistency, with Cronbach's alpha values of 0.91 for internalizing, 0.91 for fear, 0.93 for distress and 0.78 for externalizing. Participants reported approximately 1.27 stressors per day, with school-related events (not involving grade point average) and medical problems occurring most frequently (approximately once every three days), and lost or stolen property events occurring least frequently (approximately once every 100 days). An average of 11.63 out of 14 diaries (83.1%) were completed on time (that is, before 2am the day after they were mailed), a rate comparable to that of previous studies in college student samples [21]. Compliance was not related to genotype or the YASR scales ($P>0.10$), and the pattern and significance of results were unaltered when participants who missed more than three surveys were omitted. Therefore, all results presented below reflect analyses conducted for the full sample.

Table 1 Descriptive statistics for daily variables

Variable	Mean	Standard deviation	Minimum	Maximum
Daily life stressors	1.27	1.07	0.00	5.57
Internalizing symptoms	17.47	5.14	11.00	38.21
Fear symptoms	7.06	2.07	5.00	16.21
Distress symptoms	10.42	3.40	6.00	22.00
Externalizing symptoms	9.98	1.19	9.00	17.79

Note. The scale for each symptom ranged from 1 to 5, with 11 items indexing internalizing symptoms and 9 items indexing externalizing symptoms. The scale for each stressor ranged from 0 to 3. Descriptive statistics were computed by first calculating the within-person value for each participant across time-points and then averaging across participants.

Stress, 5-HTTLPR, and same-day internalizing and externalizing symptoms

We first examined the direct effects of daily life stress on reports of same-day internalizing and externalizing symptoms. Stress on Day *t* was strongly associated with elevations in internalizing symptoms ($b=1.35$, standard error (SE) = 0.19, $P<0.001$) and externalizing symptoms ($b=0.20$, $SE=0.04$, $P<0.001$) on Day *t*. As can be seen in Table 2, genotype and gender did not predict daily symptom levels, with the exception of women reporting significantly higher levels of daily distress symptoms. Prior to investigating G × E effects, we examined the association between genotype and daily stress to rule out the possibility of gene-environment correlation. This analysis demonstrated that 5-HTTLPR genotype was unrelated to daily stress exposure ($b=-0.02$, $SE=0.24$, $P=0.95$), thus ruling out gene-environment correlation.

A significant interaction between daily stress and 5-HTTLPR was detected in the prediction of internalizing symptoms ($\chi^2(2)=7.77$, $P<0.05$). Daily life stress was more strongly related to internalizing symptoms for individuals with the SS and SL genotypes compared to L homozygotes (see genotype contrasts in Table 2). Simple slopes computed for each genotype group revealed that, as hypothesized, the stress-internalizing association was significant for individuals with both the SS genotype ($b=1.63$, $SE=0.34$, $P<0.001$) and SL genotype ($b=1.52$, $SE=0.26$, $P<0.001$), but not for L homozygotes ($b=0.44$, $SE=0.36$, $P=0.22$). Figure 1 depicts the form of the 5-HTTLPR G × E interaction effect for internalizing symptoms. Regarding the interaction of genotype and daily life stress in predicting daily externalizing symptoms, the omnibus significance test of the two genotype contrasts was not indicative of a G × E effect ($\chi^2(2)=2.89$, $P=0.23$), although the comparison between SS and LL group slopes was marginally significant (see Table 2).

Table 2 Hierarchical linear models of 5-HTTLPR × daily life stress interactions: genotype coding

	Internalizing symptoms$_t$			Fear symptoms$_t$			Distress symptoms$_t$			Externalizing symptoms$_t$		
Predictors	*b*	*SE*	*P*	*b*	*SE*	*P*	*b*	*SE*	*P*	*b*	*SE*	*P*
For overall intercept, π_0												
Intercept, β_{00}	16.71	0.86	<0.001	6.63	0.32	<0.001	10.08	0.57	<0.001	10.05	0.39	<0.001
Gender, β_{01}	−1.96	1.11	0.081	−0.35	0.45	0.445	−1.61	0.69	0.021	−0.22	0.23	0.356
SS versus LL, β_{03}	1.46	1.17	0.216	0.75	0.47	0.110	0.71	0.76	0.356	−0.03	0.38	0.921
SL versus LL, β_{04}	1.49	1.11	0.184	0.52	0.43	0.232	0.96	0.73	0.190	0.00	0.39	0.994
For stress$_t$ slope, π_1												
Intercept, β_{10}	0.63	0.23	0.008	0.10	0.08	0.192	0.54	0.17	0.002	0.05	0.08	0.487
Gender, β_{11}	−0.85	0.30	0.006	−0.26	0.11	0.026	−0.58	0.22	0.010	0.09	0.13	0.464
SS versus LL, β_{12}	1.24	0.46	0.008	0.50	0.16	0.002	0.71	0.34	0.040	0.18	0.10	0.083
SL versus LL, β_{13}	1.18	0.36	0.002	0.36	0.13	0.007	0.77	0.28	0.007	0.16	0.10	0.139
For symptom$_{t-1}$ slope, π_2												
Intercept, β_{20}	0.10	0.03	0.003	0.07	0.04	0.062	0.14	0.03	<0.001	0.01	0.05	0.753

Note. For gender, male = 1, female = 0. LL, 5-HTTLPR long allele homozygosity; SL, 5-HTTLPR heterozygosity; SE, standard error; SS, 5-HTTLPR short allele homozygosity.

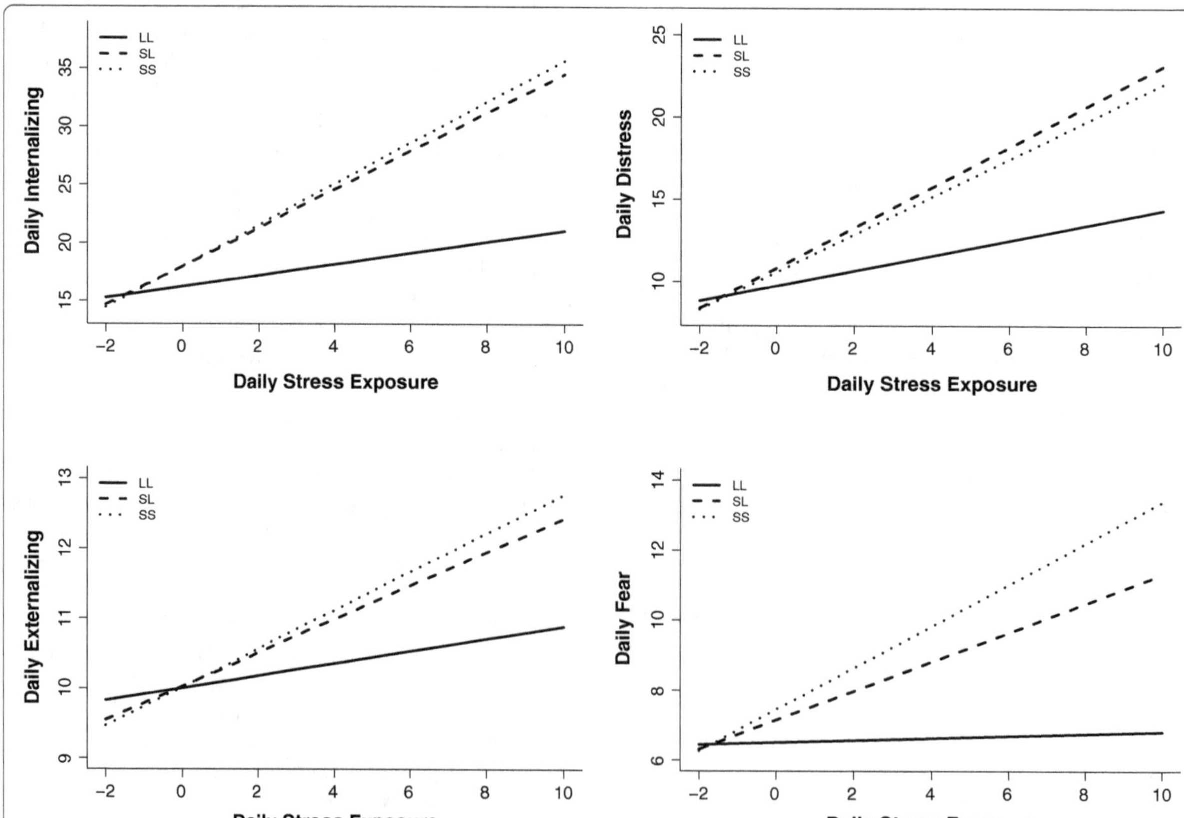

Figure 1 Within-person associations between daily life stress exposure and transdiagnostic symptoms as a function of 5-HTTLPR genotype. On the *x*-axis, the count of daily stressors is person-centered, such that 0 represents an average amount of daily stress for a given individual. LL, 5-HTTLPR long allele homozygosity; SL, 5-HTTLPR heterozygosity; SS, 5-HTTLPR short allele homozygosity.

Given the close correspondence between SS and SL groups in terms of internalizing and externalizing reactivity to daily stressors (see Figure 1), follow-up analyses were conducted collapsing across SS and SL genotypes to compare the stress-symptom association for S carriers versus L homozygotes. As seen in Table 3, a significant G × E effect was observed for internalizing symptoms, whereby S allele carriers demonstrated greater internalizing reactivity to daily life stress than L homozygotes. Simple effects analyses revealed that daily exposure to stress was associated with higher levels of internalizing symptoms for S carriers ($b = 1.57$, $SE = 0.21$, $P < 0.001$) but not L homozygotes ($b = 0.44$, $SE = 0.36$, $P = 0.22$).

Analyses also revealed some evidence that daily life stress exposure interacted with genotype to predict externalizing symptoms when the SS and SL genotype groups were combined ($b = 0.16$, $SE = 0.09$, $P = 0.08$). Simple effects analyses revealed that the magnitude of the daily stress-externalizing symptoms association for S carriers ($b = 0.23$, $SE = 0.05$, $P < 0.001$) was approximately three times greater than the corresponding association for L homozygotes ($b = 0.08$, $SE = 0.09$, $P = 0.35$).

Consistent with the large literature showing that women are at significantly higher risk for depression relative to men, and that they also exhibit greater internalizing responses to stressful life events [22], women in the present study tended to report greater increases in internalizing symptoms, but not externalizing symptoms, in response to daily life stress (Table 2). However, gender did not moderate the strength of G × E effects for either internalizing or externalizing symptoms ($t < 1.00$, $P > 0.10$). Additionally, the strength of the G × E effects did not vary across Caucasian versus Latino ethnic groups (which collectively made up approximately 93% of our sample) for either the internalizing ($b = -0.08$, $SE = 0.57$, $P = 0.88$) or externalizing ($b = -0.02$, $SE = 0.19$, $P = 0.93$) dimensions. Likewise, ethnicity was not related to 5-HTTLPR genotype, stress exposure or any daily symptom outcome ($P > 0.10$).

Stress, 5-HTTLPR and fear and distress symptoms

We observed strong effects of stress on both same-day distress symptoms ($b = 0.98$, $SE = 0.15$, $P < 0.001$) and fear symptoms ($b = 0.35$, $SE = 0.06$, $P < 0.001$). As hypothesized, and paralleling results found for the broader internalizing domain, we also found that daily stressors interacted with 5-HTTLPR genotype to predict both same-day fear symptoms ($\chi^2(2) = 7.13$, $P < 0.05$) and same-day distress symptoms ($\chi^2(2) = 4.90$, $P = 0.08$), with SS and SL groups showing stronger stress-symptom associations than L homozygotes (Table 2). These effects of daily stressors and 5-HTTLPR on fear and distress symptoms were stronger when the SS and SL genotypes were grouped and compared to L homozygotes (that is, fear, $P < 0.001$; distress, $P < 0.01$; Table 3).

Stress, 5-HTTLPR and next-day internalizing and externalizing symptoms

Consistent with prior research, HLM analyses indicated that stress was not associated with next-day reports of internalizing symptoms ($b = -0.08$, $SE = 0.08$, $P = 0.32$) or externalizing symptoms ($b = -0.01$, $SE = 0.03$, $P = 0.71$). In addition, 5-HTTLPR genotype did not moderate the lagged stress-symptom association for internalizing symptoms ($\chi^2(2) = 0.76$, $P = 0.68$) or externalizing symptoms ($\chi^2(2) = 2.69$, $P = 0.26$).

Discussion

The validity of the 5-HTTLPR stress sensitivity hypothesis has been challenged by inconsistent results in the literature on life stress, the 5-HTTLPR genotype, and depression. To address this issue, we examined stress exposure and emotional reactivity in 'high resolution' using

Table 3 Hierarchical linear models of 5-HTTLPR × daily life stress interactions: allele coding

	Internalizing symptoms$_t$			Fear symptoms$_t$			Distress symptoms$_t$			Externalizing symptoms$_t$		
Predictors	b	SE	P	b	SE	P	b	SE	P	b	SE	P
For overall intercept, π_0												
Intercept, β_{00}	16.71	0.86	<0.001	6.62	0.31	<0.001	10.09	0.57	<0.001	10.05	0.39	<0.001
Gender, β_{01}	−1.96	1.11	0.079	−0.32	0.44	0.470	−1.63	0.70	0.020	−0.22	0.23	0.345
5-HTTLPR, β_{03}	1.48	0.97	0.132	0.61	0.37	0.109	0.87	0.64	0.178	−0.01	0.37	0.967
For stress$_t$ slope, π_1												
Intercept, β_{10}	0.62	0.23	0.008	0.10	0.08	0.194	0.54	0.17	0.002	0.05	0.08	0.485
Gender, β_{11}	−0.84	0.30	0.006	−0.26	0.12	0.029	−0.59	0.22	0.009	0.09	0.12	0.466
5-HTTLPR, β_{12}	1.20	0.32	<0.001	0.41	0.12	<0.001	0.75	0.24	0.003	0.16	0.09	0.079
For symptom$_{t-1}$ slope, π_2												
Intercept, β_{20}	0.10	0.03	0.003	0.07	0.04	0.060	0.14	0.03	<0.001	0.01	0.05	0.757

Note. For gender, male = 1, female = 0. 5-HTTLPR represents the contrast between S allele carriers and L allele homozygotes, with S allele carriers coded as 1 and LL as 0. SE, standard error.

a daily diary methodology. We also evaluated the specificity of 5-HTTLPR G × E effects to depressive symptoms with the use of a novel measure of transdiagnostic emotional phenotypes. Consistent with hypotheses and prior research, we found that daily stress levels were associated with severity of internalizing symptoms, but only for 5-HTTLPR S allele carriers. Going beyond existing work on this topic, however, we also found that this interaction effect extended to both the fear and distress subdomains of internalizing symptoms, suggesting that 5-HTTLPR G × E effects are not unique to depression. Yet, there was only weak support for the hypothesis that stress-induced externalizing behaviors are more common among S allele carriers. These data are in accord with the general hypothesis that variation at 5-HTTLPR plays a role in regulating emotional reactivity to daily life stress.

In line with new dimensional approaches to psychiatric classification, such as the National Institute of Mental Health Research Domain Criteria initiative [23], these results suggest that genetic variation at 5-HTTLPR may influence transdiagnostic stress reactivity mechanisms that contribute to the onset or development of a variety of anxiety and depressive disorders, not just unipolar depression (cross-reference [1,8]). One implication of this transdiagnostic formulation is that studies on 5-HTTLPR could be more efficiently designed by selecting outcomes that are theorized to be common to several categorically defined internalizing syndromes. For instance, in longitudinal G × E studies, 5-HTTLPR may be more closely linked to intermediate phenotypes, such as a latent distress trait, than to the unipolar depression syndrome. We speculate that such an approach may be appropriate for other candidate genes in psychopathology research as well [24].

The present findings also suggest that internalizing risk associated with the S allele can be detected by observing emotional responses to everyday stressors. Through the use of genetically informed daily process studies, it may be possible - even in nonclinical populations - to identify genotypes that confer risk for clinically significant emotional disorders that are provoked by negative life events. Fear and distress responses to daily negative life events may therefore represent useful intermediate phenotypes on the causal pathway from genes to full-blown internalizing disorder.

The present results are consistent with other data showing that the interactive effects of 5-HTTLPR and stress on emotional outcomes are most robust when sophisticated stress assessment methods are used [25]. Indeed, a major strength of the present study was that stress was measured daily, on a within-person basis. Put another way, the degree of stress exposure on a given day was compared to each participant's average level of stress over the 14-day study period and not to the average level of stress exposure in the full sample. As a result, participants served as their own control when determining the magnitude of day-to-day fluctuations in stress reporting, thereby limiting the potentially confounding effects of state affect or personality traits on self-reported stress exposure.

The relatively modest sample size of the present study ($n = 104$) must be taken into account when evaluating the present results. We reasoned that a test of our hypotheses based on a smaller sample was justified because our theory was based on an existing nomological net of relations between 5-HTTLPR and stress reactivity phenotypes [7]. In other words, the established construct validity of the phenomenon under study was assumed to reduce the danger of false positive findings [26]. Nevertheless, conclusions regarding genetic reactivity to everyday stressors should be considered tentative until large-scale replication projects are available.

Several other limitations should also be noted. First, daily stress exposure, emotions and behaviors were reported at the same time by the same informant; therefore, it was not possible to confirm that the occurrence of stressors preceded the development of symptoms each day. Second, given that fear, distress and externalizing phenotypes have not been investigated previously in within-subjects research, the questionnaires in this study were novel and would benefit from validation in future work. Related, the validity of daily stress assessments for determining genetic differences in stress reactivity has yet to be established in the G × E literature. Future studies should examine whether the same genotype confers risk to both short- and long-term stress reactions in the same sample. Third, our analyses were focused on transitory changes in mood and behavior as a potential intermediate phenotype for emotional disorders; additional research is needed to determine the social and neurobiological processes involved in the activation of more severe and sustained symptomatology. Fourth, we did not correct for multiple testing given strong *a priori* hypotheses and limited sample size, and this analytic decision should be kept in mind when interpreting significance values. Fifth, the prevalence of individual stressor types was relatively low and did not permit analyses to determine whether the magnitude of G × E varied across types of stress. Determining the features of life stress that are most relevant to 5-HTTLPR G × E may ultimately lead to more effective prevention and intervention efforts. Finally, although the 5-HTTLPR G × E effects in our sample were equivalent across the two main ethnic groups, we did not use genetic controls for ethnic heterogeneity (see [27] for potential dangers of ethnic heterogeneity in genetic research).

Conclusions

The present data demonstrate for the first time that 5-HTTLPR interacts with experiences of daily life stress to predict transdiagnostic internalizing dimensions. Specifically, stress was associated with severity of internalizing symptoms on a day-to-day basis for 5-HTTLPR S allele carriers but not for L allele homozygotes. Additionally, this G × E effect was present across fear and distress dimensions, two subdomains of internalizing symptomatology identified in previous studies of the latent structure of internalizing disorders. These results are consistent with between-subjects research documenting associations of 5-HTTLPR with risk for diverse internalizing syndromes, but extend prior findings by showing that the S allele confers vulnerability to transdiagnostic emotion dysregulation phenotypes, as compared to specific psychiatric disorders. Further research on transdiagnostic emotional phenotypes may help elucidate connections between life stress, candidate genes, and the fundamental components of psychopathology.

Appendix

Daily fear symptoms

My heart was racing or pounding
I was afraid that I might think or do something bad
I felt self-conscious knowing that others were watching me
I had disturbing thoughts of something bad that happened to me
I felt panicky

Daily distress symptoms

I worried
I felt depressed
I felt discouraged about things
I felt nervous
I felt inadequate
I had little interest in my usual hobbies or activities

Daily externalizing symptoms

I was mean to others
I used drugs (e.g., marijuana) for nonmedical purposes
I broke or threw things
I screamed or yelled
I broke rules at school, work, or elsewhere
I drank too much alcohol or got drunk
I spread rumors or gossiped about someone
I intentionally ignored someone
I lied to get what I wanted

Daily stressful life events

Did not have enough money to do something or buy something
Lost money or something important
Property was damaged or stolen
Was sick or had a medical issue
Did poorly on, or failed, an important exam or major project
Failed to achieve an important school related goal that does not involve GPA
Problems at work (e.g. didn't get the schedule that you requested, couldn't find someone to fill in for you)
Problems with co-workers or boss (if different from above)
An event that happened today related to a family member or close friend having a medical or emotional problem
Had an argument/problem with significant other
Had an argument/problem with a friend
Had an argument/problem with family member
Had an argument/problem with a professor, or project group
Fight or argument among social group to which you belong
Was rejected or excluded by others (group, significant other, friend, etc.)
Was criticized by others (project group, significant other, friend, professor, etc.)

Competing interests

The authors declare that they have no competing interests.

Authors' contributions

All authors conceived of the study and participated in its design and coordination. CCC collected the data, performed statistical analyses, and wrote the first draft of the manuscript. GMS and CH edited the manuscript and approved the final version. All authors read and approved the final manuscript.

Acknowledgments

This research was supported by a National Institutes of Health Training Grant in Genomic Analysis and Interpretation (T32 HG002536) and by an American Psychological Association Dissertation Research Award to CCC, and by a Society in Science – Branco Weiss Fellowship to GMS.

Author details

[1]Department of Psychology, University of California, Los Angeles, Box 951563, Los Angeles, CA 90095-1563, USA. [2]Department of Psychology, Cousins Center for Psychoneuroimmunology, University of California, Los Angeles CA, USA. [3]Department of Psychiatry and Biobehavioral Sciences, University of California Los Angeles, CA, USA.

References

1. Caspi A, Sugden K, Moffitt TE, Taylor A, Craig IW, Harrington H, McClay J, Mill J, Martin J, Braithwaite A, Poulton R: **Influence of life stress on depression: moderation by a polymorphism in the 5HTT gene.** *Science* 2003, **301**:386–389.

2. Risch N, Herell R, Lehner T, Liang KY, Eaves L, Hoh J, Griem A, Kovacs M, Ott J, Merikangas KR: **Interaction between the serotonin transporter gene (5-HTTLPR), stressful life events, and risk of depression: a meta-analysis.** *JAMA* 2009, **30123:**2462–2471.
3. Karg K, Burmeister M, Shedden K, Sen S: **The serotonin transporter promoter variant (5 HTTLPR), stress, and depression meta-analysis revisited: evidence of genetic moderation.** *Arch Gen Psychiatry* 2011, **68:**444–454.
4. Munafò MR, Brown SM, Hariri AR: **Serotonin transporter (5-HTTLPR) genotype and amygdala activation: a meta-analysis.** *Biol Psychiatry* 2008, **63:**852–857.
5. Pergamin-Hight L, Bakermans-Kranenburg MJ, van Ijzendoorn MH, Bar-Haim Y: **Variations in the promoter region of the serotonin transporter gene and biased attention for emotional information: a meta-analysis.** *Biol Psychiatry* 2012, **71:**373–379.
6. Way BM, Taylor SE: **The serotonin transporter promoter polymorphism is associated with cortisol response to psychosocial stress.** *Biol Psychiatry* 2010, **67:**487–492.
7. Caspi A, Hariri AR, Holmes A, Uher R, Moffitt TE: **Genetic sensitivity to the environment: the case of the serotonin transporter gene and its implications for studying complex diseases and traits.** *Am J Psychiatry* 2010, **167:**509–527.
8. Kendler KS, Kuhn JW, Vittum J, Prescott CA, Riley B: **The interaction of stressful life events and a serotonin transporter polymorphism in the prediction of episodes of major depression: a replication.** *Arch Gen Psychiatry* 2005, **62:**529–535.
9. Hariri AR, Holmes A: **Genetics of emotional regulation: the role of the serotonin transporter in neural function.** *Trends Cogn Sci* 2006, **10:**182–191.
10. Wright AG, Krueger RF, Hobbs MJ, Markon KE, Eaton NR, Slade T: **The structure of psychopathology: toward an expanded quantitative mode.** *J Abnorm Psychol* 2013, **122:**281–294.
11. Ofrat S, Krueger RF: **How research on the meta-structure of psychopathology aids in understanding biological correlates of mood and anxiety disorders.** *Biol Mood Anxiety Disord* 2012, **2:**13–17.
12. Achenbach TM: *Manual for the Young Adult Self-Report and Young Adult Behavior Checklist.* Burlington: University of Vermont Department of Psychiatry; 1997.
13. Seidlitz L, Diener E: **Memory for positive versus negative life events: theories for the differences between happy and unhappy persons.** *J Pers Soc Psychol* 1993, **64:**654–663.
14. Shahar G, Henrich CC, Reiner IC, Little TD: **Development and initial validation of the brief adolescent life event scale (BALES).** *Anxiety Stress Coping* 2003, **16:**119–128.
15. Gunthert KC, Conner TS, Armeli S, Tennen H, Covault J, Kranzler HR: **Serotonin transporter gene polymorphism (5-HTTLPR) and anxiety reactivity in daily life: a daily process approach to gene-environment interaction.** *Psychosom Med* 2007, **69:**762–768.
16. Watson D, O'Hara MW, Simms LJ, Kotov R, Chmielewski M, McDade-Montez EA, Gamez W, Scott S: **Development and validation of the Inventory of Depression and Anxiety Symptoms (IDAS).** *Psychol Assess* 2007, **19:**253–268.
17. Wendland JR, Lesch KP, Newman TK, Timme A, Gachot-Neveu H, Thierry B, Suomi SJ: **Differential functional variability of serotonin transporter and monoamine oxidase a genes in macaque species displaying contrasting levels of aggression-related behavior.** *Behav Genet* 2006, **36:**163–172.
18. Wray NR, James MR, Gordon SD, Dumenil T, Ryan L, Coventry WL, Statham DJ, Pergadia ML, Madden PA, Heath AC, Montgomery GW, Martin NG: **Accurate, large-scale genotyping of 5HTTLPR and flanking single nucleotide polymorphisms in an association study of depression, anxiety, and personality measures.** *Biol Psychiatry* 2009, **66:**468–476.
19. Dasch KB, Cohen LJ, Sahl JC, Gunthert KC: **Moderating effects of sociotropy and autonomy on affective and self-esteem reactivity to daily stressors.** *Cognit Ther Res* 2008, **32:**177–195.
20. Hox J: *Multilevel Analysis: Techniques and Applications.* New York: Routlage; 2010.
21. Sahl JC, Cohen LH, Dasch KB: **Hostility, interpersonal competence, and daily dependent stress: a daily model of stress generation.** *Cognit Ther Res* 2009, **33:**199–210.
22. Shih JH, Eberhart NK, Hammen CL, Brennan PA: **Differential exposure and reactivity to interpersonal stress predict sex differences in adolescent depression.** *J Clin Child Adolesc Psychol* 2006, **35:**103–115.
23. Cuthbert BN, Insel TR: **Toward the future of psychiatric diagnosis: the seven pillars of RDoC.** *BMC Med* 2013, **11:**126–134.
24. Kendler KS: **'A gene for…': the nature of gene action in psychiatric disorders.** *Am J Psychiatry* 2005, **162:**1243–1252.
25. Uher R, McGuffin P: **The moderation by the serotonin transporter gene of environmental adversity in the etiology of depression: 2009 update.** *Mol Psychiatry* 2010, **15:**18–22.
26. Strauss ME, Smith GT: **Construct validity: advances in theory and methodology.** *Annu Rev Clin Psychol* 2009, **5:**1–25.
27. Cardon LR, Palmer LJ: **Population stratification and spurious allelic association.** *Lancet* 2003, **361:**598–604.

10

Investigating the genetic and environmental bases of biases in threat recognition and avoidance in children with anxiety problems

Jennifer Y F Lau[1*], Kevin Hilbert[1], Robert Goodman[2], Alice M Gregory[3], Daniel S Pine[4], Essi M Viding[5] and Thalia C Eley[2]

Abstract

Background: Adults with anxiety show biased categorization and avoidance of threats. Such biases may emerge through complex interplay between genetics and environments, occurring early in life. Research on threat biases in children has focuses on a restricted range of biases, with insufficient focus on genetic and environmental origins. Here, we explore differences between children with and without anxiety problems in under-studied areas of threat bias. We focused both on associations with anxious phenotype and the underlying gene-environmental correlates for two specific processes: the categorisation of threat faces and avoidance learning.

Method: Two-hundred and fifty 10-year old MZ and DZ twin pairs (500 individuals) completed tasks assessing accuracy in the labelling of threatening facial expressions and in the acquisition of avoidant responses to a card associated with a masked threatening face. To assess whether participants met criteria for an anxiety disorder, parents of twins completed a self-guided computerized version of the Development and Well-being Assessment (DAWBA). Comparison of MZ and DZ twin correlations using model-fitting were used to compute estimates of genetic, shared and non-shared environmental effects.

Results: Of the 500 twins assessed, 25 (5%) met diagnostic criteria for a current anxiety disorder. Children with anxiety disorders were more accurate in their ability to recognize disgust faces than those without anxiety disorders, but were commensurate on identifying other threatening face emotions (angry, fearful, sad). Children with anxiety disorders but also more strongly avoided selecting a conditioned stimulus than non-anxious children. While recognition of socially threatening faces was moderately heritable, avoidant responses were heavily influenced by the non-shared environment.

Conclusion: These data add to other findings on threat biases in anxious children. Specifically, we found biases in the labelling of some negative-valence faces and in the acquisition of avoidant responses. While non-shared environmental effects explained all of the variance on threat avoidance, some of this may be due to measurement error.

Keywords: Childhood anxiety, Threat biases, Face emotion recognition, Behavioural avoidance, Genetic, Environmental

* Correspondence: jennifer.lau@psy.ox.ac.uk
[1]Department of Experimental Psychology, University of Oxford, South Parks Road, Oxford OX1 3UD, UK
Full list of author information is available at the end of the article

Background

Anxiety disorders are common [1], disabling and costly for society [2]. As most adult anxiety disorders have their roots in childhood [1], there is an urgent need to understand the mechanisms by which child anxiety develops. Interventions administered in childhood may also have longer-lasting benefits on anxiety outcomes [3]. Nevertheless, childhood anxiety remains under-studied [4]. Threat biases are a key component of adult anxiety. Such threat biases may arise from inherited perturbations in brain circuitry functioning [5-7], yet are also relatively plastic, developing in response to environmental experiences [8]. Compared to adults, the few available studies on threat biases in anxious children have focused on a more restricted range of processing biases. Less is also known about the origins of processing biases in children as compared to adults. Given vast biological, cognitive and social differences between children and adults [9,10], one cannot simply extrapolate data on adults to children with anxiety. In this manuscript we: (i) follow-up cross-sectional links between less frequently-studied threat biases in our own sample of children with and without anxiety disorders; and (ii) investigate the genetic and environmental origins of some of these anxiety-based threat biases.

Threat bias research in adults and children

Extensive data from anxious adults suggest biases at various stages of information-processing. Studies have identified biases in the initial orienting towards threat cues, i.e. attention capture e.g. [11] and in the inability to disengage attention away from threat cues i.e. attention control e.g. [12,13], using both word and picture (including face) stimuli. Studies have also focused on the tendency to label neutral materials as threatening, for example by drawing threatening interpretations of ambiguous stories or words, and showing greater recognition of threatening facial expressions [14,15]. An emergent body of work has also considered biases in associative learning, particularly in the acquisition, generalisation, and extinction of fear from aversive unconditioned stimuli to neutral cues that signal threat, but also cues that signal safety [16]. These biases in threat-learning shape other biases, as they relate to subsequent behavioural responses [17,18], in which avoidant responses are acquired to attenuate aversive fear-states associated with the threat cue [19]. In summary, adult data document anxiety-based threat biases at various stages of information-processing, from attention to behaviour.

In contrast to the wealth of data on biased threat processing in adults with anxiety, pediatric studies have focused on a restricted range of processing biases. These are presented in Tables 1,2,3. To our knowledge, over 30 studies (Table 1) have measured biases in attention-capture and control to threatening words and pictures (including faces) in children and adolescents. These studies have capitalized on a range of experimental tasks tapping distinct attention processes. The largest number of studies has used the visual probe task, followed by the emotional Stroop task, then the visual search and affective Go/No-Go tasks. Results from the visual probe task generally support robust effects of anxiety on vigilance for threatening words/pictures, with only four out of 18 published studies finding no effects of anxiety (n = 1 study) or an opposite pattern of attentional-avoidance (n = 3 studies). While the reasons for these discrepancies remain unclear, preliminary data from adults may be informative. Specifically, these data suggest that conditions of acute stress can lead some individuals to shift their attention *away* from threats, perhaps to minimize prolonged stress exposure, resulting in a pattern of attentional-avoidance on tasks such as the visual-probe [20]. Given these data, it is noteworthy that among two of the studies finding contradictory results, one sampled children with PTSD following maltreatment [21] and the other was conducted during an anxiety-provoking brain scan [22]. These hypotheses, while intriguing, require further investigation. Studies using the visual search design find signs of hypervigilance to threat amongst children with anxiety problems, and most studies using the emotional Stroop have found interference effects from salient threat cues. Similarly, while the Go/No-Go task is primarily used as a measure of response inhibition, the inclusion of emotional stimuli as 'No Go' cues has also yielded anxiety-based interference effects from threats. In sum, studies of attention-capture and control are generally supportive of disruptions in attention resources in the presence of threat, manifesting as vigilance towards threat or interference that is associated with the presence of threat.

Nearly as many studies (n = 30 in Table 2) have explored biases in the labelling of material as threatening. These studies draw on many different methodologies, including presenting participants with ambiguous scenarios, words and pictures, to which participants' tendency to select threat or benign interpretations is assessed. Other tasks require participants to label face-emotions displays. Studies assessing the evaluation of ambiguous scenarios are clear in suggesting that children with anxiety draw more threatening interpretations of hypothetical situations than their peers with fewer anxiety problems, mirroring adult data. Similarly, there is generally good support for these patterns in the endorsement of threat-meanings of ambiguous words and pictures, such as in homophones or homographs. Data regarding the labelling of threatening facial expressions can be divided into those assessing the rating of fear towards face emotions and those measuring the misclassification of different expressions. The data suggest that children with anxiety do not rate negative faces as more fear-provoking than children without anxiety. Nevertheless, between-group differences

Table 1 Studies of biased attention to threat in anxious youth with studies presenting conflicting results to adult data italicised

Authors	Sample size and age information	Anxiety measure	Nature of anxiety effect reported
Visual Probe Task			
Waters et al., [23]	Anxious group = 23 *(9–12 yrs)* Healthy group = 23 *(9–12 yrs)*	Clinical diagnosis	Anxious group showed greater attention towards **threat and pleasant pictures**
Waters et al., [24]	Anxious group = 29 *(9–12 yrs)* Healthy group = 24 *(9–12 yrs)*	Clinical diagnosis	Anxious group showed greater attention towards **threat faces** but only those with more severe anxiety *(η_p^2=0.17)*
Waters et al., [25]	Anxious group = 19 *(9.8 yrs)* Healthy group = 19 *(10.1 yrs)*	Clinical diagnosis	Anxious group showed greater attention towards **threat pictures** *(η_p^2 = .13)*
Pine et al., [21]	*PTSD group = 29 (10.3 yrs)* *Healthy group = 17 (9.9 yrs)*	*Clinical diagnosis*	*PTSD group showed greater avoidance of **angry faces** (cohen's d = 0.58)*
Roy et al. [26]	Anxious group = 101 *(11.5 yrs)* Healthy group = 51 *(13.6 yrs)*	Clinical diagnosis	Anxious group showed greater attention towards **threat faces** *(cohen's d = 0.53)*
Vasey et al., [27]	Anxious group = 12 *(11.9 yrs)* Healthy group = 12 *(11.8 yrs)*	Clinical diagnosis	Anxious group showed greater attention towards **threat words** but only appearing in lower probed positions *(cohen's d = 0.35)*
Dalgleish et al. [28]	PTSD group = 24 *(12.8 yrs)* Healthy group = 24 *(12.8 yrs)*	Clinical diagnosis	Anxious group showed greater attention towards **social threat and depression related words** *(cohen's d = 0.56 and 0.60)*
Dalgleish et al. [28]	PTSD group = 24, *(12.8 yrs)* GAD group = 24 *(13.6 yrs)* Healthy group = 26 *(15.2 yrs)*	Clinical diagnosis	Anxious groups showed greater attention towards **threat words** *(cohen's d = 0.24 and 0.59)*
Monk et al., [22]	*GAD group = 18 (13.5 yrs)* *Healthy group = 15 (12.3 yrs)*	*Clinical diagnosis*	*Anxious group showed greater avoidance of **angry faces** (cohen's d = 0.64*
Dalgleish et al., [29]	GAD group = 24 *(13.6 yrs)* Healthy group = 24 *(13.2 yrs)*	Clinical diagnosis	Anxious group showed greater attention towards **threat words** *(cohen's d = 0.72)*
Monk et al.,[30]	*GAD group = 17 (14.3 yrs)* *Healthy group = 12 (13.1 yrs)*	*Clinical diagnosis*	*No group differences in attention towards **negative faces***
Keogh et al., [31]	High Anxious group = 23 *(8–10 yrs)* Low Anxious group = 16 *(8–10 yrs)*	Physical Anxiety Sensitivity	High anxious group showed greater attention towards **emotional (threat + positive) words** (η_p^2 = .099)
Heim-Dreger et al., [32]	Whole sample = 112 *(9.0 yrs)*	Trait Anxiety	Trait anxiety correlated with greater attention towards **threat faces**
Stirling et al., [33]	*Whole sample = 79 (9.67 yrs)*	*Anxiety Symptoms*	*Trait anxiety correlated with greater attention away from **threat faces***
Vasey et al., [34]	High Anxious group = 20 *(11–14 yrs)* Low Anxious group = 20 *(11–14 yrs)*	Test Anxiety	High anxious group showed greater attention towards **threat words**
Helzer et al., [35]	Whole sample = 121 *(11.4 yrs)*	Anxiety Symptoms	Anxious symptoms correlated with attention towards **social threat words** but only in those with high fearful temperament
Lonigan et al., [36]	High NA high EC group = 26 *(14.7 yrs)* High NA low EC group = 25 *(14.2 yrs)* Low NA high EC group = 27 *(14.8 yrs)*	Negative Affectivity (NA) and Effortful Control (EC)	High NA group showed greater attention towards **threat words** but only in those with low EC

Table 1 Studies of biased attention to threat in anxious youth with studies presenting conflicting results to adult data italicised *(Continued)*

	Low NA low EC group = 26 *(13.8 yrs)*		
Telzer et al., [37]	Whole sample = 16 *(15.3 yrs)*	Trait Anxiety	Trait anxiety predicted greater attention towards **angry faces** *($\beta = 0.52$, $R^2 = 0.38$)*
Emotional Stroop Task			
Kindt et al., [38]	*Anxious group = 40 (11.5 yrs)* *Healthy group = 14 (13.6 yrs)*	*Clinical diagnosis*	*No group differences in interference effects from* ***threat words***
Kindt et al., [39]	*High Anxious group = 25 (8–9 yrs)* *Low Anxious group = 22 (8–9 yrs)*	*Trait Anxiety*	*No group differences in interference effects from* ***threat faces***
Kindt et al., [40]	*High Phobic group = 72 (8–12 yrs)* *Low Phobic group = 73 (8–12 yrs)*	*Spider Phobia*	*No group differences in interference effects from* ***threat faces***
Martin et al., [41]	Phobic group = 71 *(4–9 yrs)* Healthy group = 72 *(4–9 yrs)*	Spider Phobia	High Anxious group showed a greater interference from **threat pictures**
Martin et al., [42]	Phobic group = 24 *(6–13 yrs)* Healthy group = 24 *(6–13 yrs)*	Spider Phobia	High Anxious group showed a greater interference from **threat words**
Kindt et al., [43]	High Phobic group = 29 *(8–12 yrs)* Low Phobic group = 30 *(8–12 yrs)*	Spider Phobia	High Anxious group showed a greater interference from **threat words**
Heim-Dreger et al., [32]	Whole sample = 82 *(8.6 yrs)*	State Anxiety, Trait Anxiety	Trait and state anxiety correlated with greater interference from **threat faces**
Heim-Dreger et al., [32]	Whole sample = 112 *(9.0 yrs)*	State Anxiety, Trait Anxiety	Trait and state anxiety correlated with greater interference from **threat faces**
Hadwin et al., [44]	*Whole sample = 74 (9.1 yrs)*	*Trait Anxiety*	*No correlation between trait anxiety and interference from* ***threat faces***
Richards et al., [45]	High Anxious group = 24 *(11.9 yrs)* Low Anxious group = 26 *(11.0 yrs)*	Trait Anxiety	High Anxious group showed a greater interference from **threat faces** *($\eta_p^2 = .12$)*
Richards et al., [46]	High Anxious group = 15 *(16.9 yrs)* Low Anxious group = 15 *(16.0 yrs)*	Anxiety Symptoms	High Anxious group showed a greater interference from **threat words**
Visual Search Task			
Hadwin et al., [47]	Whole sample = 53 *(7–10 yrs)*	Trait Anxiety	Trait anxiety correlated with faster search times for **threat cartoons** when the threat-target was absent
Hadwin et al., [47]	Whole sample = 38 *(6–10 yrs)*	Trait Anxiety	Trait anxiety correlated with faster search times for **threat face** when the threat-target was absent
Emotional Go/No-Go Task			
Waters et al., [48]	Anxious group = 20 *(9.9 yrs)* Healthy group = 20 *(10.0 yrs)*	Clinical diagnosis	Anxious girls were slower in responding to 'neutral face' Go trials when embedded in 'angry face' No-Go trials
Ladouceur et al., [49]	Anxious group = 23 *(12.5 yrs)* Healthy group = 26 *(12.5 yrs)*	Clinical diagnosis	Anxious group were slower in responding to 'neutral face' Go trials when embedded in 'angry face' No-Go trials

GAD Generalized anxiety disorder, *PTSD* Post-traumatic stress disorder, *SAD* Separation anxiety disorder, *SP* social phobia, *ADHD* Attention deficit hyperactivity disorder, *MDD* Major Depressive Disorder, *SCR* skin conductance responses.

arise in the categorisation of various negative but also positive facial expressions. These data, while intriguing are few. Moreover, these results contrast with data in adults with anxiety, who are superior at identifying angry and fearful faces than adults without anxiety [14,85]. However, they require further clarification in other samples.

Finally, a handful of studies (n = 6, Table 3) have begun to explore biases in the acquisition and extinction of fear and avoidance of conditioned threat stimuli (CS+), paired with an aversive unconditioned stimulus (UCS), and of conditioned safety stimuli (CS-) not paired with the UCS. Together these studies tentatively suggest that there are anxiety-based differences in the learning and retention of fear to neutral stimuli paired with UCSs (i.e. the CS+). Moreover, these persistent fears can generalize to neutral stimuli that are unpaired with the UCS (i.e. the CS-). Only

Table 2 Studies of biased selection of threat interpretations in anxious youth with studies presenting conflicting results to adult data italicised

Authors	Sample size and age information	Anxiety measure	Nature of anxiety effect reported
Ambiguous Scenarios			
Dodd et al., [50]	Anxious group = 57 *(4.0 yrs)* Healthy group = 74 *(4.0 yrs)*	Clinical diagnosis	Anxious group selected more threatening interpretations *(cohen's d = 0.51)*
Schneider et al., [51]	*SAD/SP groups = 102 (8.8 yrs)* *Healthy group = 42 (9.3 yrs)*	*Clinical diagnosis*	*No group difference in selection of threat interpretations*
Waters et al., [52]	Anxious group = 15 *(9.5 yrs)* Healthy group = 14 *(9.4 yrs)*	Clinical diagnosis	Anxious group selected more threatening interpretations *($\eta_p^2 = .35$)*
Waters et al., [25]	Anxious group = 19 *(9.8 yrs)* Healthy group = 19 *(10.1 yrs)*	Clinical diagnosis	Anxious group selected more threatening interpretations *($\eta_p^2 = .15$)*
Hughes et al., [53]	Anxious group = 34 *(9.9 yrs)* Healthy group = 34 *(10.8 yrs)*	Clinical diagnosis	Anxious group selected more threatening interpretations *($\eta 2 = .09$)*
Barrett et al., [54]	Anxious group = 152 *(7–14 yrs)* Clinical control group = 27 *(10.0 yrs)* Healthy group = 26 *(10.2 yrs)*	Clinical diagnosis	Anxious group and clinical control group selected more threatening interpretations
Creswell et al., [55]	*Anxious group = 27 (11.0 yrs)* *Healthy group = 33 (10.8 yrs)*	*Clinical diagnosis,* *Anxiety Symptoms*	*No group difference but anxiety symptoms correlated with number of threat interpretations ($\eta 2 = .09$)*
Bögels et al., [56]	Anxious group = 15 *(12.2 yrs)* Clinical control group = 15 *(13.5 yrs)* Healthy group = 15 *(11.9 yrs)*	Clinical diagnosis	Anxious group selected more threatening interpretations
Dalgleish et al., [57]	Anxious group = 2 *(14.0 yrs)* Depression group = 15 *(15.1 yrs)* Healthy group = 43 *(13.6 yrs)*	Clinical diagnosis	Anxious group selected more threatening expectations for the future, but only for other people
Dineen et al., [58]	Whole sample = 50 *(8.4 yrs)*	Trait Anxiety	High levels of anxiety correlated with more threatening interpretations of intentions (when asked about other people)
Eley et al., [59]	*Whole sample = 600 twins (8.0 yrs)*	*Anxiety Symptoms*	*High levels of anxiety correlated with threat interpretations; no significant correlation once depressive scores regressed out*
Bell-Dolan, [60]	*High Anxious group = 52 (4th-5th grade)* *Low Anxious group = 38 (4th-5th grade)*	*Anxiety Symptoms*	*No group difference in selection of threat interpretations*
Creswell et al., [61]	Whole sample = 65 *(8–10 yrs)*	Anxiety Symptoms	High levels of anxiety symptoms correlated with threat interpretations at 2 out of 3 time-points of their study
Muris et al., [62]	High Anxious group = 28 *(9.6 yrs)* Low Anxious group = 224 *(10.2 yrs)*	Social Anxiety	High anxious group selected more threatening interpretations
Muris et al., [63]	Whole sample = 299 *(9.8 yrs)*	Anxiety Symptoms	High levels of anxiety correlated with more threat interpretations
Bögels et al., [64]	High Anxious group = 55 *(9.9 yrs)* Low Anxious group = 41 *(10.0 yrs)*	Anxiety Symptoms	High anxious group selected more threatening interpretations
Muris et al., [65]	Whole sample = 157 *(10.1 yrs)*	Anxiety Symptoms	High levels of anxiety correlated with more threat interpretations
Muris et al., [66]	Whole sample = 76 *(10.4 yrs)*	Social Anxiety, Trait Anxiety	High levels of anxiety correlated with more threat interpretations

Table 2 Studies of biased selection of threat interpretations in anxious youth with studies presenting conflicting results to adult data italicised *(Continued)*

Morren et al., [67]	Whole sample = 122 *(10.5 yrs)*	Anxiety Symptoms	High levels of anxiety symptoms correlated with more threat interpretations at 1 out of 2 time-points of their study
Muris et al., [68]	Whole sample = 105 *(10.5 yrs)*	Anxiety Symptoms	High levels of anxiety correlated with more threat interpretations
Vassilopoulos et al., [69]	Whole sample = 109 *(11.3 yrs)*	Social Anxiety	High levels of social anxiety correlated with more threat interpretations
Higa et al., [70]	Whole sample = 175 *(11.5 yrs)*	Social Anxiety	High levels of social anxiety predicted more threatening interpretations *($\beta = 0.49$, cohen's $d = 1.06$)*
Miers et al., [71]	High Anxious group = 37 *(13.7 yrs)* Low Anxious group = 36 *(13.6 yrs)*	Social Anxiety	High anxious group selected more negative interpretations *($\eta_p{}^2 = .31$.)*
Salemink etal., [72]	Whole sample = 170 *(14.5 yrs)*	State Anxiety, Trait Anxiety	High levels of state and trait anxiety correlated with more threat interpretations
Ambiguous Words			
Taghavi et al., [73]	GAD group = 17 *(13.7 yrs)* Healthy group = 40 *(13.3 yrs)*	Clinical diagnosis	Anxious group selected more threatening interpretations of **homographs** *(cohen's $d = 0.84$)*
Hadwin et al., [74]	Whole sample = 40 *(8.5 yrs)*	Trait Anxiety	High levels of trait anxiety predicted more threatening interpretations of **homophones**
Eley et al., [59]	*Whole sample = 300 twin pairs (8.0 yrs)*	*Anxiety Symptoms*	*No significant correlation between anxiety symptoms and selection of threatening interpretations of* ***homophones*** *once depressive symptoms were regressed out*
Face emotion recognition and ratings			
Simonian et al., [75]	SP group = 15 *(12.2 yrs)* Healthy group = 14 *(11.0 yrs)*	Clinical diagnosis	Anxious group made more errors recognizing **happy, sad and disgust faces** *(cohen's $d = -1.55$)*
McClure et al., [76]	*Anxious group = 10 (12.9 yrs)* *Healthy group = 25 (13.5 yrs)*	*Clinical diagnosis*	*No group difference in fearful ratings of negative* ***faces***
Beesdo et al., [77]	*Anxious group = 16 (12.8 yrs)* *Healthy group = 45 (13.9 yrs)*	*Clinical diagnosis*	*No group difference in fearful ratings of negative* ***faces***
Easter et al., [78]	Anxious group = 15 *(13.1 yrs)* Healthy group = 11 *(12.5 yrs)*	Clinical diagnosis	Anxious group made more errors recognizing **happy, sad, angry, and fearful faces** of adults, but not of children
Richards et al., [45]	High Anxious group = 24 *(11.9 yrs)* Low Anxious group = 26 *(11.0 yrs)*	Trait Anxiety	High anxious group labelled **positive faces** significantly more often as angry

GAD Generalized anxiety disorder, *PTSD* Post-traumatic stress disorder, *SAD* Separation anxiety disorder, *SP* social phobia, *ADHD* Attention deficit hyperactivity disorder, *MDD* Major Depressive Disorder, *SCR* skin conductance responses.

one study has investigated anxiety links with the acquisition of avoidant responses to neutral cues associated with the UCS [84]. This study demonstrated that children with anxiety were more likely to avoid selecting the CS+, a red (or yellow) coloured card that was paired with a masked threatening face, when asked to choose one of two cards to win points. These differences associated with high levels of anxiety were of moderately large effect size (Table 3) but await further verification in other samples.

At first, the findings on avoidant-learning may seem to contradict other data showing that children with anxiety are more vigilant for threat cues in visual probe tasks, compared to their peers with fewer anxiety problems (Table 1). However, the tasks from which these two sets of findings arise may tap different stages in processing. Thus, one could consider the visual probe task to measure biases in 'attention capture', the initial, automatic attention-orienting towards threat cues. In contrast, the avoidance paradigm used here may tap response-selection or even behavioral enactment, that is, the degree to which children act to deselect a cue that has an acquired threat value. Given these differences between tasks, the data may instead point to a pattern of initial vigilance (demonstrated by visual probe tasks that present threat stimuli briefly) followed by avoidance (demonstrated by the avoidance-learning task where children either select or

Table 3 Studies of biased fear and avoidance learning in anxious children with studies presenting conflicting results to adult data italicised

Authors	Sample size and age information	Anxiety measure	Nature of anxiety effect reported
Acquisition and extinction			
Craske et al., [79]	Anxious group = 23 *(9.4 yrs)* Healthy group = 11 *(9.4 yrs)*	Clinical diagnosis	Anxious group showed larger anticipatory skin conductance responses (SCR) to CS + and CS- cues during acquisition and extinction
Lipp et al., [80]	Anxious group = 53 *(9.7 yrs)* Healthy group = 30 *(10.1 yrs)*	Clinical diagnosis	Anxious group rated the CS + as more fear provoking after extinction *(cohen's d = 0.68)* but as less fear provoking after acquisition *(cohen's d = 0.63)*.
Pliszka et al., [81]	*ADHD/anxious group = 11 (9.9 yrs)* *Healthy group = 22 (10.2 yrs)*	*Clinical diagnosis*	*No group differences in SCR and cardiac responses to CS + and CS- during acquisition or extinction*
Waters et al., [82]	Anxious group = 17 *(10.2 yrs)* Healthy group = 18 *(10.2 yrs)*	Clinical diagnosis	Anxious group showed larger SCRs to CS + and CS- and rated the CS + as more arousing during acquisition; and showed greater SCRs during extinction
Lau et al., [83]	Anxious group = 16 *(12.8 yrs)* Healthy group = 38 *(14.0 yrs)*	Clinical diagnosis	Anxious group rated CS + and CS- as more fear-provoking after acquisition *(cohen's d = 0.60)* but only to the CS + after extinction *(cohen's d = 0.85)*
Lau et al., [84]	High Anxious group = 18 *(10.6 yrs)* Low Anxious group = 18 *(10.6 yrs)*	Anxiety Symptoms	High Anxious group showed greater acquisition of avoidant responses to the CS + (threat face) *(cohen's d* = 0.19-0.91*)*

GAD Generalized anxiety disorder, *PTSD* Post-traumatic stress disorder, *SAD* Separation anxiety disorder, *SP* social phobia, *ADHD* Attention deficit hyperactivity disorder, *MDD* Major Depressive Disorder, *SCR* skin conductance responses.

deselect a cue signalling threat) among children with anxiety. Such a pattern has also been described in adult data (see [86] for a review), in which individuals with anxiety problems tend to be hypervigilant to briefly presented threat cues, and avoidant of threat cues presented under longer durations.

In summary, there is a large corpus of data investigating attentional mechanisms in children with anxiety. While there are also many studies focusing on interpretations of ambiguous scenarios and words, far fewer studies have measured anxiety-based differences in the categorisation of non-verbal threatening stimuli, such as negative face-emotions. There is also a dearth of research investigating threat-learning difficulties in general and the acquisition of avoidance learning in particular. Given these gaps, the current study aimed to verify the direction of less well-studied anxiety-linked processing biases in youth by comparing children with and without anxiety problems in the *categorisation* of threatening faces, including angry, fearful, sad, and disgust facial expressions; and in the acquisition of *avoidance* of cues signaling threat. Mixed results precluded specific hypotheses on the direction and nature of recognition biases, but enhanced tendencies to engage avoidant response styles were predicted from one other prior study [84].

Developmental origins of threat biases

Very few studies have clarified the origins of putative information-processing biases in children with anxiety. In adults, threat biases may arise from genetic variation, as revealed through preliminary candidate-gene studies [5] and family studies [54] of anxiety-based biases. However threat biases can clearly be shaped by exposure to environmental experiences, as illustrated by individuals who have recently experienced a traumatic event. Data from cognitive bias modification studies also show that external training paradigms can be used to manipulate threat biases in attention and interpretation [87]. Given that there may be changes in the expression of particular anxiety-genes across development [10], and in the salience of particular environmental factors between children and adults [88], simple extrapolation of adult data to understanding anxiety in children is not valid.

Many models of child anxiety suggest that threat biases arise from *both* family and child characteristics [54,89-91]. In spite of this, empirical work has typically focused on the so-called 'nurture' aspect, noting that family interaction patterns in general and parenting styles in particular predict response strategies among anxious offspring [54,92-94]. Apart from work on associations between temperamental traits and information-processing, very few studies have examined the role of 'nature' on threat biases in children. In one study, we found moderate genetic effects on threat interpretation of ambiguous words and scenarios [59]. In another study of the same sample, moderate genetic contributions were also found for labelling of various threatening facial expressions, including fearful, sadness, and disgust [95]. In the current manuscript, we extended exploration of genetic and environmental effects to another information-processing factor relevant to anxiety, acquisition of avoidance to a threat cue, also in the sample. Consistent with existing theories of childhood anxiety and our previous findings, we predicted joint roles of environmental and genetic factors.

Present article

The present study had two goals. The focus of the first set of analysis reported here was to identify whether there were anxiety-based group differences on under-studied threat biases: the categorisation of threat faces and in avoidance learning. While both sets of analyses were conducted in a twin sample, we focused our comparison on children with anxiety disorders (specifically, those meeting symptom-threshold and reporting clinical distress and impairment) and those who had never met criteria for an anxiety disorder and who reported low levels of anxiety symptoms. We compared these 'extreme' groups to maximize anxiety group differences, and to make our findings maximally relevant to clinical samples. Our second set of analyses estimated genetic and environmental influences on threat biases that appeared to play a role in child anxiety. These analyses were conducted in a larger twin sample because analyses that partition individual variability into several sources of influence rely on larger samples that include both MZ and DZ twins, with a full range of scores on these measures. The smaller sub-sample in the first set of analysis would not have yielded enough power to detect genetic and environmental influences with confidence.

Method

Participants

Subjects were 250 pairs of 10 year-old twins from Wave 2 of the Emotions, Cognitions, Heredity and Outcomes (ECHO) study. Participants of this study were initially selected using an extremes design from a large longitudinal sample of twins born in England and Wales [96] to target children with high levels of emotional symptoms. The Wave 1 sample comprised: 247 8 year-old twin pairs selected for high scores on parent-reported anxiety at age 7 years; and 53 randomly selected 'control twin pairs' [97], in which neither of the children within the pair scored in the top 5% of the anxiety score distribution in TEDS at age 7. These control pairs were included to ensure coverage of the full range of scores on test measures. A total of 250 twin pairs returned for Wave 2 [98], forming the subject pool for the current analyses. The reduction in numbers between Waves 1 and 2 was because of attrition and because 11 families were considered unusable at Wave 1, due to autistic spectrum disorders, severe receptive language impairments, and persistent attention problems in at least one of the twins (2 of these 11 families were control pairs). Of these twin pairs, 203 pairs were those selected for high scores on parentreported anxiety at age 7, and the remaining 47 pairs were those initially selected as 'control' pairs. At the time of the Wave 2 visit, twins were aged between 9 years 7 months and 10 years 10 months (mean: 10 years 1 month). A total of 56.4% of the sample was female, with 83 monozygotic (MZ) and 167 dizygotic (DZ) twin pairs. Informed consent was obtained from parents of twins. Ethical approval for this study was given by the Research Ethics Committee of the Institute of Psychiatry and South London and Maudsley NHS Trust.

To assess current psychiatric status, parents of twins completed a self-guided computerized version of a structured interview concerning their child's behaviour at age 10 years: Development and Well-being Assessment (DAWBA, [99]). This interview was conducted at the Wave 2 visit, and contained items assessing not only the presence but also severity and impairment of psychiatric symptoms. Computer algorithms generated preliminary DSM-IV diagnoses. In addition to these items, free text boxes allowed parents to include supplementary details. Together with computer-generated diagnoses, these were used by one of the authors of this study (RG), who was also the first author of the DAWBA interview, and a highly experienced clinician, to make the final diagnosis, blind to all other information. In another study, inter-rater reliability for the presence of any DSM-IV diagnosis was =0.86 across 500 subjects [100], with = 0.67 for agreement between DAWBA diagnoses and diagnoses from casenotes [99]. No other diagnostic instruments were employed to validate diagnoses. However, subjects meeting criteria for an anxiety diagnosis had significantly higher scores on the Screen for Anxiety Related Emotional Disorders (SCARED) [101] than subjects who did not meet criteria (mean scores = 30.00 versus 24.89, Δ 2 (1) = 9.46, $p < 0.01$ when comparing sub-modelsthat tested mean differences).

Of the 500 twins (250 twin pairs) seen at Wave 2, 25 (5%) met criteria for a current anxiety disorder, while 437 received no diagnoses for any psychiatric disorder. Of the 25 anxious subjects, 2 had generalized anxiety, 7 had separation anxiety, 8 had specific phobia and 10 had an anxiety disorder not otherwise specified; one met criteria for a comorbid depressive disorder and 5 other met criteria for externalizing disorders. Because of the extremes design used at Wave 1 to select symptomatic subjects to the study, some of the 437 individuals who did not receive anxiety diagnoses could still manifest high levels of anxiety symptoms even though they did not meet clinical criteria. Indeed, as reported above, these individuals had an overall mean score of 24.89 on the SCARED, which approaches the clinical cut-off on this measure (total score > 25). As such, using these individuals does not comprise an appropriate comparison group for testing anxiety-linked differences on test variables. Instead, we removed those individuals who were initially selected for having high scores on the age 7 parent-reported anxiety measure, leaving only subjects who were initially designated 'control pairs' at Wave 1 as comparison subjects in our group analysis of threat measures. Of the original 106 control twins (53 twin pairs), only 94 (47 twin pairs) were retained at Wave 2. This was because of attrition (4 families) and because 2 families were not followed up due to presence of autistic spectrum disorders, severe receptive language impairments, and persistent attention problems in at least one of the twins. One individual from these 94 children met criteria for an anxiety disorder at Wave 2 and was grouped in the anxious group; their co-twin was also removed as a comparative subject in these analyses. The mean score on the SCARED for the remaining 92 'control twins' was 21.86 (SD = 9.95). As such, these comparison individuals reflected those who had: (i) not fallen in the top 5% of age 7 anxiety scores, (ii) did not meet diagnostic criteria for an anxiety disorder at age 10 years, and (iii) had fewer anxiety symptoms, as measured by the SCARED than those in the diagnostic group at age 10.

Tasks

Two tasks assessing biases in the interpretation of face emotions and in avoidance learning were administered.

The recognition of facial affect task measured ability to correctly label five face emotions: happiness, anger, fear, sad and disgust. However, because of our interest in threat faces, trials in which happy faces were presented were excluded from these data analysis. On each trial, subjects were instructed to label each facial expression by selecting one of five labels that corresponded to the different emotions (happy, anger, sad, fear, disgust) with their computer mouse. Once the subject had clicked on a label, the next trial was presented. The task was therefore self-pacing with variable inter-stimulus intervals across trials and across participants. Facial expression morphs were displayed as animations changing from the neutral expression (0%) to one of four levels of intensity (25%, 50%, 75% or 100%). Accurate responses were scored 1, and inaccurate responses were scored 0. The task comprised 160 trials. Thus, there were 32 trials of each face-emotion, with 8 trials for each of the four intensity levels. These 8 trials were further divided into 4 trial-types (Figure 1). Specifically, head orientation (facing i.e. frontal or sideways i.e. profile to the camera) and eye-gaze direction (towards or away from the camera) of faces was manipulated to create these 4 trial-types: head facing-eyes towards; head facing-eyes away; head sideways-eyes towards; and head sideways-eyes away. The manipulations were used to increase task difficulty, ensuring greater individual variability on accuracy scores for subsequent twin analysis and to avoid ceiling effects (i.e. with all participants correctly identifying all expressions). As expected, across all

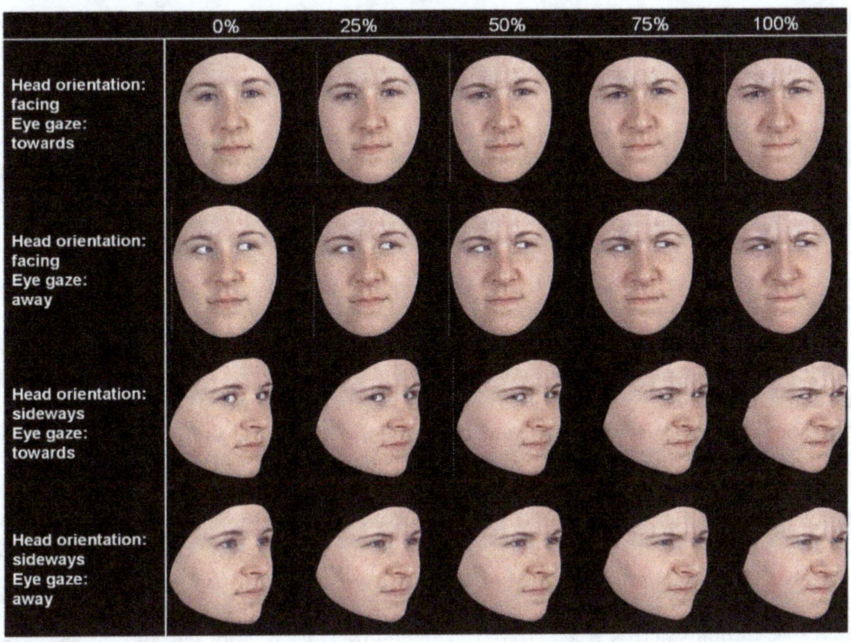

Figure 1 Schematic of the face emotion recognition task with the different expression intensities and eye gaze and head orientation conditions; only angry faces are shown for brevity.

participants in the whole sample trials in which the head faced the subject yielded greater accuracy relative to when the head was presented from a side angle ($F(1,247) = 8.28$, $p < .01$). Similarly, greater accuracy characterized trials in which the eyes appeared toward rather than away from the subject across all participants in the whole sample ($F(1,247) = 22.93$ $p < .001$). Finally, half of the images were drawn from one male actor, and the other half, from one female actor. In summary, trials varied across a number of variables: gender of the face, facial expression, intensity, head orientation and eye gaze direction with equal numbers of each combination, randomly ordered.

Prior to commencing the task, subjects were read standardized instructions. To ensure all subjects were familiar with the 5 emotions, they were asked to provide a definition of each emotion. Subjects were also given 5 practice trials consisting of the faces of two individuals (one male and one female) not used elsewhere in the experiment, demonstrating the five expressions animated from neutral to full-blown intensity. Accuracy scores were summed separately for angry, fear, sad and disgust facial expressions comprising the dependent variables for these analyses. As each face emotion was presented across 32 trials, a score of 32 reflects 100% accuracy. Similar tasks employing computer-generated animation of facial expressions have differentiated anxious from non-anxious adults [14].

Variations of the present task have been used to study face emotion recognition in a variety of populations, ranging from normal volunteers (of different ages) to individuals with psychopathology, genetic disorders or medical conditions. These results suggest that the paradigm is sensitive to subtle age-related trajectories and disorder-linked impairments of emotion perception, compared to tasks employing static images (see [102] for details). The facial expressions of the male and female actor used in the present study were also drawn from these same studies [103,104]. In brief, these individuals were selected from 26 individuals as having the most recognizable expressions of the four basic emotions see [103]; in this same study, which also presented computer generated morphs of the 'intermediate' expressions (i.e. displaying different intensities), healthy adults' accuracy scores ranged from approximately 70-100%, suggesting that facial expressions were valid. Facial expressions were presented in colour. The actors were young adults of Caucasian ethnicity.

The avoidance learning task was designed to assess whether participants associated a neutral stimulus (a colored card) with a threatening stimulus (an angry face) and subsequently avoided this stimulus across trials [105]. On each trial, subjects were presented with two packs of cards (red and yellow). Standardized instructions indicated that the goal was to choose between the coloured packs to win points. Subjects were led to believe that one colour was associated with more points and advised to sample from both packs to decide which was more advantageous. Once they were reasonably sure, subjects were encouraged to continue with that pack for the remainder of the task. In reality subjects' choice of colored card was systematically associated with the subsequent presentation of an angry or neutral facial expression, rather than being associated with high or low reward points. In fact, reward points were either 2358, 2361, 2459, or 2463, chosen to increase the difficulty in tracking points. The face expression followed card-color choice and was presented for 30 ms, which was then followed by a gray face-shaped oval mask (200 ms). Prior studies have found that these presentation conditions can result in a reduced awareness of the facial expression, that is, subjects only report seeing the mask but not the face [106].

This task consisted of five blocks of 32 trials. The number of responses to the color card associated with the angry face in each block formed the dependent test variable indexing avoidance. As each block contained 32 trials, a score of 32 reflects 100% avoidant responses, whereas 50% reflects chance-responding. Color-face pairings were counterbalanced across subjects: for some subjects, the yellow card presented on the left side was always paired with the angry face while the red card, presented on the right side was paired with the neutral face. Other subjects received reversed pairings such that the red card on the left was paired with the angry face and the yellow card on the right with the neutral face. Facial expressions were taken from a standard set of pictures of facial affect, presented in black and white [107].

Data analysis

The structural equation modeling package Mx [108] was used to conduct two sets of analyses on our sample of twins. First, we analyzed differences between children with and without anxiety problems on threat measures, by comparing children who met diagnostic criteria for an anxiety disorder and those who did not meet criteria and who did not experience high levels of anxiety symptoms. Second we explored genetic and environmental influences on threat measures that showed significant differences in the first set of analysis. While the first set of analysis used a sub-sample of ECHO, the second set focussed on all twins in Wave 2. In the first set of analyses, we compared the 25 individuals meeting criteria for current anxiety diagnoses with the 92 individuals selected as control twins at age 7 years. We used a model-fitting approach to test for differences between children with and without anxiety problems because these analyses can control for the non-independence of data from related individuals. Specifically, we compared nested models that either assumed that means for a variable were the same or different for children with and without anxiety. Thus, anxiety-linked differences on threat measures were ascertained by comparing a model that estimated separate means for each group, with a sub-model equating means across the sample. The fit of a model, i.e. the extent to which estimated parameters reflect observed statistics, is indexed by the Chi-square (^{2}) value relative to the degrees of freedom. This ^{2} value is derived from the difference in the loglikelihood (−2LL) statistic generated from comparison of tested models with saturated models (which estimate the means, variances and covariances of all data). Lower, non-significant ^{2} values indicate good model-fit. Another consideration of model-fitting is parsimony, which means that of two models of equal fit the one with fewer parameters is preferred. The Akaike's Information Criterion (AIC), which is calculated as ^{2}-2df is an index of both fit and parsimony, with more negative values indicating a well-fitting and parsimonious model.

Differences between children with and without anxiety problems were therefore reflected by assessing whether there were significant differences in model-fit between models that estimated separate or the same mean across groups for a particular measure indexed through changes in ^{2} relative to changes in degrees of freedom (df). Model-fitting techniques to assess between group differences can control for shared variance between family members by estimating the covariance between twin 1 and twin 2 variables. Complementary mixed design ANOVA analyses were also performed to ensure similar results as those found from model-fitting approaches. For the face emotion recognition responses, 'emotion' was included as a within-subjects factor and 'anxiety group' as a between-subjects factor. For the avoidance learning data, we included 'block' as the within-subject factor and again anxiety-group as the between-subjects factor. Groups did not differ on key demographic variables of age, gender and ethnicity ratio, and socioeconomic status (SES) (Table 4). SES was assessed using the TEDS composite score based on qualifications and current employment for both parents, and mother's age at the birth of her first child.

The second set of analyses used data from the entire Wave 2 sample ($n = 500$) to explore genetic and environmental influences on threat measures that showed significant differences in our first set of analysis. As we have already reported on genetic and environmental influences on classification of face-emotions in this sample, here, we just focused on avoidance acquisition. As this sample over-selected for children with high anxiety scores, it is likely that means are increased, while variances and covariance of correlated variables are decreased [109]. Thus in estimating genetic and environmental influences on threat measures, a weighting system was used. A weight controlling for ascertainment bias was first constructed using the ratio of the selection probability of families of children with high symptom scores to that of 'control' families of children with lower symptom scores among ECHO participants. A second weight controlling for attrition bias was then made using significant predictors of the probability of families remaining at Wave 2. Significant predictors included individuals with mothers reporting higher levels of emotional symptoms and who experienced greater negative life events being less likely to participate. These weights were multiplied and included in analyses to compensate for unequal response rates among individuals from different population strata. During model-fitting procedures, which use maximum likelihood methods to estimate parameters, less weight is applied to individuals from categories overrepresented and more weight to individuals from categories underrepresented in the ECHO sample, relative to the larger more representative, TEDS sample.

Genetic, shared environmental and non-shared environmental effects are estimated through comparisons of within-pair similarity among MZ twins, who share 100% of their genetic makeup and DZ twins who share on average 50% of segregating genes. Within-pair similarity is typically indexed by twin correlations. Higher MZ compared to DZ similarity is attributed to the increased genetic resemblance among MZ twins, and used to estimate heritability (a^2). Within-pair similarity not due to genetic factors is assigned as shared environmental variance (c^2), which contributes towards resemblance among individuals reared in the same family. Finally, non-shared environmental influences (e^2) are individual-specific experiences differing among individuals from the same family, and are estimated from within-pair differences between MZ twins (1 - MZ twin correlations). This term also includes measurement error. As before ^{2} and AIC values were used to assess fit and parsimony of these models.

Results

Anxiety-based differences in recognition of facial affect

Table 4 presents for each group, the total number of correct responses to each face-emotion across all trials, with a total number of 32 trials of each face-emotion. Equivocal evidence arose for an anxiety-related deficit in face-emotion identification. Subjects with and without anxiety problems were comparable in recognizing angry, fear and sad faces (Table 4 for comparison of fit statistics across models). However children with an anxiety diagnosis were better than children without an anxiety ^{2} diagnosis at identifying disgust faces (comparison of fit statistics across models: Δ $(1) = 6.52$, $p < 0.05$). Complementary repeated measures ANOVA did find a main effect of emotion ($F(3,348) = 11.08$, $p < .001$) but a non-significant emotion-

Table 4 Demographic, diagnostic and threat measure variables across children with anxious problems (n = 25) and without (n = 92) subjects

	Anxiety diagnosis	Control subjects with no anxiety problems	Change in model-fit Δχ2(Δdf)	Effect sizes Cohen's d
Demographics				
Mean age	10 years 0 mo.	10 years 1 mo.		
% females	56%	47%		
Mean SES	0.26 (0.76)	0.35 (0.61)		
% Caucasian	91%	98%		
Measures of threat processing				
Recognition of threat (mean no. correct, SD)				
Angry faces	18.63 (3.73)	17.72 (5.89)	$\Delta\chi^2(1) = 0.51$, p = n.s.	
Fear faces	21.29 (6.88)	20.75 (7.15)	$\Delta\chi^2(1) = 0.10$, p = n.s.	
Sad faces	16.08 (5.15)	16.47 (5.90)	$\Delta\chi^2(1) = 0.09$, p = n.s.	
Disgust faces	19.88 (5.11)	16.43 (6.44)	$\Delta\chi^2(1) = 6.52$,	0.59
			$p < 0.05$	
Avoidance of threat	104.88	90.51		0.41
(mean no. of avoidant responses, SD)	(33.41)	(36.40)	$\Delta\chi^2(1) = 6.89$, $p < 0.01$	
Block 1				
Block 2	18.08	17.14 (3.87)	$\Delta\chi^2(1) = 0.56$, p = n.s.	
Block 3	(4.90)	17.53 (6.66)	$\Delta\chi^2(1) = 1.71$, p = n.s.	
Block 4	20.00	18.32	$\Delta\chi^2(1) = 3.56$, p = n.s.	0.39
Block 5	(6.25)	(.93)	$\Delta\chi^2(1) = 5.42$, $p < 0.01$	0.33
	20.56 (8.38)	18.40	$\Delta\chi^2(1) = 6.02$, $p < 0.05$	
	23.36 (9.42)	(10.90)		
	22.88	19.11		
	(10.74)	(11.80)		

The recognition of threat measures corresponds to the mean number and standard deviation of correct responses across 32 trials for each face emotion across groups; the avoidance of threat measure corresponds to the mean number and standard deviation of avoidant responses across the 160 trials of the whole task, and across each 32 trials in each Block at Block 2; p = n.s. at Block 3; at Block 4; and at Block 5.

by-anxiety-group interaction ($F(3,348) = 2.17$, $p = .1$). We next examined group differences associated with anxiety problems for each emotion separately. As with the model-fitting data, independent sample t-tests showed that children with anxiety problems made fewer errors when labelling disgust but were similar in their accuracy in identifying other facial expressions ($t(116) = 2.61$, $p < .05$ for group comparison to disgust faces). Effect sizes of these group differences, calculated using the standardised difference between the means (Cohen's d), were moderate (Table 4).

Anxiety-based differences in avoidance learning

Table 4 reports, for each group, the total number of responses corresponding to avoidance in each block, with a total number of 32 trials presented in each block. A clear association between anxiety and avoidance emerged: subjects with anxiety disorders were less likely than subjects without anxiety disorders to choose [2] a cue paired with the angry face (comparison of fit statistics across models: Δ (1) = 6.89, $p < 0.01$). Moreover, differences in these 'avoidant' responses emerged across blocks (Table 4). Again, we repeated these analyses using ANOVAs. A main effect of block emerged ($F(4,464) = 5.06$, $p < .01$). However the main effect of anxiety only approached a non-significant trend ($F(1,116) = 3.18$, $p = .08$). Examining avoidant choices in each block separately yielded main effects of anxiety-group in Block 4 only ($t(116) = 2.07$, $p < .05$). These discrepancies in results between model-fitting approaches and mixed design ANOVAs may reflect the use of sampling weights in model-fitting approaches. Effect sizes of these group differences, calculated using the standardised difference between the means (Cohen's d), were moderate (Table 4).

Of note, to assess *when* children with and without anxiety problems began to consistently select specific cues, we conducted in each group a series of one sample t tests comparing whether total responses for the card associated with the angry face, per block deviated significantly from 16 trials (i.e. chance responding). For children with anxiety problems, responses from Block 1 and 5 were all significantly below 16 (indicating selection of the card associated with the neutral face); for children without anxiety problems, responses from all blocks were significantly greater than 16 (indicating selection of the card associated with the angry face). This suggests that differential responses are selected between children with and without anxiety problems in the first 32 trials.

Genetic and environmental influences on avoidance learning

Next, we explored genetic and environmental influences on avoidance acquisition. MZ and DZ twin correlations were -.08 and -.03 respectively for avoidance. As both of these were close to zero, they suggested sole influence of non-shared environmental variance/measurement error on avoidance. Model-fitting confirmed these interpretations where a model with non-shared environmental variance at 100% (92-100%) and no genetic (0-7%) or shared environmental effects (0-6%) provided good fit: $-2LL = 1021.20$, $df = 456$, $2\ (12) = 4.46$, $AIC = -19.44$. A previous study found support for genetic effects with non-shared environmental contributions on disgust recognition in this sample [97]. As only one pair of DZ twins were concordant on having an anxiety disorder, inadequate power precluded estimating genetic and environmental influences on diagnostic data.

Discussion

Biased information-processing for threat material is a key component of anxiety, with many data suggesting biases in attention towards threat and in the interpretation of ambiguous (verbal) material (Tables 1,2,3). Prior studies have demonstrated anxiety-based disruptions on attentional mechanisms, and in the interpretation of verbal ambiguous material, such as words and scenarios. However, there are gaps in the literature with fewer studies measuring differences in the evaluation of non-verbal threatening stimuli, such as negative face-emotions, and in the acquisition of fear and avoidance to potential threat cues.

Here, we aimed to follow up some gaps identified in our knowledge of anxiety-based threat biases in children, by exploring differences in the classification of threatening facial expressions and in the acquisition of avoidant responses to a masked threatening face.

Specifically, within our sample of 10-year old twins, we compared those who had been selected for high anxiety symptoms at age 7 and who also met criteria for an anxiety disorder at age 10, with those who did not meet diagnostic criteria and reported lower anxiety scores at age 7 or 10 years. Clear support for one of our hypotheses was found: subjects with an anxiety problem were more likely to avoid a cue paired with a masked angry facial expression, compared to children without anxiety problems. This replicates a prior study using this task in another sample of children [84]. Interestingly in both studies, this tendency appeared to emerge over the course of the task across blocks between children with and without anxiety problems. Results were less clear for another hypothesis: while the ability to recognize angry, fear, and sad facial expressions was not associated with anxiety, children with an anxiety problem were significantly better than those without problems at identifying disgust faces. Contrary to our predictions on the origins of threat biases, no support was found for genetic effects, and all of the variance was explained by non-shared environmental effects, which could include measurement error. This contrasted with the ability to identify disgust faces, which in a previous study of the same sample showed moderate genetic and large environmental contributions [96], consistent with joint roles for nature and nurture.

These data are subject to various limitations. First, it is possible that the avoidance task is less reliable than the facial recognition task, and that this reduced the twin correlations. This may explain the lack of heritability on threat avoidance, while artificially inflating non-shared environmental contributions which includes measurement error. More particularly, different methodologies for assessing threat biases are likely to have different levels of reliability; an experimental task is likely to be less reliable than a questionnaire measure, resulting in greater non-shared environmental and subsequently smaller genetic influences. Investigating the genetic and environmental origins of such threat biases using experimental tasks rather than questionnaires would therefore benefit from attempts to quantify and improve on the psychometrics of such tasks.

A second set of caveats concerns methods used to ascertain diagnostic status of our 'anxious' subjects. While we relied on a version of a well-validated structured interview [99] -the DAWBA - its' application of the functional impairment criterion described in DSM, as well as meeting symptom-threshold may have under-identified those with anxiety problems reported in the present sample. Indeed other studies have often reported discrepancies in prevalence rates of anxiety disorders depending on whether clinically-significant distress and impairment are incorporated in the diagnostic procedures [110,111], with far lower rates reported when 'clinical impact' is considered. In the present study, using both clinical impact and symptoms to determine diagnosis, 5% of the sample met criteria for an anxiety disorder. While this figure is not particularly low when considered against other reported prevalence rates of this age range, which can vary between 2.6% to 41.2% [4], it is lower than expected given that most children in the sample were selected for high anxiety. This allows the possibility that many more children in our sample had high anxiety, but only some also experienced distress and impairment. Indeed as a group, non-diagnosed children in the ECHO sample reported a mean anxiety score on the SCARED that approached clinical cut-off for that measure. As we were interested in assessing anxiety-based differences in threat biases, it was even more important for us to compare children who met clinical diagnosis with children who not only did not meet clinical diagnosis, but who also reported fewer anxiety problems at age 7 and at age 10. Thus, we selected our original control twin pairs as the comparison subjects for this analysis (rather than simply those who did not meet anxiety disorder at age 10 years). A second issue relates to the use of parent-reported data to generate computerized algorithms to detect children meeting criteria for an anxiety disorder. This approach raises issues on the accuracy of parents as informants, in the absence of clinical interview. Future research should employ multi-method, multi-informant measures to increase the validity of reported associations between anxiety and information-processing biases.

A final issue concerns heterogeneity in diagnostic subtypes and co-morbid conditions within the group meeting criteria for at least one current anxiety disorder. Although collapsing across subtypes is sub-optimal, adequate numbers precluded examination of more specific links with biases in information-processing. Nevertheless studies of anxiety subtypes in children typically yield strong cross-sectional and longitudinal comorbidity; similar mental health histories; and large overlap in genetic liability [112,113], lending justification to analyzing anxiety disorders as a single group in the first instance.

Despite these limitations, our data offer some interesting extensions into cognitive phenotypes of child anxiety. One key finding relates to the association between anxiety and avoidance. Prior studies examining avoidance in anxiety have used questionnaires or observational measures that do not correspond closely to definitions of established theories [105]. According to such theories, through associative learning, a neutral conditioned stimulus (e.g. color card, CS+) acquires fear-eliciting properties of an aversive unconditioned stimulus (e.g. angry face, UCS). Avoidance is then employed and reinforced through its fear-reducing capacity. The paradigm in the current study was designed to model the acquisition of avoidance learning. Both the current and a prior study using this paradigm [84] show that children with anxiety problems, defined by questionnaire and diagnostic measures, are more likely than children with fewer anxiety problems to 'avoid' a cue associated with a threatening face in favor of a cue associated with a neutral face. These data fit in well with suggestions that anxiety in childhood can be characterised by a pattern of initial vigilance (as suggested by visual probe studies showing attention-orienting towards threats) followed by subsequent avoidance in response-selection. Interestingly, this vigilance-avoidance pattern has also been described in adults with anxiety [86]. These findings are not too surprising when placed in the context of clinical features of anxiety disorders in children and adults, which often involve marked fear and avoidance of the feared object in tandem. Indeed avoidant strategies are thought to maintain the marked fear. Finally, using model-fitting estimates, the current study does not support the role of inherited factors in shaping these avoidant behaviours but instead points to the importance of non-shared environmental variance. Future studies should try to assess the contribution of specific, measured environmental influences that account for this source of variance.

A second interesting finding was the association between anxiety and biased recognition of disgust faces, a bias that we previously reported to be influenced by genetic factors [95]. This bias in the recognition of disgust among children with anxiety problems occurred in the context of similar abilities to identify angry, fear and sad expressions relative to children without anxiety. There is some support from pediatric samples corroborating the relationship between trait anxiety and disgust sensitivity [114]. Preliminary data also finds greater sensitivity to disgust in adults with high levels of social anxiety, relative to adults with lower levels. This sensitivity is manifest through behavioral ratings and reaction times to disgust faces as well as in patterns of brain activation [115]. Why would anxious individuals be more sensitive to disgust stimuli? Given that biases associated with threat are a characteristic of children with anxiety, disgust could reflect a social threat (e.g. rejection). Disgust could also signal a physical threat (e.g. contamination). Further work is needed to clarify the role of disgust in children's anxiety problems. It would also be interesting to explore whether disgust faces similarly affect other stages of information-processing, such as by capturing or interfering with attentional resources.

Increased avoidance of feared stimuli and sensitivity to disgust stimuli may contribute to pathological anxiety in the long-term by maintaining anxious states. Thus therapeutic interventions that aim to *extinguish* acquired fear and avoidant associations, or *modify* biases in the processing of threats may be particularly helpful in combating anxiety. Exposure based interventions, which capitalize on fear reduction through extinction learning have been used effectively to treat adult anxiety and to some extent in children with anxiety problems. As fear to the CS + declines via extinction, avoidance will no longer be needed to attenuate fear. Alternatively, children could be taught counter strategies to terminate conditioned fear, such as the use of approach-based strategies. For disgust sensitivity, new bias modification programs could be developed and implemented to train children to re-evaluate initial impressions based on other evidence, such as the presence of positive emotional expressions. While cognitive bias modification training tasks appear effective in manipulating attention away from threats, or leading to the re-appraisal of ambiguous scenarios, these training tasks have not yet been extended to manipulate the labelling of ambiguous non-verbal cues, such as face-emotions. If children with high anxiety do show greater recognition of disgust faces, this could be a new target for such computerized training paradigms - with the aim to reduce negative perceptions and thus anxious mood-states.

Conclusion

In the present study, we systematically examined anxiety-based threat biases in children. Through a brief review of studies, we identified gaps in the range of processing biases explored. To extend this literature, we assessed threat biases in the tendency to label ambiguous face-emotions as threatening, and in the acquisition of avoidance responses to threat cues. Our data showed that children with anxiety problems were more likely to correctly identify disgust faces and to avoid a conditioned stimulus paired with a masked angry face. We also investigated the genetic and environmental origins of these threat biases. While disgust sensitivity, as reported by a previous study was shaped both by inherited characteristics and by individual-specific aspects of the environment, data tentatively suggested that the tendency to acquire avoidance to a threat was heavily influenced by non-shared environmental experiences. These data add to existing findings showing linkages between anxiety in children and the tendency to favour threatening information during information-processing. More generally, they also support the role of nurture on generating these threat biases.

Competing interests

The authors declare that they have no competing interests.

Authors' contributions

JL, AG and TE conceived of the study design and carried out the testing of participants. EV and DP contributed to the design of the experimental tasks used. JL conducted the statistical analysis. RG rated all diagnostic data from the DAWBA. JL and KH conducted the brief review of studies in the article and drafted the manuscript. All authors read and approved the final manuscript.

Acknowledgements

The authors would like to thank all participants from the ECHO study. We are also grateful to Jeanette Augustin, James Blair, Pippa Carter, David Clark, Orla Jordan, Helen Mathews, Peter McGuffin, Maria Napolitano, Robert Plomin and Nina Shiffrin for their assistance on various aspects of the study. We would also like to acknowledge Michael Burt who developed and programmed the task on facial expression recognition. Data collection for this study was supported by a Career Development Award from the UK MRC to TE. JL was supported by a MRC Studentship during the data collection phase of this research. AG is currently supported by a Leverhulme Trust Fellowship.

Author details

[1]Department of Experimental Psychology, University of Oxford, South Parks Road, Oxford OX1 3UD, UK. [2]Institute of Psychiatry, King's College London, London, UK. [3]Psychology Department, Goldsmiths, London, UK. [4]Mood and Anxiety Program, National Institute of Mental Health, Bethesda, USA. [5]Department of Psychology, University College London, London, UK.

References

1. Kessler RC, *et al*: **Lifetime prevalence and age-of-onset distributions of mental disorders in the World Health Organization's World Mental Health Survey Initiative.** *World Psychiatry* 2007, **6**(3):168–176.
2. Greenberg PE, *et al*: **The economic burden of anxiety disorders in the 1990s.** *JClin Psychiatry* 1999, **60**(7):427–435.
3. Leonardo ED, Hen R: **Anxiety as a developmental disorder.** *Neuropsychopharmacology* 2008, **33**(1):134–140.
4. Cartwright-Hatton S, McNicol K, Dobbleday E: **Anxiety in a neglected population.** *Clin Psychol Rev* 2006, **26**:817–833.
5. Fox E, Ridgewell A, Ashwin C: **Looking on the bright side: biased attention and the human serotonin transporter gene.** *Proc Biol Sci* 2009, **276**(1663):1747–1751.
6. Fox E, *et al*: **The serotonin transporter gene alters sensitivity to attention biasmodification (ABM): Evidence for a plasticity gene.** *Biological Psychiatry*, . inpress.
7. Hariri AR, *et al*: **Serotonin transporter genetic variation and the response of thehuman amygdala.** *Science* 2002, **297**(5580):400–403.
8. Bar-Haim Y, Holoshitz Y, Eldar S, Frenkel TI, Muller D, Charney DS, Pine DS, Fox NA, Wald I: **Life-threatening danger suppresses attention bias to threat.** *Am J Psychiatry* 2010, **167**:694–698.
9. Scerif G, Karmiloff-Smith A: **The dawn of cognitive genetics? Crucial developmental caveats.** *Trends Cogn Sci* 2005, **9**(3):126–135.
10. Bergen SE, Gardner CO, Kendler KS: **Age-related changes in heritability of behavioral phenotypes over adolescence and young adulthood: a metaanalysis.** *Twin Res Hum Genet* 2007, **10**(3):423–433.
11. Mogg K, Garner M, Bradley BP: **Anxiety and orienting of gaze to angry and fearful faces.** *Biol Psychol* 2007, **76**(3):163–169.
12. Georgiou GA, *et al*: **Focusing on fear: Attentional disengagement from emotional faces.** *Vis Cogn* 2005, **12**(1):145–158.
13. Bishop SJ: **Trait anxiety and impoverished prefrontal control of attention.** *Nat Neurosci* 2009, **12**(1):92–98.
14. Joormann J, Gotlib IH: **Is this happiness I see? Biases in the identification of emotional facial expressions in depression and social phobia.** *J Abnorm Psychol* 2006, **115**(4):705–714.
15. Huppert JD, *et al*: **Interpretation biases in social anxiety: response generation, response selection, and self-appraisals.** *Behav Res Ther* 2007, **45**(7):1505–1515.
16. Lissek S, *et al*: **Classical fear conditioning in the anxiety disorders: a meta-analysis.** *Behav Res Ther* 2005, **43**(11):1391–1424.
17. Rinck M, *et al*: **Social anxiety predicts avoidance behaviour in virtual encounters.** *Cognition & Emotion* 2010, **24**(7):1269–1276.
18. Roelofs K, Ly V: **Social anxiety and cognitive expectancy of aversive outcome in avoidance conditioning.** *Behav Res Ther* 2009, **47**(10):840–847.
19. Mowrer OH: **Two-factor learning theory reconsidered, with special reference to secondary reinforcement and the concept of habit.** *Psychol Rev* 1956, **63**(2):114–128.
20. Wald I, *et al*: **Battlefield-like stress following simulated combat and suppression of attention bias to threat.** *Psychol Med* 2011, **41(4)**:699–707.
21. Pine DS, *et al*: **Attention bias to threat in maltreated children: implications for vulnerability to stress-related psychopathology.** *Am J Psychiatry* 2005, **162**(2):291–296.
22. Monk CS, *et al*: **Ventrolateral prefrontal cortex activation and attentional bias in response to angry faces in adolescents with generalized anxiety disorder.** *Am J Psychiatry* 2006, **163**(6):1091–1097.

23. Waters AM, Lipp OV, Spence SH: **Attentional bias toward fear-related stimuli: an investigation with nonselected children and adults and children with anxiety disorders.** *J Exp Child Psychol* 2004, **89**(4):320–337.
24. Waters AM, *et al*: **Attentional bias towards angry faces in childhood anxiety disorders.** *J Behav Ther Exp Psychiatry* 2010, **41**(2):158–164.
25. Waters AM, *et al*: **Threat-based cognitive biases in anxious children: comparison with non-anxious children before and after cognitive behavioural treatment.** *Behav Res Ther* 2008, **46**(3):358–374.
26. Roy AK, *et al*: **Attention bias toward threat in pediatric anxiety disorders.** *J Am Acad Child Adolesc Psychiatry* 2008, **47**(10):1189–1196.
27. Vasey MW, *et al*: **Biased attention in childhood anxiety disorders: a preliminary study.** *J Abnorm Child Psychol* 1995, **23**(2):267–279.
28. Dalgleish T, *et al*: **Patterns of processing bias for emotional information across clinical disorders: A comparison of attention, memory, and prospective cognition in children and adolescents with depression, generalized anxiety, and posttraumatic stress disorder.** *J Clin Child Adolesc Psychol* 2003, **32**(1):10–21.
29. Dalgleish T, *et al*: **An experimental investigation of hypervigilance for threat in children and adolescents with post-traumatic stress disorder.** *Psychol Med* 2001, **31**(3):541–547.
30. Monk CS, *et al*: **Amygdala and ventrolateral prefrontal cortex activation to masked angry faces in children and adolescents with generalized anxiety disorder.** *Arch Gen Psychiatry* 2008, **65**(5):568–576.
31. Keogh E, Hunt C, French CC: **Anxiety sensitivity, conscious awareness and selective attentional biases in children.** *Behav Res Ther* 2007, **45**(3):497–509.
32. Heim-Dreger U, *et al*: **Attentional biases for threatening faces in children: Vigilant and avoidant processes.** *Emotion* 2006, **6**(2):320–325.
33. Stirling L, Eley TC, Clark DM: **Preliminary evidence for an association between social anxiety symptoms and avoidance of negative faces in school-age children.** *J Clin Child Adolesc Psychol* 2006, **35**(3):440–445.
34. Vasey MW, ElHag N, Daleiden EL: **Anxiety and the processing of emotionally threatening stimuli: Distinctive patterns of selective attention among high- and low-test-anxious children.** *Child Dev* 1996, **67** (3):1173–1185.
35. Helzer EG, Connor-Smith JK, Reed MA: **Traits, states, and attentional gates: Temperament and threat relevance as predictors of attentional bias to social threat.** *Anxiety Stress Coping* 2009, **22**(1):57–76.
36. Vasey MW, Lonigan CJ: **Negative Affectivity, Effortful Control, and Attention to Threat-Relevant Stimuli.** *J Abnorm Child Psychol* 2009, **37** (3):387–399.
37. Telzer EH, *et al*: **Relationship between trait anxiety, prefrontal cortex, and attention bias to angry faces in children and adolescents.** *Biol Psychol* 2008, **79**(2):216–222.
38. Kindt M, Bogels S, Morren M: **Processing bias in children with separation anxiety disorder, social phobia and generalised anxiety disorder.** *Behav Chang* 2003, **20**(3):143–150.
39. Kindt M, Brosschot JF, Everaerd W: **Cognitive processing bias of children in a real life stress situation and a neutral situation.** *J Exp Child Psychol* 1997, **64**(1):79–97.
40. Kindt M, Bierman D, Brosschot JF: **Cognitive bias in spider fear and control children: Assessment of emotional interference by a card format and a single-trial format of the Stroop task.** *J Exp Child Psychol* 1997, **66**(2):163–179.
41. Martin M, Jones GV: **Integral Bias in the Cognitive Processing of Emotionally Linked Pictures.** *Br J Psychol* 1995, **86**:419–435.
42. Martin M, Horder P, Jones GV: **Integral Bias in Naming of Phobia-Related Words.** *Cognition & Emotion* 1992, **6**(6):479–486.
43. Kindt M, Brosschot JF: **Cognitive bias in spider-phobic children: Comparison of a pictorial and a linguistic spider Stroop.** *J Psychopathol Behav Assess* 1999, **21**(3):207–220.
44. Hadwin JA, *et al*: **Childhood anxiety and attention to emotion faces in a modified stroop task.** *Br J Dev Psychol* 2009, **27**:487–494.
45. Richards A, *et al*: **A comparison of selective attention and facial processing biases in typically developing children who are high and low in self-reported trait anxiety.** *Dev Psychopathol* 2007, **19**(2): 481–495.
46. Richards A, Richards LC, McGeeney A: **Anxiety-related stroop interference in adolescents.** *J Gen Psychol* 2000, **127**(3):327–333.
47. Hadwin JA, *et al*: **The influence of children's self-report trait anxiety and depression on visual search for emotional faces.** *J Child Psychol Psychiatry* 2003, **44**(3):432–444.
48. Waters AM, Valvoi JS: **Attentional bias for emotional faces in paediatric anxiety disorders: An investigation using the emotional go/no go task.** *J Behav Ther Exp Psychiatry* 2009, **40**(2):306–316.
49. Ladouceur CD, *et al*: **Processing emotional facial expressions influences performance on a Go/NoGo task in pediatric anxiety and depression.** *J Child Psychol Psychiatry* 2006, **47**(11):1107–1115.
50. Dodd HF, *et al*: **Interpretation bias in preschool children at risk for anxiety: A prospective study.** *J Abnorm Psychol* 2011, .
51. Schneider S, *et al*: **Forced choice reaction time paradigm in children with separation anxiety disorder, social phobia, and nonanxious controls.** *Behav Res Ther* 2009, **47**(12):1058–1065.
52. Waters AM, *et al*: **Threat interpretation bias as a vulnerability factor in childhood anxiety disorders.** *Behav Res Ther* 2008, **46**(1):39–47.
53. Hughes AA, Kendall PC: **Effect of a positive emotional state on interpretation bias for threat in children with anxiety disorders.** *Emotion* 2008, **8**(3):414–418.
54. Barrett PM, *et al*: **Family enhancement of cognitive style in anxious and aggressive children.** *J Abnorm Child Psychol* 1996, **24**(2):187–203.
55. Creswell C, Schniering CA, Rapee RM: **Threat interpretation in anxious children and their mothers: comparison with nonclinical children and the effects of treatment.** *Behav Res Ther* 2005, **43** (10):1375–1381.
56. Bogels SM, Zigterman D: **Dysfunctional cognitions in children with social phobia, separation anxiety disorder, and generalized anxiety disorder.** *J Abnorm Child Psychol* 2000, **28**(2):205–211.
57. Dalgleish T, *et al*: **Information processing in clinically depressed and anxious children and adolescents.** *J Child Psychol Psychiatry* 1997, **38**(5):535–541.
58. Dineen KA, Hadwin JA: **Anxious and depressive symptoms and children's judgements of their own and others' interpretation of ambiguous social scenarios.** *J Anxiety Disord* 2004, **18**(4):499–513.
59. Eley TC, *et al*: **In the face of uncertainty: A twin study of ambiguous information, anxiety and depression in children.** *J Abnorm Child Psychol* 2008, **36**(1):55–65.
60. Belldolan DJ: **Social Cue Interpretation of Anxious Children.** *J Clin Child Psychol* 1995, **24**(1):2–10.
61. Creswell C, O'Connor TG: **Interpretation Bias and Anxiety in Childhood: Stability, Specificity and Longitudinal Associations.** *Behav Cogn Psychother* 2011, **39**(2):191–204.
62. Muris P, Merckelbach H, Damsma E: **Threat perception bias in nonreferred, socially anxious children.** *J Clin Child Psychol* 2000, **29**(3):348–359.
63. Muris P, *et al*: **Threat perception abnormalities in children: the role of anxiety disorders symptoms, chronic anxiety, and state anxiety.** *J Anxiety Disord* 2003, **17**(3):271–287.
64. Bogels SM, Snieder N, Kindt M: **Specificity of dysfunctional thinking in children with symptoms of social anxiety, separation anxiety and generalised anxiety.** *Behav Chang* 2003, **20**(3):160–169.
65. Muris P, *et al*: **Threat perception distortions and psychopathological symptoms in typically developing children.** *Infant Child Dev* 2005, **14** (3):273–285.
66. Muris P, *et al*: **"Danger is lurking everywhere". The relation between anxiety and threat perception abnormalities in normal children.** *J Behav Ther Exp Psychiatry* 2000, **31**(2):123–136.
67. Morren M, *et al*: **Emotional Reasoning and Parent-Based Reasoning in Non- Clinical Children, and Their Prospective Relationships with Anxiety Symptoms.** *Child Psychiatry Hum Dev* 2008, **39**(4):351–367.
68. Muris P, *et al*: **Anxiety and threat perception abnormalities in normal children.** *J Psychopathol Behav Assess* 2000, **22**(2):183–199.
69. Vassilopoulos SP, Banerjee R: **Interpretations and judgments regarding positive and negative social scenarios in childhood social anxiety.** *Behav Res Ther* 2008, **46**(7):870–876.
70. Higa CK, Daleiden EL: **Social anxiety and cognitive biases in non-referred children: The interaction of self-focused attention and threat interpretation biases.** *J Anxiety Disord* 2008, **22**(3):441–452.
71. Miers AC, *et al*: **Interpretation bias and social anxiety in adolescents.** *J Anxiety Disord* 2008, **22**(8):1462–1471.
72. Salemink E, Wiers RW: **Modifying Threat-related Interpretive Bias in Adolescents.** *J Abnorm Child Psychol* 2011, **39**(7):967–976.
73. Taghavi MR, *et al*: **Interpretation of ambiguous emotional information in clinically anxious children and adolescents.** *Cognition & Emotion* 2000, **14** (6):809–822.

74. Hadwin J, *et al*: **Cognitive processing and trait anxiety in typically developing children: Evidence for an interpretation bias.** *J Abnorm Psychol* 1997, **106**(3):486–490.
75. Simonian SJ, *et al*: **Recognition of facial affect by children and adolescents diagnosed with social phobia.** *Child Psychiatry Hum Dev* 2001, **32**(2):137–145.
76. McClure EB, *et al*: **Facial expression recognition in adolescents with mood and anxiety disorders.** *Am J Psychiatry* 2003, **160**(6):1172–1174.
77. Beesdo K, *et al*: **Common and Distinct Amygdala-Function Perturbations in Depressed vs Anxious Adolescents.** *Arch Gen Psychiatry* 2009, **66**(3):275–285.
78. Easter J, *et al*: **Emotion recognition deficits in pediatric anxiety disorders: Implications for amygdala research.** *J Child Adolesc Psychopharmacol* 2005, **15**(4):563–570.
79. Craske MG, *et al*: **Is aversive learning a marker of risk for anxiety disorders in children?** *Behav Res Ther* 2008, **46**(8):954–967.
80. Lipp OV, *et al*: **Evidence for retarded extinction of aversive learning in anxious children.** *Behav Res Ther* 2006, **44**(10):1491–1502.
81. Pliszka SR, *et al*: **Classical-Conditioning in Children with Attention-Deficit Hyperactivity Disorder (Adhd) and Anxiety Disorders - a Test of Quays Model.** *J Abnorm Child Psychol* 1993, **21**(4):411–423.
82. Waters AM, Henry J, Neumann DL: **Aversive Pavlovian Conditioning in Childhood Anxiety Disorders: Impaired Response Inhibition and Resistance to Extinction.** *J Abnorm Psychol* 2009, **118**(2):311–321.
83. Lau JYF, *et al*: **Fear conditioning in adolescents with anxiety disorders: Results from a novel experimental paradigm.** *J Am Acad Child Adolesc Psychiatry* 2008, **47**(1):94–102.
84. Lau JY, Viding EM: **Anxiety-related biases in children's avoidant responses to a masked angry face.** *Behav Res Ther* 2007, **45**(7):1639–1645.
85. Codispoti M, *et al*: **Facial emotion recognition in trait anxiety.** *J Anxiety Disord* 2006, **20**(1):110–117.
86. Bögels SM, Mansell W: **Attention processes in the maintenance and treatment of social phobia: hypervigilance, avoidance and self-focused attention.** *Clin Psychol Rev* 2004, **24**(7):827–856.
87. Mathews A, MacLeod C: **Cognitive vulnerability to emotional disorders.** *Annu Rev Clin Psychol* 2005, **1**:167–195.
88. Gardner M, Steinberg L: **Peer influence on risk taking, risk preference, and risky decision making in adolescence and adulthood: an experimental study.** *Dev Psychol* 2005, **41**(4):625–635.
89. Barlow DH: *Anxiety and Its Disorders: The Nature and Treatment of Anxiety and Panic.* New York: Guilford Press; 1988.
90. Krohne HW, Hock M: **Relationships Between Restrictive Mother-Child Interactions and Anxiety of the Child.** *Anxiety Research* 1991, **4**:109–124.
91. Rapee RM: **The development of generalized anxiety disorder.** In *The developmental psychopathology of anxiety.* Edited by Vasey MW, Dadds MR. New York: Oxford University Press; 2001:481–504.
92. Creswell C, Schniering CA, Rapee RM: **Threat interpretation in anxious children and their mothers: comparison with nonclinical children and the effects of treatment.** *Behavior Research and Therapy* 2005, **43**: 1375–1381.
93. Barrett DE: **The Three Stages of Adolescence.** *High Sch J* 1996, **79**(4): 333–339.
94. Hadwin JA, Garner M, Perez-Olivas G: **The development of information processing biases in childhood anxiety: a review and exploration of its origins in parenting.** *Clin Psychol Rev* 2006, **26**(7):876–894.
95. Lau JYF, *et al*: **Individual Differences in Children's Facial Expression Recognition Ability: The Role of Nature and Nurture.** *Dev Neuropsychol* 2009, **34**(1):37–51.
96. Plomin R, Trouton A, Spinath FM: **Twins Early Development Study (TEDS): A multivariate, longitudinal genetic investigation of language, cognition and behavior problems in childhood.** *Twin Res* 2002, **5**(5):444–448.
97. Gregory AM, *et al*: **Genetic and environmental influences on interpersonal cognitions and associations with depressive symptoms in 8-year-old twins.** *J Abnorm Psychol* 2007, **116**(4):762–775.
98. Lau JY, *et al*: **Assessing gene-environment interactions on anxiety symptom subtypes across childhood and adolescence.** *Dev Psychopathol* 2007, **19**(4):1129–1146.
99. Goodman R, *et al*: **The Development and Well-Being Assessment: Description and initial validation of an integrated assessment of child and adolescent psychopathology.** *J Child Psychol Psychiatry* 2000, **41** (5):645–655.
100. Fombonne E, *et al*: **Prevalence of pervasive developmental disorders in the British nationwide survey of child mental health.** *J Am Acad Child Adolesc Psychiatry* 2001, **40**(7):820–827.
101. Birmaher B, *et al*: **The screen for child anxiety related emotional disorders (SCARED): Scale construction and psychometric characteristics.** *J Am Acad Child Adolesc Psychiatry* 1997, **36**(4):545–553.
102. Kessels RPC, *et al*: **The emotion recognition task: A paradigm to measure the perception of facial emotional expressions at different intensities.** *Percept Mot Skills* 2007, **104**(2):589–598.
103. Gagliardi C, *et al*: **Facial expression recognition in Williams syndrome.** *Neuropsychologia* 2003, **41**(6):733–738.
104. Frigerio E, *et al*: **Facial affect perception in alcoholics.** *Psychiatry Res* 2002, **113**(1–2):161–171.
105. Mowrer OH: **On the dual nature of learning-a re-interpretation of "conditioning" and "problem-solving".** *Harv Educ Rev* 1947, **17**:102–148.
106. Morris JS, Ohman A, Dolan RJ: **Conscious and Unconscious Emotional Learning in the Human Amygdala.** *Nature* 1998, **393**:467–470.
107. Elkman P: *Freisen WV: Facial Action Coding System: A Technique for the Measurement of Facial Movement.* Palo Alto, California: Consulting Psychologists; 1978.
108. Neale MC, *et al*: *Mx: Statistical Modeling.* 5th edition. VCU Box 900126, Richmond, VA 23298: Department of Psychiatry; 1999.
109. Felsenfeld S, *et al*: **A Study of the Genetic and Enviromental Etiology of Stuttering in a Selected Twin Sample.** *Behav Genet* 2000, **30**:359–366.
110. Simonoff E, *et al*: **The Virginia Twin Study of Adolescent behavioral development - Influences of age, sex, and impairment on rates of disorder.** *Arch Gen Psychiatry* 1997, **54**(9):801–808.
111. Merikangas KR, *et al*: **Lifetime prevalence of mental disorders in U.S. adolescents: results from the National Comorbidity Survey Replication--Adolescent Supplement (NCS-A).** *J Am Acad Child Adolesc Psychiatry* 2010, **49**(10):980–989.
112. Eley TC, *et al*: **A Twin Study of Anxiety-Related Behaviours in Pre-school Children.** *J Child Psychol Psychiatry* 2003, **44**(7):945–960.
113. Gregory AM, *et al*: **Juvenile Mental Health Histories of Adults with Anxiety Disorders.** *Am J Psychiatry* 2007, **164**(2):301–308.
114. Muris P, *et al*: **Disgust sensitivity, trait anxiety and anxiety disorders symptoms in normal children.** *Behav Res Ther* 1999, **37**(10):953–961.
115. Amir N, *et al*: **Increased activation of the anterior cingulate cortex during processing of disgust faces in individuals with social phobia.** *Biol Psychiatry* 2005, **57**(9):975–981.

Altered amygdala activation during face processing in Iraqi and Afghanistani war veterans

Alan N Simmons[1,2,3*], Scott C Matthews[1,2,3,4], Irina A Strigo[2,3], Dewleen G Baker[1,2,3], Heather K Donovan[1,2,3], Arame Motezadi [1,2,3,4], Murray B Stein[1,2] and Martin P Paulus[1,2,3]

Abstract

Background: Exposure to combat can have a significant impact across a wide array of domains, and may manifest as post-traumatic stress disorder (PTSD), a debilitating mental illness that is associated with neural and affective sequelae. This study tested the hypothesis that combat-exposed individuals with and without PTSD, relative to healthy control subjects with no history of PTSD or combat exposure, would show amygdala hyperactivity during performance of a well-validated face processing task. We further hypothesized that differences in the prefrontal cortex would best differentiate the combat-exposed groups with and without PTSD.

Methods: Twelve men with PTSD related to combat in Operations Enduring Freedom and/or Iraqi Freedom, 12 male combat-exposed control patients with a history of Operations Enduring Freedom and/or Iraqi Freedom combat exposure but no history of PTSD, and 12 healthy control male patients with no history of combat exposure or PTSD completed a face-matching task during functional magnetic resonance imaging.

Results: The PTSD group showed greater amygdala activation to fearful versus happy faces than both the combat-exposed control and healthy control groups. Both the PTSD and the combat-exposed control groups showed greater amygdala activation to all faces versus shapes relative to the healthy control group. However, the combat-exposed control group relative to the PTSD group showed greater prefrontal/parietal connectivity with the amygdala, while the PTSD group showed greater connectivity with the subgenual cingulate. The strength of connectivity in the PTSD group was inversely related to avoidance scores.

Conclusions: These observations are consistent with the hypothesis that PTSD is associated with a deficiency in top-down modulation of amygdala activation by the prefrontal cortex and shows specific sensitivity to fearful faces.

Background

Soldiers exposed to combat in Operations Iraqi Freedom (OIF) and Enduring Freedom (OEF) are at high risk for post-traumatic stress disorder (PTSD) [1]. PTSD is an aversive reaction to a life-threatening, emotionally salient event [2] that is associated with increased mortality and morbidity [3]. The majority of those who experience such an event have a substantial stress response [4] that is characterized by activation in physiological and neuroendocrine systems [5-8]. Such stress responses are associated with hyperactivation in the insula and amygdala [9,10] brain structures that are involved in processing emotional information. Amygdala activation has been strongly linked to negative affective states in fear processing [11-13] and PTSD [14-17]. A number of studies have successfully used face tasks to probe affective circuits such as the amygdala to better understand affective symptomology in PTSD [18-23]. However, amygdala activation has not been as consistent in PTSD as in other anxiety groups [10]. While a number of studies have shown amygdala hyperactivation in individuals with combat-related PTSD versus healthy controls (HC) with no history of PTSD or combat exposure [20,23-25], a similar number of studies have shown amygdala hyperactivation in individuals with combat-related PTSD versus individuals with combat exposure but no PTSD [21,26-28]. Other studies have shown amygdala hyperactivation in individuals with combat exposure but not PTSD relative to individuals with no history of combat exposure or PTSD [29]. Although these findings suggest strongly that

* Correspondence: ansimmons@ucsd.edu
[1]Veterans Affairs San Diego Healthcare System, 3350 La Jolla Village Drive, San Diego, CA 92161, USA
Full list of author information is available at the end of the article

PTSD is related to amygdala hyperactivation, it can also be suggested that the experience of emotional trauma in and of itself may relate to significant differences in the functioning of emotional processing circuits.

Exposure to combat where there is a risk of death (in other words, Criterion A for the diagnosis of PTSD; [30]) can have significant psychiatric or cognitive repercussions [31] even when it does not result in PTSD. However, one important difference between those exposed to trauma who develop PTSD versus those who do not may be in the increased avoidance of aversive experiences and emotions [32]. This maladaptive response to aversive emotions following trauma may enhance and maintain symptoms of PTSD [33] by diminishing the likelihood of fear extinction [34].

Recent neural models of PTSD and trauma exposure suggest that the functional networks associated with the amygdala may be of similar importance to understanding emotional processing as the amygdala itself [35]. These theories posit that PTSD is, in part, a manifestation of ineffective top-down modulation of the amygdala and limbic circuitry by the prefrontal cortex [15,35]. This model has been proposed as a mechanism for the depersonalization seen in PTSD [36]. For example, it has been shown that reduced functional connections between the amygdala and prefrontal cortex relate to increased levels of depersonalization following emotional trauma, suggesting that impaired functioning of this prefrontal modulatory network may be related to clinical symptoms in traumatized individuals [37].

The use of multiple control groups can be effective in separating the contributions of combat exposure and PTSD. Specifically, a multiple control group design is useful for testing the hypothesis that trauma disrupts emotional circuits relevant to face processing, and that the subsequent development of PTSD is related to less engagement of frontal top-down circuitry [15,35].

Two recent papers investigated the effects of trauma and PTSD during functional magnetic resonance imaging (fMRI) through comparison of PTSD, trauma-exposed and HC subjects. Using a cognitive inhibition task, Falconer and colleagues found greater frontal activation in the trauma-exposed and HC individuals versus the PTSD subjects, and greater parahippocampal activation in PTSD versus HC (but not trauma control) individuals [38]. New and colleagues compared how these three groups relate when downregulating emotion during performance of a negative cognitive reappraisal task and found that both HC and trauma controls relative to PTSD subjects showed greater activation of frontal circuitry. However, they did not find significant differences in amygdala activation between the groups [39]. The authors of this paper posit that the 'trauma-exposed groups may engage a more distributed cortical network in the control of emotion' (p. 662) than HCs, suggesting that trauma-exposed controls show greater limbic and frontal activation in the control of emotion. Both of these studies used cognitive tasks in groups with non-combat trauma exposure. In addition, positron emission tomography (PET) studies have used the three-group model to dissociate the biomarkers of PTSD and trauma. Phan and colleagues suggest that both trauma and PTSD groups show activations in the amygdala but that the PTSD group differentially modulates the ventral medial frontal gyrus [40]. Britton and colleagues showed that the dorsal medial frontal gyrus was less active in patients with PTSD while was there was greater ventromedial prefrontal activation [41]. These findings suggest the importance of frontal circuitry in trauma response and resilience. However, the degree to which these findings translate to a sample with combat trauma during performance of a task that probes affective brain circuits is unknown. Delineation of the effects of combat exposure and PTSD will help increase understanding of possible mechanisms of resilience or vulnerability to PTSD after exposure to trauma.

In prior studies, using a simple face-matching task, we and others have identified clinically meaningful differences in amygdala activation in groups with mood and anxiety disorders [42-44], and shown significant changes in response to psychopharmacological intervention [45,46]. This simple face-matching task has also been successful in delineating differences in functionally connected networks in psychiatric populations [43]. While face tasks do not use trauma-related stimuli and do not directly provoke re-experiencing symptoms in PTSD, they do require appraisal of social emotions, thus they appear to provide a method to measure affective circuitry in a theoretically and clinically meaningful way.

In the current study, we collected fMRI data in combat-exposed veterans with and without PTSD, as well as in healthy participants, during performance of a face-matching task that reliably activates the amygdala [43,44] in an effort to understand how neural response in affective circuitry could help delineate the effects of trauma from PTSD. Based on the literature described above, we hypothesized that PTSD individuals would show greater amygdala activation during a face matching task relative to HC participants with no history of PTSD or combat exposure. Furthermore, functional connectivity between the amygdala and frontoparietal structures, including the dorsal lateral and medial prefrontal cortex, involved in emotion modulation would be reduced in the PTSD group in contrast to the trauma-exposed groups.

Results

Demographic, psychiatric and behavioral results

After correcting for multiple comparisons, the groups did not differ on several demographic variables (Table 1).

Table 1 Demographic, psychiatric and behavioral variables

	PTSD		CEC		HC			
Variable	Mean	SD	Mean	SD	Mean	SD	F-statistic	*p*
Age	32.3	6.9	28.7	4.5	27.3	6.2	2.193	0.128
Education	13.9	1.7	13.8	2.2	13.5	2.0	0.065	0.938
Ethnicity (n)								
Caucasian	6		10		5		$\chi^2 = 6.20$	0.185
Hispanic	3		2		5			
Black	3		0		2			
CTQ	39.8	5.4	42.6	6.5	-	-	0.858	0.371
CES	22.7	7.2	19.1	9.9	-	-	0.623	0.444
BDI	14.6	9.5	5.5	5.9	-	-	5.083	0.042
CAPS-B[a]	19.0	7.3	3.9	6.9	-	-	20.194	< 0.001
CAPS-C	25.8	5.3	4.8	8.0	-	-	40.163	< 0.001
CAPS-D	25.0	3.9	11.0	8.4	-	-	18.584	< 0.001
CAPS Total	69.8	13.2	19.7	22.2	-	-	31.497	< 0.001
Task reaction time (ms)							70.974[b]	< 0.001[b]
Shape	1029	317	965	278	919	188	1.146[c]	0.384[c]
Angry	1458	435	1470	455	1347	251		
Fear	1652	369	1625	532	1395	336		
Happy	1257	289	1185	336	1009	161		

[a] CAPS was measured in eight out of twelve of the PTSD group and ten out of twelve of the CEC group; [b]task effect; [c]group effect. BDI = Beck Depression Inventory; CAPS = Clinician-Administered PTSD Scale; CEC = combat exposed control; CES = Combat Exposure Scale; CTQ = Childhood Trauma Questionnaire; HC = healthy control; PTSD = post traumatic stress disorder.

The PTSD and combat-exposed control (CEC) groups did not differ on combat exposure, childhood trauma severity or depression. However, the PTSD had significantly higher scores on the Clinician-Administered PTSD Scale (CAPS) total and on several subscales of the CAPS relative to the CEC group. A significant difference of condition was seen in the reaction time, but not accuracy, from the face-matching task. This difference was largely powered by the shorter reaction time to the shapes versus the faces, and mirrored results from prior analysis. No group, or group by condition, differences were seen for reaction time or accuracy (see Table 1; Supplementary Tables 2-4 in Additional File 1).

Neuroimaging results (region of interest analyses)

Clusters of significant activation were found for all three contrasts of interest. These were the effect of PTSD, measured as the task-related activity in PTSD versus CEC individuals; the effect of combat exposure, or task-related activity in PTSD and CEC individuals versus HCs; and the effect of task, which was the activity for face-matching minus shape-matching trials in all groups (PTSD, CEC and HC; see Table 2). In the PTSD-CEC contrast, the right insula was significantly more active in the PTSD group and the anterior cingulate was significantly more active in the CEC group. In the PTSD+CEC-HC contrast, we found significantly greater activation for the PTSD +CEC group in the right amygdala, whereas the left anterior cingulate was significantly more active in the HC group (see Figure 1). In the task effect, we found significant activation in the right and left amygdala, the right and left insula and right hippocampus, as well as significant deactivations in numerous clusters throughout the anterior cingulate, and insula (see Table 2). Additional post-hoc analysis was done contrasting the three groups on the fearful-happy contrast. The PTSD group had significantly greater activation in the amygdala than both groups (Table 3) while the CEC and HC groups did not differ significantly.

Brain-behavior correlations

When inspected in the PTSD group alone, a significant inverse correlation was observed between the avoidance subscale ("C") of the CAPS and right amygdala activation in the group (PTSD+CEC-HC) contrast (Spearman's rho = -0.976, $P < 0.001$; n = 8) and the task (faces-shapes) contrast (Spearman's rho = -0.796, $P = 0.026$; n = 8). No other subscales of the CAPS correlated significantly with amygdala activations. It should be noted the fearful-happy contrast did not correlate in the group or task contrast regions of interest (ROIs; Spearman's rho = -.228, $P = 0.588$, n = 8; and Spearman's rho = -0.132, $P = 0.756$, n = 8, respectively). The avoidance subscale was selected based on prior findings within our group [47].

Functional connectivity results

In order to examine differences within functional amygdala networks between the combat-exposed groups

Table 2 Region of interest analysis for all faces versus shapes.

Volume	x	y	z	Region	t-statisic	df	*p*
PTSD-CEC							
320	40	-23	3	Right insula	4.03	22	< 0.001
320	2	12	20	Right anterior cingulate	-2.48	22	< 0.05
(PTSD+CEC)-HC							
320	-9	27	23	Left anterior cingulate	-3.11	34	< 0.005
256	24	-5	-18	Right amygdala	2.71	34	< 0.01
PTSD+CE+HC							
3712	5	45	0	Right anterior cingulate	-5.57	35	< 0.001
1536	23	-6	-18	Right amygdala	6.14	35	< 0.001
1472	-22	-5	-18	Left amygdala	5.30	35	< 0.001
896	13	33	22	Right anterior cingulate	-3.30	35	< 0.005
576	-39	-36	20	Left insula	-3.16	35	< 0.005
512	-17	41	-5	Left anterior cingulate	-3.64	35	< 0.001
512	-3	31	-5	Left anterior cingulate	-3.05	35	< 0.005
448	-40	-22	6	Left posterior insula	3.89	35	< 0.001
384	53	-35	18	Right insula	-4.62	35	< 0.001
320	41	-24	3	Right posterior insula	3.25	35	< 0.005
256	15	39	14	Right anterior cingulate	-3.35	35	< 0.005
192	44	6	-8	Right anterior cingulate	-2.46	35	< 0.05
192	-10	31	8	Left anterior cingulate	-2.23	35	< 0.05
192	12	30	12	Right anterior cingulate	-2.30	35	< 0.05
192	51	-20	16	Right insula	-3.26	35	< 0.005

CEC, combat exposed control; HC, healthy control; PTSD; post traumatic stress disorder group.

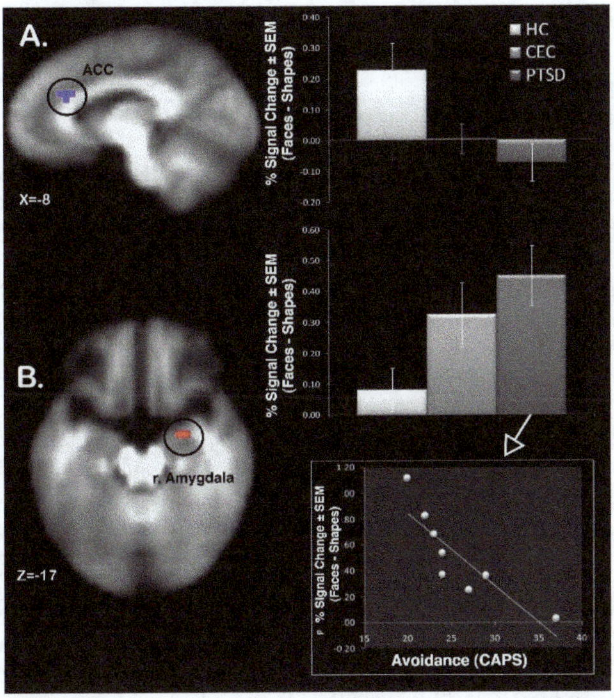

Figure 1 Faces versus shape activation differences for the combat groups versus healthy controls. (A) Anterior cingulate cortex and **(B)** amygdala. **(C)** Contrasts for angry-shape, fear-shape, and happy-shape for the amygdala region. **(D)** Correlation in the PTSD group between avoidance on the CAPS and face-shape. Details for the associated clusters provided in Table 2.

Table 3 Region of interest analysis for fearful versus happy faces

vol	x	y	z	Region	BA	t-statistic	p
PTSD > HC							
1152	-36	5	2	Left insula	13	3.13	0.01
576	36	10	14	Right insula	13	2.38	0.05
320	-23	-5	-15	Left parahippocampal Gyrus/amygdala		2.56	0.05
320	-44	10	-3	Left insula	13	2.38	0.05
320	-3	21	21	Left anterior cingulate	33	2.56	0.05
192	-21	-1	-12	Left parahippocampal Gyrus/amygdala		2.72	0.05
PTSD > CEC							
7616	40	-3	5	Right insula	13	2.93	0.01
7424	1	36	14	Right anterior cingulate	32	2.93	0.01
5376	-39	-2	1	Left insula	13	3.09	0.01
448	-36	-2	16	Left insula	13	3.53	0.005
384	-19	-3	-14	Left parahippocampal Gyrus/amygdala		3.03	0.01
192	18	-8	-15	Right parahippocampal Gyrus/amygdala		3.10	0.01
HC > CEC							
512	45	-22	8	Right posterior insula	13	2.84	0.01
448	36	7	6	Right insula	13	2.69	0.05
384	-35	2	16	Left insula	13	2.67	0.05
320	10	31	24	Right anterior cingulate	32	2.71	0.05
320	-7	30	24	Left anterior cingulate	32	2.32	0.05
PTSD+CEC+HC							
2624	38	16	-1	Right insula	13	2.96	0.01
896	-34	19	1	Left insula	13	2.77	0.05
640	7	49	-4	Right anterior cingulate	32	-4.42	0.001
384	20	-4	-17	Right parahippocampal Gyrus/amygdala		2.62	0.05
384	-13	41	-3	Left anterior cingulate	32	-2.52	0.05
384	48	5	2	Right insula	13	2.88	0.01
320	-6	30	22	Left anterior cingulate	32	2.82	0.01

CEC = combat exposed control; HC = healthy control; PTSD = post traumatic stress disorder group; BA = Brodmann Area.

(PTSD versus CEC), we performed a functional connectivity analysis with the bilateral amygdala as seed regions. This analysis revealed that the sole area that the PTSD group showed greater connectivity with the right amygdala, compared to the CEC group, was in the subgenual cingulate cortex. There was no area where PTSD showed greater connectivity using the left amygdala seed. However, the CEC compared to the PTSD group showed numerous areas with significantly greater functional connections with bilateral amygdala, such as the posterior cingulate, inferior frontal, middle occipital, and superior temporal gyri (Table 4; Supplementary Figures 1 and 2 in Additional File 1).

Discussion

This experiment yielded three main findings. First, individuals with PTSD and CECs without PTSD showed significantly greater right amygdala activation during an affective face-matching task when compared to HCs without PTSD or combat exposure in the all faces minus shapes contrast, while only the PTSD group had significantly higher activation in the amygdala for the fearful-happy contrast when contrasted with the CEC and HC groups. Second, in the PTSD group, task-related amygdala activation showed a significant inverse correlation with the severity of avoidance symptoms (as measured by the CAPS). Third, in the CEC compared to the PTSD group, the amygdala showed greater functional connectivity with frontal and parietal regions. Taken together, these findings are consistent with the hypothesis that individuals with combat exposure show a generalized increased limbic activation (in other words, in the amygdala) versus controls without combat exposure; and that among combat-exposed individuals, greater connectivity between the amygdala and frontal cortex may be associated with greater resilience to the development of PTSD. Furthermore, these findings suggest that those with PTSD may attempt to 'turn down' amygdala activation through avoidance.

Increased emotional reactivity in the amygdala has been linked to depression [48], anxiety [49,50], PTSD [14] and genetic vulnerability to psychiatric disorders [51,52]. Using the same task that was administered in the

Table 4 Functional connectivity results from amygdala task seed regions of interest differences between PTSD and CEC

Seed	vol	x	y	z	Region	BA	t-statistic	p
Right amygdala								
PTSD > CEC								
	1728	6	16	2	Subgenual cingulate gyrus/caudate	25	3.027	< 0.01
CEC > PTSD								
	59200	2	-46	28	posterior cingulate gyrus	31	-3.814	< 0.001
	11200	-49	2	4	Left superior temporal gyrus	22	-5.137	< 0.001
	5248	34	37	12	Right middle frontal gyrus	10	-4.162	< 0.001
	2624	30	-70	13	Right middle occipital gyrus	30	-3.527	< 0.005
	2368	51	-35	-5	Right middle temporal gyrus	20	-3.727	< 0.001
	2240	-36	23	-26	Left superior temporal gyrus	38	-5.271	< 0.001
	1280	-35	-38	-33	Left cerebellum		-3.281	< 0.005
	1152	-26	46	2	Left superior frontal gyrus	10	-3.699	< 0.001
	1152	-12	-21	4	Left thalamus		-2.290	< 0.05
	1024	9	-38	14	Right posterior cingulate	29	-3.107	< 0.005
	1024	50	-39	26	Right inferior parietal lobule	13	-3.539	< 0.005
	832	28	0	-37	Right uncus	20	-3.207	< 0.005
Left amygdala								
PTSD > CEC								
	-	-	-	-	-	-	-	-
CEC > PTSD								
	4096	-4	-76	26	Left occipital gyrus	18	-2.983	< 0.01
	3840	48	21	18	Right inferior frontal gyrus	45	-2.714	< 0.05
	2496	4	1	41	Right cingulate gyrus	24	-2.375	< 0.05
	1664	-49	8	12	Left precentral gyrus	44	-3.668	< 0.001
	1600	58	-50	2	Right middle temporal gyrus	21	-3.450	< 0.005
	1536	48	-47	30	Right supramarginal gyrus	40	-3.156	< 0.005
	1408	-28	13	-24	Left superior temporal gyrus	38	-2.558	< 0.05
	1408	-3	-50	31	Left precuneus	31	-2.464	< 0.05
	1408	13	-41	39	Right posterior cingulate gyrus	31	-3.087	< 0.005
	1024	32	-74	16	Right middle occipital gyrus	19	-2.601	< 0.05
	896	-6	-79	-15	Left occipital gyrus	18	-2.809	< 0.01
	832	-47	0	25	Left inferior frontal gyrus	9	-2.971	< 0.01

CEC = combat exposed control; HC = healthy control; PTSD = post traumatic stress disorder group; BA = Brodmann Area.

current study, we observed similar findings in major depressive disorder [42,43], trait anxiety [44] and victims of domestic violence [19]. The amygdala has been a relatively robust measure of trauma-related reactivity, especially in studies using PET scans [41,53-56]. However, amygdala findings have been somewhat split in the PTSD literature in fMRI studies, potentially due to avoidance or similar mechanisms associated with PTSD [9,10] and/or the exact contrasts used in the analysis. In the current study, we found that amygdala activation was greater in the PTSD group in the fearful-happy contrast. This suggests that this contrast does have specific relevance to PTSD. However, this activation did not correlate to symptom severity. In contrast, we found that combat exposure was associated with amygdala hyperactivation irrespective of PTSD in the faces versus shape contrast. Despite similarly increased amygdala activation to face-shape processing in both combat-exposed groups in the current study; it may be that different functional mechanisms and neural networks are utilized in the PTSD and CEC groups to modulate amygdala hyperactivation. Specifically, the PTSD group may potentially use a psychological mechanism (such as avoidance) while preliminary evidence suggests that the CECs use a cognitive or neural regulatory mechanism (in other words, top-down modulation). These findings further extend previous work, showing weaker connectivity with amygdala functioning in PTSD versus HCs [19,57], into the comparison with trauma-exposed controls. Even though amygdala activation was similar across trauma groups for when all faces were taken together, when fearful faces were separately contrasted with happy faces the PTSD group showed a significant difference with both control groups in more dorsal regions of the amygdala. These findings replicate prior data in PTSD literature [19-21,24,27] and suggest that PTSD individuals show a specific sensitivity to fearful faces that is not seen in trauma controls. These findings are in line with relative consistency of greater sensitivity in the amygdala with regard to aversive versus positive stimuli (such as fearful versus happy faces). The capacity to modulate the amygdala can therefore be an effective way to control affective responses to aversive stimuli.

There is strong evidence of a reciprocal relationship between activation in the medial prefrontal cortex and amygdala in PTSD in combat veterans [54]. This work also showed that regional blood flow in the amygdala correlated positively with PTSD symptom severity while blood flow in the medial prefrontal cortex correlated negatively with PTSD symptom severity. A similar reciprocal relationship between the subgenual cingulate and amygdala has been shown in depression [58], as well as in normal controls where the rostral cingulate and lateral prefrontal cortex in conjunction appear to regulate the amygdala during processing of faces [59,60]. Furthermore, animal and human data appear to converge on a model in which successful fear extinction depends on the functionality of this network [61]. Taken together, these studies suggest that this amygdala-prefrontal cortex network may play an important role in trauma exposure such that those who experience trauma and have more robust connections between the amygdala and the prefrontal cortex are less likely to develop PTSD [11,15,35].

It is important to note that, although the CEC group showed greater functional connections between the amygdala and numerous regions across the brain, only the subgenual cingulate cluster was found to be more functionally connected to the amygdala in the PTSD group. In a prior study using the same task, we observed similar patterns of functional connectivity, whereby the dorsal cingulate was less functionally connected with the amygdala and the subgenual cingulate was more functionally connected with the amygdala in depressed versus non-depressed individuals [43]. Decreased connectivity between the amygdala and the dorsal anterior cingulate cortex (ACC) has been observed in individuals with current depression relative to controls [62,63], and connectivity increased significantly in depressed individuals following treatment [62]. These findings are in line with evidence that altered functional activity of the amygdala and cingulate may represent a biomarker for psychiatric stress. In a separate study that investigated face processing, contrasting PTSD due to domestic violence and HCs, we found that the subgenual cingulate, in contrast to the insula, showed greater connectivity in the PTSD group [57]. We interpret these findings as an indication of a recursive connection that further fosters, rather than regulates, regional activation. In line with this hypothesis, prior research has indicated that the subgenual/rostral cingulate is an important region for modulation of amygdala reaction [60,64,65]. The subgenual cingulate has specifically been outlined as being a primary area in the response to sad faces as well as being a biomarker for negative mood [49,66-68]. Several PET and fMRI studies indicate that neural substrates such as the amygdala and subgenual cingulate, which are critical for emotion processing, are hyperactive in individuals with major depressive disorder both at rest [58] and during emotional tasks [69-72]. Conversely, brain structures such as the dorsal ACC and middle/superior frontal gyrus, which are involved in the cognitive control of behavior [73] and emotion [74], are hypoactive in individuals with depression both at rest [58] and during cognitive tasks [75]. Anatomical studies in animal have identified efferent projections from the ACC to the amygdala [76]. In connectivity studies in humans, the subgenual ACC showed strong connections with the amygdala and medial temporal lobe [77]. It has been suggested that subgenual ACC activation is observed when individuals attend to their internal emotional states [78]. Related evidence suggests that this structure is deactivated by performing difficult cognitive tasks that require an external focus of attention and prompt inhibitory control processes [79,80]. This further suggests that the CECs are enacting a more cognitive approach to the situation than the PTSD group.

Modulatory control of behavioral-affective responses such as avoidance has been posited as an important mechanism for regulating emotional responses in individuals with PTSD in both psychological [81] and neural [82] models. Avoidance symptoms inversely correlate with brain activation in task relevant emotional processing areas [83] as well as in individuals with PTSD compared to non-traumatized [47] and traumatized controls [84]. In addition, individuals with PTSD experiencing greater dissociative symptomology, as opposed to greater re-experiencing symptoms, showed attenuation of connectivity to a wide area of brain regions important in affective processing [85]. Diffusion tensor imaging studies in PTSD suggest that the anatomical integrity of connecting fibers in the medial and posterior corpus may be compromised in children with PTSD with a history of childhood maltreatment [86]. Similar reductions in posterior white matter integrity were found in the right superior longitudinal fasciculus OEF/OIF combat veterans who develop psychiatric disorders, such as major depressive disorder, after blast-related concussion [42]. Taken together, these findings support the notion that avoidance symptoms in PTSD may be associated with reduced amygdala connectivity with frontal structures. This provides confirmatory evidence for the hypothesis that individuals with PTSD may show less neural/cognitive control and resort to increased symptom avoidance.

Other important regions of differential activation were observed in the current study. Specifically, the anterior cingulate gyrus was more active in the HCs versus the CECs as well as in CECs versus the individuals with PTSD. Also, the insula was more active in the PTSD patients versus the CECs. Several prior studies have reported anterior cingulate gyrus hypoactivity in PTSD [87-89], which has been hypothesized to relate to the degree to which those with PTSD engage in emotional tasks. This hypothesis is congruent with the current findings. Increased insula activation has also been associated with PTSD [9,87]. This may suggest that individuals with PTSD have an impaired ability to maintain homeostasis via integration of physiological and emotional information [90]. Our prior work indicates that those with PTSD may have greater ability to alter insula activation in the face of a changing affective environment [91].

This study has several notable limitations. First, while a complete structured clinical interview was completed in all individuals, six of the 24 participants did not complete the CAPS. Therefore, it was not possible to determine if the correlation with avoidance symptoms remained significant across the complete sample. Second, the task used was not, nor was it intended to be, a provocation task. Thus trauma response is not being modeled in the current design; rather, everyday emotion processing patterns are being assessed. In addition, the face versus shape contrast focuses on face-processing in addition to a fearful versus happy contrast. The fearful versus happy faces contrast was done primarily to verify that the current dataset is behaving in accordance with prior literature. The faces versus shape contrast was selected due to its robust findings as well as the importance of face-processing in daily functioning. While these two conditions are very different, the group differences in areas of affective processing areas are the primary focus of this paper. This contrast is being used to probe the social affective processing of judging facial expressions without focus on valence. Third, the results of this study require replication given the modest size of the sample. Fourth, since the initiation of this study much has been learned about the importance of comorbid head injury. Unfortunately, this was not measured or controlled for in the current study.

Conclusions

PTSD, like all mental disorders, has a multifactorial etiology. The current study highlights the potential impact of trauma exposure on neural response to affectively relevant stimuli, regardless of whether or not this trauma experience results in PTSD. Prior studies investigating the neuropsychological sequelae of OEF/OIF combat suggest that trauma exposure may explain more of the variance in cognitive performance than PTSD alone [92]. Following the experience of trauma, the development and maintenance of PTSD may relate to the way in which individuals attempt to regulate this hyperactivation. Here, we find that those without PTSD activate more top-down modulatory areas, while those who acquire PTSD show less neural connectivity with emotion regulation centers but instead exhibit avoidance. It is unclear from the current findings if these effects represent vulnerabilities, or rather are results of the trauma experience.

Methods

Subjects

Twelve men with combat-related PTSD, 12 men with combat-exposure without PTSD (CEC), and 12 HC men with no history of combat exposure or PTSD completed a face-matching task during fMRI. The groups were demographically matched (Table 1). Subjects were excluded if they had a lifetime history of alcohol or substance dependence, a history of alcohol or substance abuse within 30 days of study participation, irremovable ferromagnetic material, claustrophobia, bipolar disorder or schizophrenia. PTSD subjects with other comorbid anxiety or mood disorders, such as major depressive disorder, were included as long as PTSD was the clinically predominant disorder. The CEC group had experienced a PTSD 'Criterion A' event but did not have current or past PTSD. The CEC group was free of Axis I psychiatric diagnosis. The HC group had no military experience, no history of a PTSD 'Criterion A' event, and no history of current or past Axis I psychiatric diagnoses. PTSD and CEC participants were recruited from the VA San Diego Healthcare System. All participants gave informed written consent to participate in this study, which was approved by the University of California San Diego Human Research Protection Program and the Research and Development Committee at the VA San Diego Healthcare System.

Psychiatric measures

All subjects completed a Structured Clinical Interview for Diagnostic and Statistical Manual of Mental Disorders edition 4 (SCID) [93] including the PTSD module, the Beck Depression Inventory (BDI) [94], Childhood Trauma Questionnaire [95] and the Combat Exposure Scale [96]. In addition, eight PTSD and ten CEC participants performed an additional session during which the CAPS [97] was completed. The presence of PTSD was determined by the results of the PTSD module of the SCID, and the diagnosis was confirmed by a board certified psychiatrist (DGB/MPP) and confirmed by the CAPS when available.

Stimulus and apparatus

During fMRI, participants performed a face-matching task, with a comparison condition of shape matching (described in more detail in [43,44]). Each five-second trial consisted of a target face (on the top of the computer screen) and two probe faces (on the bottom left and bottom right of the computer screen). Participants were instructed to match the emotion (angry, fearful or happy) of the target and probe faces. The trials were block designed, such that each block consisted of six consecutive trials in which the target face was angry, fearful or happy. During the shape-matching control condition, subjects were presented with an analogous configuration of ovals and circles, and were instructed to match the shape of the target and probe stimuli. Each block of the faces and shapes was presented three times in pseudorandom order, and a fixation cross was interspersed between each block. Reaction time (RT) data were obtained for each trial. Due to device errors, RT was not recorded from three participants (one from the PTSD and two from the CEC group); however this did not affect subject feedback or the subject experience.

Image acquisition

fMRI data were collected during the task using a Signa EXCITE 3.0 Tesla GE (General Electric, New York, NY, USA) scanner (T2-weighted echo planar imaging, repetition time (TR) = 2000 ms, echo time (TE) = 32 ms, field of view (FOV) = 230 × 230 mm^3, 64 × 64 matrix, yielding 30 2.6 mm axial slices with a 1.4 mm gap, 256 scans). For anatomical reference, a high resolution T1-weighted image (spoiled grass sequence; inversion time = 450 ms, TR = 8 ms, TE = 4 ms, FOV = 250 × 250 mm^3, flip angle = 12°, 172 sagittally acquired slices, approximately 1 mm^3 voxels) was obtained during the same session.

fMRI analysis pathway/image processing

Single subject

All structural and functional image processing was done with the Analysis of Functional Neuroimages software package (AFNI, Bethesda, MD, USA). The echoplanar images were realigned to a base using a Fourier transform using the AFNI program 3dvolreg and then time-corrected for slice acquisition order. Preprocessed time series data for each individual were analyzed using a multiple regression model. For this model, the four orthogonal regressors of interest were (1) happy, (2) angry, (3) fearful and (4) circle/oval sensorimotor condition. These regressors were convolved with a modified gamma variate function to account for the delay and the dispersion of the hemodynamic response of the BOLD-fMRI signal. Additionally, five nuisance regressors were used to account for residual motion (roll, pitch and yaw) and to eliminate slow signal drifts (baseline and linear trend). These nine regressors were applied to the AFNI program 3dDeconvolve in order to calculate the estimated voxel-wise response amplitude. The linear contrast of all faces versus shapes was used for maximal power in subsequent analyses. In addition, the fearful-happy faces were analyzed to provide better comparison of these results with prior literature. To account for individual variation of anatomical landmarks, a Gaussian filter with 4 mm full width at half maximum was applied to the voxelwise percent signal change data and then resampled to a 4 mm^3 voxel dimension.

Group analysis

Data for each subject were normalized to Talairach coordinates. A voxel-based two-way ANOVA was performed with group (PTSD, CEC and HC) as a fixed factor and participants as a random factor within AFNI on the faces-shapes contrast. An additional, post-hoc ANOVA was performed on the fearful-happy contrast. *A priori* ROIs, including the amygdala, hippocampus, cingulate cortex and insula, were used as masks, as these regions are of interest in PTSD [98], stress [99] and face processing [100]. Based on these four areas, a voxel-wise *a priori* probability of 0.05 was determined via simulations using the AFNI function AlphaSim [101], which resulted in a corrected cluster-wise activation probability of 0.05 using a minimum volume of 192 mm^3 and three connected voxels (for an amygdala or hippocampus cluster), or 320 mm^3 and five connected voxels (for a cingulate or insular cortex cluster). Small volume corrections were used to inspect areas that may not have been of sufficient size to meet minimum whole brain cluster size corrections. Using the thresholds and cluster sizes defined above, the corrected voxel-wise probabilities are as follows: amygdala $P < 0.002$, hippocampus $P < 0.0002$, cingulate cortex $P < 0.0008$ and insular cortex $P < 0.0008$. The areas of interest were superimposed on each individual's voxel-wise percent signal change brain image. Stereotactic coordinates of the ROIs were based on standardized atlas locations [102]. Only the activations within the regions of interest that survived the volume and voxel correction criteria were extracted and used for further analysis.

Functional connectivity analysis

To examine between-group differences in functional connectivity within the amygdala, we performed a modified Psycho-Physiological Interaction analysis that has been used previously [103]. Prior to this analysis, the individual raw signal datasets were: (a) band-pass filtered (0.009 Hz < f < 0.08 Hz), (b) corrected for slice-dependent time shifts, (c) corrected for interleaved acquisition, (d) corrected for rigid body head motion, and (e) warped to conform to the Talairach atlas. Individual time courses in the processed raw signal datasets were extracted from seed ROIs in left and right amygdala. These two seeds were identified based on the task-related activation in all 36 subjects related to all face-matching minus all shape-matching trials (see Table 2). This region was selected to provide a task relevant region that was minimally biased between groups. A total of twelve regressors were then entered into a multiple regression against the voxel-based time series: the regressors of interest being the interaction between seed region time-course and faces blocks, along with 11 nuance regressors: three movement (roll, pitch, yaw) regressors, the four task regressors described previously, the entire time course of the seed region, the entire time course of the white matter, and baseline and linear trend regressors. The deconvolution analyses for left and right amygdala were run separately. The resulting correlation coefficients were then calculated for each voxel, providing correlation maps of the relationships between the time courses of activation in the voxels within the seed ROI's and all voxels. The Fisher's Z transforms of these correlation maps were then warped to conform to the Talairach atlas and a Gaussian blur of 4 mm full width half maximum was applied to allow for a between-groups comparison. Data for each subject were normalized to Talairach coordinates. A voxel-based two-way ANOVA was performed with group (PTSD, CEC and HC) as a fixed factor and participants as a random factor within AFNI on the Fisher Z for each amygdala. The following planned linear contrasts were performed: (1) PTSD-CEC, to determine the effects of PTSD, (2) PTSD+CEC-HC, to determine the effects of trauma exposure and (3) PTSD+CEC+HC, to determine the task effects. A voxel-wise *a priori* probability of 0.05 was determined via simulations using the AFNI function AlphaSim, as above, which resulted in a corrected cluster-wise activation probability of 0.05 using a minimum volume of 768 mm^3 in a whole brain analysis.

Statistical analysis

All behavioral and secondary analyses were carried out with StatistiXL 1.8 (StatistiXL, Nedlands, Western Australia). Continuous demographic and performance variables such as age, education, RT and accuracy were compared between the groups in a fixed-factor ANOVA. Ethnicity was compared using a chi-squared test across all three groups. Clinical measures, such as BDI and CAPS scores, were compared between PTSD and CEC groups using a two-sample t-test.

Additional material

Additional file 1: Supplementary Data. Additional information to aid in the interpretation of the results (as listed below). Supplementary Table 1. Whole brain group contrasts for the faces versus shape. Supplementary Table 2. Task accuracy data group by condition. Supplementary Table 3. Within subjects analysis of task performance data. Supplementary Table 4. Between subject analysis of task performance data. Supplementary Figure 1. Functional connectivity results from left amygdala task seed region of interest differences between PTSD and CEC. Supplementary Figure 2. Functional connectivity results from right amygdala task seed region of interest differences between PTSD and CEC.

List of abbreviations

ACC: anterior cingulate cortex; AFNI: analysis of functional neuroimages; ANOVA: analysis of variance; BDI: Beck Depression Inventory; CAPS: Clinician-Administered PTSD Scale; CEC: combat exposed control; fMRI: functional magnetic resonance imaging; FOV: field of view; HC: healthy control; OEF: Operation Enduring Freedom; OIF: Operation Iraqi Freedom; PET: positron emission tomography; PTSD: post-traumatic stress disorder; ROI: region of interest; RT: reaction time; SCID: Structured Clinical Interview for DSM-IV; TE: echo time; TR: repetition time.

Acknowledgements

Some of this work was supported by the VA Center of Excellence for Stress and Mental Health (CESAMH; ANS, MPP) and a VA Merit (ANS and MPP), which is supported by the Department of Veterans Affairs. CESAMH is affiliated with VISN 22, the Veterans Affairs San Diego Healthcare System and the University of California, San Diego. Dr Matthews' VA salary is supported by a Career Development Award through the VA Clinical Science Research and Development Service. We appreciate the feedback of the reviewers towards improving this manuscript.

Author details

[1]Veterans Affairs San Diego Healthcare System, 3350 La Jolla Village Drive, San Diego, CA 92161, USA. [2]University of California San Diego, 9500 Gilman Drive, La Jolla, CA 92093, USA. [3]Center of Excellence in Stress and Mental Health, VASDHS, 3350 La Jolla Village Drive, San Diego, CA 92161, USA. [4]Research Service & VA Mental Illness Research, Education and Clinical Center, VASDHS, 3350 La Jolla Village Drive, San Diego, CA 92161, USA.

Authors' contributions

ANS was involved in the conception and design of the study as well as acquisition, analysis and interpretation of data. SCM was involved in interpretation of the data. IAS was involved in analysis and interpretation of the data. DBG was involved in the acquisition of the study data. HKD and AM were involved in the acquisition of the data for the study. MBS and MPP participated in the conception and design of the study. All authors read, contributed to and approved the final manuscript.

Competing interests

The authors declare that they have no competing interests.

References

1. Hoge CW, Auchterlonie JL, Milliken CS: **Mental health problems, use of mental health services, and attrition from military service after returning from deployment to Iraq or Afghanistan.** *JAMA* 2006, **295**:1023-1032.
2. Breslau N: **The epidemiology of posttraumatic stress disorder: what is the extent of the problem?** *J Clin Psychiatry* 2001, **62(Suppl 17)**:16-22.
3. Boscarino JA: **Posttraumatic stress disorder and mortality among U.S. Army veterans 30 years after military service.** *Ann Epidemiol* 2006, **16**:248-256.
4. North CS, Nixon SJ, Shariat S, Mallonee S, McMillen JC, Spitznagel EL, Smith EM: **Psychiatric disorders among survivors of the Oklahoma City bombing.** *JAMA* 1999, **282**:755-762.
5. Geracioti TD Jr, Carpenter LL, Owens MJ, Baker DG, Ekhator NN, Horn PS, Strawn JR, Sanacora G, Kinkead B, Price LH, Nemeroff CB: **Elevated cerebrospinal fluid substance p concentrations in posttraumatic stress disorder and major depression.** *Am J Psychiatry* 2006, **163**:637-643.
6. Bremner JD, Vythilingam M, Anderson G, Vermetten E, McGlashan T, Heninger G, Rasmusson A, Southwick SM, Charney DS: **Assessment of the hypothalamic-pituitary-adrenal axis over a 24-hour diurnal period and in response to neuroendocrine challenges in women with and without**

childhood sexual abuse and posttraumatic stress disorder. *Biol Psychiatry* 2003, **54**:710-718.
7. Liberzon I, Abelson JL, Flagel SB, Raz J, Young EA: **Neuroendocrine and psychophysiologic responses in PTSD: a symptom provocation study.** *Neuropsychopharmacology* 1999, **21**:40-50.
8. Bremner JD, Licinio J, Darnell A, Krystal JH, Owens MJ, Southwick SM, Nemeroff CB, Charney DS: **Elevated CSF corticotropin-releasing factor concentrations in posttraumatic stress disorder.** *Am J Psychiatry* 1997, **154**:624-629.
9. Simmons AN, Paulus MP, Thorpe SR, Matthews SC, Norman SB, Stein MB: **Functional activation and neural networks in women with posttraumatic stress disorder related to intimate partner violence.** *Biol Psychiatry* 2008, **64**:681-690.
10. Etkin A, Wager TD: **Functional neuroimaging of anxiety: a meta-analysis of emotional processing in PTSD, social anxiety disorder, and specific phobia.** *Am J Psychiatry* 2007, **164**:1476-1488.
11. Shin LM, Liberzon I: **The neurocircuitry of fear, stress, and anxiety disorders.** *Neuropsychopharmacology* 2010, **35**:169-91.
12. Barad M, Gean PW, Lutz B: **The role of the amygdala in the extinction of conditioned fear.** *Biol Psychiatry* 2006, **60**:322-328.
13. Rudy JW, Huff NC, Matus-Amat P: **Understanding contextual fear conditioning.** *Neurosci Biobehav Rev* 2004, **28**:675-685.
14. Rauch SL, Shin LM, Phelps EA: **Neurocircuitry models of posttraumatic stress disorder and extinction: human neuroimaging research–past, present, and future.** *Biol Psychiatry* 2006, **60**:376-382.
15. Shin LM, Rauch SL, Pitman RK: **Amygdala, medial prefrontal cortex, and hippocampal function in PTSD.** *Ann N Y Acad Sci* 2006, **1071**:67-79.
16. Hull AM: **Neuroimaging findings in post-traumatic stress disorder. Systematic review.** *Br J Psychiatry* 2002, **181**:102-110.
17. Simmons AN, Matthews SC: **Neural circuitry of PTSD with or without mild traumatic brain injury: a meta-analysis.** *Neuropharmacology* 2011.
18. Bryant RA, Kemp AH, Felmingham KL, Liddell B, Olivieri G, Peduto A, Gordon E, Williams LM: **Enhanced amygdala and medial prefrontal activation during nonconscious processing of fear in posttraumatic stress disorder: An fMRI study.** *Hum Brain Mapp* 2008, **29**:517-523.
19. Fonzo GA, Simmons AN, Thorp SR, Norman SB, Paulus MP, Stein MB: **Exaggerated and disconnected insular-amygdalar blood oxygenation level-dependent response to threat-related emotional faces in women with intimate-partner violence posttraumatic stress disorder.** *Biol Psychiatry* 2010, **68**:433-441.
20. Bryant RA, Kemp AH, Felmingham KL, Liddell B, Olivieri G, Peduto A, Gordon E, Williams LM: **Enhanced amygdala and medial prefrontal activation during nonconscious processing of fear in posttraumatic stress disorder: an fMRI study.** *Hum Brain Mapp* 2008, **29**:517-523.
21. Shin LM, Wright CI, Cannistraro PA, Wedig MM, McMullin K, Martis B, Macklin ML, Lasko NB, Cavanagh SR, Krangel TS, Orr SP, Pitman RK, Whalen PJ, Rauch SL: **A functional magnetic resonance imaging study of amygdala and medial prefrontal cortex responses to overtly presented fearful faces in posttraumatic stress disorder.** *Arch Gen Psychiatry* 2005, **62**:273-281.
22. Armony JL, Corbo V, Clement MH, Brunet A: **Amygdala response in patients with acute PTSD to masked and unmasked emotional facial expressions.** *Am J Psychiatry* 2005, **162**:1961-1963.
23. Protopopescu X, Pan H, Tuescher O, Cloitre M, Goldstein M, Engelien W, Epstein J, Yang Y, Gorman J, LeDoux J, Silbersweig D, Stern E: **Differential time courses and specificity of amygdala activity in posttraumatic stress disorder subjects and normal control subjects.** *Biol Psychiatry* 2005, **57**:464-473.
24. Williams LM, Kemp AH, Felmingham K, Barton M, Olivieri G, Peduto A, Gordon E, Bryant RA: **Trauma modulates amygdala and medial prefrontal responses to consciously attended fear.** *Neuroimage* 2006, **29**:347-357.
25. Bryant RA, Felmingham KL, Kemp AH, Barton M, Peduto AS, Rennie C, Gordon E, Williams LM: **Neural networks of information processing in posttraumatic stress disorder: a functional magnetic resonance imaging study.** *Biol Psychiatry* 2005, **58**:111-118.
26. Morey RA, Dolcos F, Petty CM, Cooper DA, Hayes JP, LaBar KS, McCarthy G: **The role of trauma-related distractors on neural systems for working memory and emotion processing in posttraumatic stress disorder.** *J Psychiatr Res* 2009, **43**:809-817.
27. Rauch SL, Whalen PJ, Shin LM, McInerney SC, Macklin ML, Lasko NB, Orr SP, Pitman RK: **Exaggerated amygdala response to masked facial stimuli in posttraumatic stress disorder.** *Biol Psychiatry* 2000, **47**:769-776.
28. Hendler T, Rotshtein P, Yeshurun Y, Weizmann T, Kahn I, Ben-Bashat D, Malach R, Bleich A: **Sensing the invisible: differential sensitivity of visual cortex and amygdala to traumatic context.** *Neuroimage* 2003, **19**:587-600.
29. Chen S, Li L, Xu B, Liu J: **Insular cortex involvement in declarative memory deficits in patients with post-traumatic stress disorder.** *BMC Psychiatry* 2009, **9**:39.
30. American Psychiatric Association: *Diagnostic and statistical manual of mental disorders: DSM-IV-TR.* 4 edition. Washington, DC: American Psychiatric Association; 2000.
31. Vasterling JJ, Proctor SP, Amoroso P, Kane R, Heeren T, White RF: **Neuropsychological outcomes of army personnel following deployment to the Iraq war.** *JAMA* 2006, **296**:519-529.
32. Foa EB, Kozak MJ: **Emotional processing of fear: exposure to corrective information.** *Psychol Bull* 1986, **99**:20-35.
33. Krause ED, Kaltman S, Goodman LA, Dutton MA: **Avoidant coping and PTSD symptoms related to domestic violence exposure: a longitudinal study.** *J Trauma Stress* 2008, **21**:83-90.
34. Foa EB: **Psychological processes related to recovery from a trauma and an effective treatment for PTSD.** *Ann N Y Acad Sci* 1997, **821**:410-424.
35. Liberzon I, Sripada CS: **The functional neuroanatomy of PTSD: a critical review.** *Prog Brain Res* 2008, **167**:151-169.
36. Sierra M, Berrios GE: **Depersonalization: neurobiological perspectives.** *Biol Psychiatry* 1998, **44**:898-908.
37. Lanius RA, Williamson PC, Boksman K, Densmore M, Gupta M, Neufeld RW, Gati JS, Menon RS: **Brain activation during script-driven imagery induced dissociative responses in PTSD: a functional magnetic resonance imaging investigation.** *Biol Psychiatry* 2002, **52**:305-311.
38. Falconer E, Bryant R, Felmingham KL, Kemp AH, Gordon E, Peduto A, Olivieri G, Williams LM: **The neural networks of inhibitory control in posttraumatic stress disorder.** *J Psychiatry Neurosci* 2008, **33**:413-422.
39. New AS, Fan J, Murrough JW, Liu X, Liebman RE, Guise KG, Tang CY, Charney DS: **A functional magnetic resonance imaging study of deliberate emotion regulation in resilience and posttraumatic stress disorder.** *Biol Psychiatry* 2009, **66**:656-664.
40. Phan KL, Britton JC, Taylor SF, Fig LM, Liberzon I: **Corticolimbic blood flow during nontraumatic emotional processing in posttraumatic stress disorder.** *Arch Gen Psychiatry* 2006, **63**:184-192.
41. Britton JC, Phan KL, Taylor SF, Fig LM, Liberzon I: **Corticolimbic blood flow in posttraumatic stress disorder during script-driven imagery.** *Biol Psychiatry* 2005, **57**:832-840.
42. Matthews SC, Strigo IA, Simmons AN, O'Connell RM, Reinhardt LE, Moseley SA: **A multimodal imaging study in U.S. veterans of Operations Iraqi and Enduring Freedom with and without major depression after blast-related concussion.** *Neuroimage* 2011, **54(Suppl 1)**:S69-S75.
43. Matthews SC, Strigo IA, Simmons AN, Yang TT, Paulus MP: **Decreased functional coupling of the amygdala and supragenual cingulate is related to increased depression in unmedicated individuals with current major depressive disorder.** *J Affect Disord* 2008, **111**:13-20.
44. Stein MB, Simmons AN, Feinstein JS, Paulus MP: **Increased amygdala and insula activation during emotion processing in anxiety-prone subjects.** *Am J Psychiatry* 2007, **164**:318-327.
45. Arce E, Simmons AN, Lovero KL, Stein MB, Paulus MP: **Escitalopram effects on insula and amygdala BOLD activation during emotional processing.** *Psychopharmacology (Berl)* 2008, **196**:661-672.
46. Paulus MP, Feinstein JS, Castillo G, Simmons AN, Stein MB: **Dose-dependent decrease of activation in bilateral amygdala and insula by lorazepam during emotion processing.** *Arch Gen Psychiatry* 2005, **62**:282-288.
47. Strigo IA, Simmons AN, Matthews SC, Grimes EM, Allard CB, Reinhardt LE, Paulus MP, Stein MB: **Neural correlates of altered pain response in women with posttraumatic stress disorder from intimate partner violence.** *Biol Psychiatry* 2010, **68**:442-450.
48. Nestler EJ, Barrot M, DiLeone RJ, Eisch AJ, Gold SJ, Monteggia LM: **Neurobiology of depression.** *Neuron* 2002, **34**:13-25.
49. Phillips ML, Drevets WC, Rauch SL, Lane R: **Neurobiology of emotion perception I.** *Biol Psychiatry* 2003, **54**:504-514.
50. LeDoux JE: **Emotion circuits in the brain.** *Ann Rev Neurosci* 2000, **23**:155-184.
51. Hariri AR, Holmes A: **Genetics of emotional regulation: the role of the serotonin transporter in neural function.** *Trends Cogn Sci* 2006, **10**:182-191.

52. Brown SM, Hariri AR: **Neuroimaging studies of serotonin gene polymorphisms: exploring the interplay of genes, brain, and behavior.** *Cogn Affect Behav Neurosci* 2006, **6**:44-52.
53. Gilboa A, Shalev AY, Laor L, Lester H, Louzoun Y, Chisin R, Bonne O: **Functional connectivity of the prefrontal cortex and the amygdala in posttraumatic stress disorder.** *Biol Psychiatry* 2004, **55**:263-272.
54. Shin LM, Orr SP, Carson MA, Rauch SL, Macklin ML, Lasko NB, Peters PM, Metzger LJ, Dougherty DD, Cannistraro PA, Alpert NM, Fischman AJ, Pitman RK: **Regional cerebral blood flow in the amygdala and medial prefrontal cortex during traumatic imagery in male and female Vietnam veterans with PTSD.** *Arch Gen Psychiatry* 2004, **61**:168-176.
55. Seedat S, Warwick J, van Heerden B, Hugo C, Zungu-Dirwayi N, Van Kradenburg J, Stein DJ: **Single photon emission computed tomography in posttraumatic stress disorder before and after treatment with a selective serotonin reuptake inhibitor.** *J Affect Disord* 2004, **80**:45-53.
56. Liberzon I, Britton JC, Phan KL: **Neural correlates of traumatic recall in posttraumatic stress disorder.** *Stress* 2003, **6**:151-156.
57. Simmons AN, Paulus MP, Thorp SR, Matthews SC, Norman SB, Stein MB: **Functional activation and neural networks in women with posttraumatic stress disorder related to intimate partner violence.** *Biol Psychiatry* 2008, **64**:681-690.
58. Mayberg HS, Liotti M, Brannan SK, McGinnis S, Mahurin RK, Jerabek PA, Silva JA, Tekell JL, Martin CC, Lancaster JL, Fox PT: **Reciprocal limbic-cortical function and negative mood: converging PET findings in depression and normal sadness.** *Am J Psychiatry* 1999, **156**:675-682.
59. Egner T, Etkin A, Gale S, Hirsch J: **Dissociable neural systems resolve conflict from emotional versus nonemotional distracters.** *Cereb Cortex* 2008, **18**:1475-1484.
60. Etkin A, Egner T, Peraza DM, Kandel ER, Hirsch J: **Resolving emotional conflict: a role for the rostral anterior cingulate cortex in modulating activity in the amygdala.** *Neuron* 2006, **51**:871-882.
61. Hartley CA, Phelps EA: **Changing fear: the neurocircuitry of emotion regulation.** *Neuropsychopharmacology* 2010, **35**:136-146.
62. Chen CH, Suckling J, Ooi C, Fu CH, Williams SC, Walsh ND, Mitterschiffthaler MT, Pich EM, Bullmore E: **Functional coupling of the amygdala in depressed patients treated with antidepressant medication.** *Neuropsychopharmacology* 2008, **33**:1909-1918.
63. Anand A, Li Y, Wang Y, Wu J, Gao S, Bukhari L, Mathews VP, Kalnin A, Lowe MJ: **Activity and connectivity of brain mood regulating circuit in depression: a functional magnetic resonance study.** *Biol Psychiatry* 2005, **57**:1079-1088.
64. Etkin A, Prater KE, Schatzberg AF, Menon V, Greicius MD: **Disrupted amygdalar subregion functional connectivity and evidence of a compensatory network in generalized anxiety disorder.** *Arch Gen Psychiatry* 2009, **66**:1361-1372.
65. Straube T, Glauer M, Dilger S, Mentzel HJ, Miltner WH: **Effects of cognitive-behavioral therapy on brain activation in specific phobia.** *Neuroimage* 2005.
66. Mayberg HS, Lozano AM, Voon V, McNeely HE, Seminowicz D, Hamani C, Schwalb JM, Kennedy SH: **Deep brain stimulation for treatment-resistant depression.** *Neuron* 2005, **45**:651-660.
67. Seminowicz DA, Mayberg HS, McIntosh AR, Goldapple K, Kennedy S, Segal Z, Rafi-Tari S: **Limbic-frontal circuitry in major depression: a path modeling metanalysis.** *Neuroimage* 2004, **22**:409-418.
68. Phillips ML, Drevets WC, Rauch SL, Lane R: **Neurobiology of emotion perception II.** *Biol Psychiatry* 2003, **54**:515-528.
69. Drevets WC, Price JL, Simpson JR, Todd RD, Reich T, Vannier M, Raichle ME: **Subgenual prefrontal cortex abnormalities in mood disorders.** *Nature* 1997, **386**:824-827.
70. Sheline YI, Barch DM, Donnelly JM, Ollinger JM, Snyder AZ, Mintun MA: **Increased amygdala response to masked emotional faces in depressed subjects resolves with antidepressant treatment: an fMRI study.** *Biol Psychiatry* 2001, **50**:651-658.
71. Siegle GJ, Steinhauer SR, Thase ME, Stenger VA, Carter CS: **Can't shake that feeling: event-related fMRI assessment of sustained amygdala activity in response to emotional information in depressed individuals.** *Biol Psychiatry* 2002, **51**:693-707.
72. Siegle GJ, Thompson W, Carter CS, Steinhauer SR, Thase ME: **Increased amygdala and decreased dorsolateral prefrontal BOLD responses in unipolar depression: related and independent features.** *Biol Psychiatry* 2007, **61**:198-209.
73. Aron AR, Behrens TE, Smith S, Frank MJ, Poldrack RA: **Triangulating a cognitive control network using diffusion-weighted magnetic resonance imaging (MRI) and functional MRI.** *J Neurosci* 2007, **27**:3743-3752.
74. Ochsner KN, Gross JJ: **The cognitive control of emotion.** *Trends Cogn Sci* 2005, **9**:242-249.
75. George MS, Ketter TA, Parekh PI, Rosinsky N, Ring HA, Pazzaglia PJ, Marangell LB, Callahan AM, Post RM: **Blunted left cingulate activation in mood disorder subjects during a response interference task (the Stroop).** *J Neuropsychiatry Clin Neurosci* 1997, **9**:55-63.
76. Paus T: **Primate anterior cingulate cortex: where motor control, drive and cognition interface.** *Nat Rev Neurosci* 2001, **2**:417-424.
77. Margulies DS, Kelly AM, Uddin LQ, Biswal BB, Castellanos FX, Milham MP: **Mapping the functional connectivity of anterior cingulate cortex.** *Neuroimage* 2007, **37**:579-588.
78. Lane RD, Fink GR, Chau PM, Dolan RJ: **Neural activation during selective attention to subjective emotional responses.** *Neuroreport* 1997, **8**:3969-3972.
79. Kennedy DP, Redcay E, Courchesne E: **Failing to deactivate: resting functional abnormalities in autism.** *Proc Natl Acad Sci USA* 2006, **103**:8275-8280.
80. Marsh R, Zhu H, Schultz RT, Quackenbush G, Royal J, Skudlarski P, Peterson BS: **A developmental fMRI study of self-regulatory control.** *Hum Brain Mapp* 2006, **27**:848-863.
81. Foa EB, Stein DJ, McFarlane AC: **Symptomatology and psychopathology of mental health problems after disaster.** *J Clin Psychiatry* 2006, **67(Suppl 2)**:15-25.
82. Krystal JH, Bennett AL, Bremner JD, Southwick SM, Charney DS: **Toward a cognitive neuroscience of dissociation and altered memory functions in post-traumatic stress disorder.**Edited by: Friedmen MJ, Charney DS, Deutsch AY. Neurobiological and clinical consequences of stress: from normal adaptions to PTSD. New York: Raven Press; 1995:239-68.
83. Hopper JW, Frewen PA, van der Kolk BA, Lanius RA: **Neural correlates of reexperiencing, avoidance, and dissociation in PTSD: symptom dimensions and emotion dysregulation in responses to script-driven trauma imagery.** *J Trauma Stress* 2007, **20**:713-725.
84. Lanius RA, Williamson PC, Densmore M, Boksman K, Gupta MA, Neufeld RW, Gati JS, Menon RS: **Neural correlates of traumatic memories in posttraumatic stress disorder: a functional MRI investigation.** *Am J Psychiatry* 2001, **158**:1920-1922.
85. Lanius RA, Williamson PC, Bluhm RL, Densmore M, Boksman K, Neufeld RW, Gati JS, Menon RS: **Functional connectivity of dissociative responses in posttraumatic stress disorder: a functional magnetic resonance imaging investigation.** *Biol Psychiatry* 2005, **57**:873-884.
86. Jackowski AP, Douglas-Palumberi H, Jackowski M, Win L, Schultz RT, Staib LW, Krystal JH, Kaufman J: **Corpus callosum in maltreated children with posttraumatic stress disorder: a diffusion tensor imaging study.** *Psychiatry Res* 2008, **162**:256-261.
87. Werner NS, Meindl T, Engel RR, Rosner R, Riedel M, Reiser M, Fast K: **Hippocampal function during associative learning in patients with posttraumatic stress disorder.** *J Psychiatr Res* 2009, **43**:309-318.
88. Shin LM, Whalen PJ, Pitman RK, Bush G, Macklin ML, Lasko NB, Orr SP, McInerney SC, Rauch SL: **An fMRI study of anterior cingulate function in posttraumatic stress disorder.** *Biol Psychiatry* 2001, **50**:932-942.
89. Kim MJ, Chey J, Chung A, Bae S, Khang H, Ham B, Yoon SJ, Jeong DU, Lyoo IK: **Diminished rostral anterior cingulate activity in response to threat-related events in posttraumatic stress disorder.** *J Psychiatr Res* 2008, **42**:268-277.
90. Craig AD: **Interoception: the sense of the physiological condition of the body.** *Curr Opin Neurobiol* 2003, **13**:500-505.
91. Simmons A, Strigo IA, Matthews SC, Paulus MP, Stein MB: **Initial evidence of a failure to activate right anterior insula during affective set shifting in posttraumatic stress disorder.** *Psychosom Med* 2009, **71**:373-377.
92. Hoge CW: **Deployment to the Iraq war and neuropsychological sequelae.** *Jama* 2006, **296**:2678-2679, author reply 2679-2680.
93. First MB, Spitzer RL, Gibbon M, Williams JBW: *Structured Clinical Interview for DSM-IV-TR Axis I Disorders, Research Version, Non-patient Edition. (SCID-I/NP)* New York: New York Biometrics Research, New York State Psychiatric Institute; 2002.
94. Beck AT, Ward CH, Medelson M, Mock J, Erbaugh J: **An inventory for measuring depression.** *Arch Gen Psychiatry* 1961, **4**:561-571.

95. Bernstein DP, Fink L, Handelsman L, Foote J, Lovejoy M, Wenzel K, Sapareto E, Ruggiero J: **Initial reliability and validity of a new retrospective measure of child abuse and neglect.** *Am J Psychiatry* 1994, **151**:1132-1136.
96. Breslau N, Davis GC: **Posttraumatic stress disorder: the etiologic specificity of wartime stressors.** *Am J Psychiatry* 1987, **144**:578-583.
97. Blake DD, Weathers FW, Nagy LM, Kaloupek DG, Gusman FD, Charney DS, Keane TM: **The development of a Clinician-Administered PTSD Scale.** *J Trauma Stress* 1995, **8**:75-90.
98. Liberzon I, Phan KL: **Brain-imaging studies of posttraumatic stress disorder.** *CNS Spectr* 2003, **8**:641-650.
99. Admon R, Lubin G, Stern O, Rosenberg K, Sela L, Ben-Ami H, Hendler T: **Human vulnerability to stress depends on amygdala's predisposition and hippocampal plasticity.** *Proc Natl Acad Sci USA* 2009, **106**:14120-14125.
100. Cardinal RN, Parkinson JA, Hall J, Everitt BJ: **Emotion and motivation.** *Neurosci Biobehav Rev* 2002, **26**:321-352.
101. Boynton GM, Engel SA, Glover GH, Heeger DJ: **Linear systems analysis of functional magnetic resonance imaging in human V1.** *J Neurosci* 1996, **16**:4207-4221.
102. Talairach J, Tournoux P: *Co-planar stereotaxic atlas of the human brain: 3-dimensional proportional system: an approach to cerebral imaging* New York, NY: Thieme Medical Publishers, Inc; 1998.
103. Morris JS, Friston KJ, Buchel C, Frith CD, Young AW, Calder AJ, Dolan RJ: **A neuromodulatory role for the human amygdala in processing emotional facial expressions.** *Brain* 1998, **121**(Pt 1):47-57.

12

Structural abnormality of the corticospinal tract in major depressive disorder

Matthew D Sacchet[1,2*], Gautam Prasad[2,3], Lara C Foland-Ross[2], Shantanu H Joshi[4], J Paul Hamilton[5], Paul M Thompson[3] and Ian H Gotlib[1,2]

Abstract

Background: Scientists are beginning to document abnormalities in white matter connectivity in major depressive disorder (MDD). Recent developments in diffusion-weighted image analyses, including tractography clustering methods, may yield improved characterization of these white matter abnormalities in MDD. In this study, we acquired diffusion-weighted imaging data from MDD participants and matched healthy controls. We analyzed these data using two tractography clustering methods: automated fiber quantification (AFQ) and the maximum density path (MDP) procedure. We used AFQ to compare fractional anisotropy (FA; an index of water diffusion) in these two groups across major white matter tracts. Subsequently, we used the MDP procedure to compare FA differences in fiber paths related to the abnormalities in major fiber tracts that were identified using AFQ.

Results: FA was higher in the bilateral corticospinal tracts (CSTs) in MDD (p's < 0.002). Secondary analyses using the MDP procedure detected primarily increases in FA in the CST-related fiber paths of the bilateral posterior limbs of the internal capsule, right superior *corona radiata*, and the left external capsule.

Conclusions: This is the first study to implicate the CST and several related fiber pathways in MDD. These findings suggest important new hypotheses regarding the role of CST abnormalities in MDD, including in relation to explicating CST-related abnormalities to depressive symptoms and RDoC domains and constructs.

Keywords: Major depressive disorder (MDD), Diffusion tensor imaging (DTI), Tractography, Clustering, Automated fiber quantification (AFQ), Maximum density path (MDP), Corticospinal tract (CST), Fractional anisotropy (FA)

Background

Major depressive disorder (MDD) is the most common psychiatric disorder in the United States [1], accounting for approximately half of disability-adjusted life years worldwide [2], with major economic and personal costs [3]. MDD involves a wide range of symptoms, including most prominently negative affect and anhedonia (loss of pleasure), as well as difficulties in psychomotor functioning, sleep, and weight changes. If we could better understand the neural basis of MDD, we may be able to better prevent and treat this debilitating disorder.

Across different areas of neuroscience, there has been growing interest in delineating brain networks, in contrast to examining specific brain regions in isolation. Networks of brain regions have been increasingly implicated in depressive pathology, underscoring the need to understand depression-related anomalies in the connections among these regions [4-6]. In this context, diffusion-weighted imaging can assess diffusion properties of white matter and can be used to infer brain connectivity. Using diffusion tensor imaging (DTI), water diffusion can be quantified using fractional anisotropy (FA), which measures the degree of directional preference in water diffusion. FA, the most commonly used diffusion metric, is influenced by intra-voxel orientation dispersion, axonal myelination and packing density, membrane permeability, the number of axons, and partial volume effects [7]. Moreover, tractography algorithms can use diffusion tensor information to estimate the location and direction of fiber tracts. DTI has been used to characterize abnormal white matter diffusion properties in a range of diseases, including psychiatric

* Correspondence: msacchet@stanford.edu
[1]Neurosciences Program, Stanford University, Stanford, CA, USA
[2]Department of Psychology, Stanford University, Jordan Hall, Building 01-420, 450 Serra Mall, Stanford, CA 94305, USA
Full list of author information is available at the end of the article

disorders involving psychosis and disturbances in mood and attention [4,5,8,9].

To our knowledge, there have been three reviews documenting diffusion abnormalities in MDD [4-6]. Across these three reviews, there has been considerable discrepancy in the direction and location of effects of white matter abnormalities in MDD. This may be because of significant heterogeneity in participant samples (e.g., half of the studies included in one review assessed elderly individuals [5]), meta-analytic methods (e.g., qualitative [5], signed differential mapping (SDM) [6], and activation likelihood estimation (ALE) [4]), individual study analysis techniques (e.g., tractography, voxel-based analysis (VBA), or tract-based spatial statistics (TBSS)), and/or study inclusion criteria (e.g., only analyzing decreases in FA [6]). Thus, our current understanding of white matter pathology in MDD is based on relatively few studies that, themselves, incorporate heterogeneous methodological approaches. Most studies of diffusion in MDD have not assessed tractography, but instead examined FA or other diffusion measures in specific regions of interest (ROIs), or, globally, using VBA or TBSS [4-6]. Tractography uses directional information from the diffusion data to extract diffusion properties from specific fiber tracts, and it may offer greater power to detect disease-related abnormalities than do VBA and TBSS [10].

Few studies have used tractography-based methods to characterize white matter connectivity in MDD. Zhang et al. first used tractography to identify the cingulum bundle and uncinate fasciculi and then estimated diffusion properties in these fiber tracts. These investigators found that FA was lower and mean diffusivity was higher in the right uncinate fasciculus in depressed individuals relative to nondepressed controls [10]. In a second study, Zhang and colleagues found MDD-related reductions in FA in tractography-identified anterior limb of the internal capsule, an important component of the cortico-striatal-pallidal-thalamic (CSPT) circuit [11]. Finally, in a connectomics framework, tractography and graph theory have been used to explicate large-scale network abnormalities in depression [12,13].

Whole-brain tractography commonly includes tens of thousands of fibers; consequently, findings using this technique in isolation can be difficult to interpret. To better understand such massive amounts of data, whole-brain tractography is often summarized. One data reduction method identifies key fiber tracts by requiring manual tracing of an ROI which is followed by algorithmic assessment of the fibers that pass through it (as in [10,11]). This manual identification of ROIs is time consuming, however, and limits the number of fascicles that can be assessed. In addition, manual tracing methods can introduce investigator bias during selection and tracing of ROIs. In contrast, clustering methods permit the automated, unbiased summarization of fiber tract information, by using anatomical and DTI information to locate important fiber tracts. Automated fiber quantification (AFQ) [14] and the maximum density path (MDP) [15] approach are two such clustering methods. Briefly, AFQ identifies important white matter tracts by assessing sets of fibers that intersect pairs of waypoint ROIs. Similarly, the MDP procedure uses a graph search method in a set of white matter ROIs to identify abnormalities in fiber paths. MDPs are smaller and more numerous than the AFQ-identified tracts and provide complementary anatomical information.

Given the likely importance of anomalies in white matter connectivity in MDD, the inconsistency in the literature concerning diffusion-related findings in this disorder, and the recent development of sensitive, automated, tractography clustering methods, the present study was designed to use the AFQ and MDP tractography clustering methods to automatically characterize properties of white matter diffusion in MDD. First, we used AFQ to identify depression-related anomalies in FA in 18 major white matter paths. MDPs allow for additional and complementary information relative to tract properties derived by AFQ, given their small size, large number, and association with major white matter tracts. After identifying abnormal white matter pathways using AFQ, we conducted secondary analyses in a subset of MDPs that were associated with these specific paths. In addition, given evidence that age of onset of depression and severity of disorder are related to abnormalities in white matter properties [6,16], we assessed the relations between these two variables as well as the level of global functioning and diffusion properties of abnormal white matter paths.

Thus, we used information from tractography and took advantage of the lower bias and higher efficiency of two automated clustering methods to study major white matter paths in MDD. We hypothesized that FA would be lower in depressed individuals in the uncinate fasciculus, which links regions associated with emotion processing (e.g., hippocampus, amygdala) with regions implicated in cognitive control (e.g., prefrontal cortex).

Methods

Participants

Participants were 14 women diagnosed with MDD and 18 healthy, age-matched, female controls (CTLs) 18–55 years of age. The Structured Clinical Interview for DSM-IV-TR Axis I (SCID-I) [17] was used to establish a psychiatric diagnosis of MDD based on DSM-IV-TR criteria. To qualify for study entry, individuals in the CTL group could not have met criteria for any past or current DSM-IV-TR Axis I disorder. Exclusion criteria for both MDD and CTL participants included current alcohol or substance abuse or dependence and head trauma resulting in loss of consciousness greater than 5 min. During the SCID-I, to assess age of onset of depression, depressed participants were asked at what age they first experienced a depressive episode. A trained interviewer also completed the Global Assessment of Functioning (GAF) scale [18]. This scale indexes, from 1 to 100 (sickest to healthiest), the level of the participants' social, occupational, and psychological functioning. Severity of depression was assessed with the Beck Depression Inventory-II (BDI-II [19]). The Stanford University Institutional Review Board approved the study and informed consent was collected from each participant.

MRI data acquisition

Whole-brain diffusion-weighted and high-resolution T1-weighted images were collected using a Discovery MR750 3.0 T MR system (GE Medical Systems, Milwaukee, WI, USA), housed at the Stanford Center for Neurobiological Imaging. The T1-weighted images were used for anatomical registration (spoiled gradient echo (SPGR) pulse sequence; repetition time (TR) = 6,240 ms; echo time (TE) = 2.34 ms; flip angle = 12°; resolution = 0.9 mm isotropic; 186 slices; scan duration = 5 min 15 s). The diffusion-weighted scan was a single-shot, dual-spin-echo, echo-planar imaging sequence (96 unique directions; $b = 2{,}000$ s/mm^2; TR = 8,500 ms; TE = 93.6 ms; resolution = 2 mm isotropic; 64 slices; scan duration = 15 min 1 s). Nine non-diffusion-weighted ($b = 0$ s/mm^2) volumes were additionally collected for anatomical localization and registration purposes.

AFQ procedure

AFQ systematically uses whole-brain tractography methods to characterize major white matter fiber tracts. Here we briefly describe the AFQ procedure (see Additional file 1 for more detail). First, diffusion data were preprocessed, including motion correction, data alignment, resampling, and trilinear interpolation [20]. Tensors were then fit at each voxel using a robust tensor fitting method [21], and FA was computed as the normalized standard deviation of the tensor's eigenvalues. FA ranges from 0 (perfectly isotropic) to 1 (perfectly anisotropic diffusion). Following this, tractography was estimated using a deterministic streamline tracing algorithm [22,23]. Then, waypoint ROIs labeled on the MNI template were warped into participant-specific diffusion space, and fibers intersecting these ROIs were identified. After a series of fiber cleaning and tract refinement steps, the central portion of each fiber tract was located and diffusion metrics were computed along this core, resulting in a "tract profile". These tract profiles permit the systematic and unbiased assessment of group differences in diffusion metrics, FA in this study. After identifying tract profiles, we computed the mean FA along each white matter tract.

MDP procedure

The MDP approach allows for the automated assessment of compact and localized white matter paths on an individual-participant basis [15] (see Additional file 1 for more detail). Because MDPs are smaller, more numerous, and associated with major white matter tracts (i.e., they are located in major tracts or in areas to which these tracts project), they offer additional information to that obtained using AFQ. We identified MDPs in 50 white matter regions described in the Johns Hopkins University white matter atlas, resulting in a total of 67 MDPs (several regions have more than one MDP). To implement this procedure, we first corrected the diffusion data for eddy current and motion effects; next, we estimated whole-brain tractography using an optimized global probabilistic tractography method [24]. Then, from the whole-brain tractography computed using the global method, we created fiber density images for each white matter ROI by identifying fibers that intersect with the ROI (AFQ-identified fibers intersected pairs of ROIs). The next step employed graph theoretical analysis. Specifically, fiber density graphs were created with nodes as voxel locations and edges as density information. Seed points identified in the white matter atlas were then warped into each fiber density graph image. Using an optimized grid search method to find the path of highest density [25], MDPs were identified between each pair of seed points. The resulting paths were compact representations of the given tract's scale/size, location, and geometry/shape. Finally, paths were registered spatially across individuals using a geodesic curve registration procedure [26,27], allowing us to conduct between-group comparisons of FA in a point-wise manner.

Analysis plan and statistical analysis

In the first stage of analysis, we used two-sample t-tests to compare the 18 AFQ-identified fiber tract core mean FA values for the MDD and CTL groups. To correct for false positive inflation as a result of multiple comparisons, we implemented a false discovery rate (FDR) procedure ($q = 0.05$) [28]. This analysis identified major fiber bundles in which there were depression-related abnormalities. Using Pearson linear partial correlation (controlling for age), we assessed the correlations between identified abnormal fiber tracts and age of onset of depression, severity of depression (BDI-II scores), and level of global functioning (GAF scores) in the MDD group.

Second, we identified MDPs that were associated (i.e., overlapping, outside of the AFQ fiber tract but in projection fibers, or spatially proximal) with the abnormal fiber tracts that were identified using AFQ. Spatially proximal MDPs were included because AFQ incorporates weighted FA values into the estimates of major fiber tract FA from fibers that are not in the fiber tract core; thus, proximal MDPs may exhibit relevant FA abnormalities. The step-wise analysis procedure was implemented because MDPs are neuroanatomically associated with the AFQ fiber tracts, and are smaller and more numerous, therefore allowing for additional but complementary information to that provided by the AFQ-identified major fiber tracts. We conducted two-sample t-tests to assess point-wise differences between the MDD and CTL groups, using FDR to correct for multiple comparisons across points for each analyzed MDP (i.e., the subset of the 67 MDPs that were included for further analysis given their relation to the abnormal fiber tracts identified using AFQ).

Results

Demographic and clinical characteristics

Means and standard deviations for demographic and clinical variables for the 14 depressed and 18 control female participants are presented in Table 1. The two groups did not differ in age ($t(30) = -1.53$, $p > 0.10$), handedness ($\chi^2(1) = 0.14$, $p > 0.10$), or level of education achieved ($t(30) = -1.34$, $p > 0.10$). As expected, the depressed participants had significantly higher BDI-II scores than did the never-depressed controls. Half of the participants in the depressed group met criteria for at least one anxiety disorder, and three depressed participants were currently taking psychotropic medications (see Table 2).

AFQ

Across the entire sample, AFQ was unable to characterize 5 of the 576 fiber tracts (i.e., $N \times$ [number of fiber tracks] = 32×18): the callosum forceps major for three participants and the callosum forceps minor for two participants. These participants were excluded from analyses involving these particular fiber tracts. The failure of AFQ to identify these fibers may be a result of crossing fibers, noise in the data, abnormal anatomy that caused problems for automated segmentation, or small fiber tracks for which it is difficult to compute statistics. Of the 18 analyzed fiber groups (Table 3), two distinguished MDD from CTL participants after correcting for multiple comparisons: the left corticospinal tract (CST) ($t(30) = 3.45$, $p < 0.002$) and the right CST ($t(30) = 3.79$, $p < 0.001$) (Table 4, Figure 1). Both CSTs were characterized by greater FA in the MDD than in the CTL group (Table 4). As an exploratory analysis, we divided the group of MDD participants into two subgroups based on the presence or absence of comorbid anxiety; these two subgroups did not differ in FA for either the left or the right CST (p's > 0.10). In addition, the group differences in CST were unchanged after removing the three MDD participants who were taking psychotropic medications (left CST: $t(27) = 3.45$, $p < 0.002$; right CST: $t(27) = 3.11$, $p < 0.005$). Finally, in the MDD group, we correlated age of onset and severity of depression, and level of global functioning, with mean FA individually for both left and right CST. No significant correlations were obtained ($p > 0.10$).

MDPs

For the second stage of the analysis plan, we identified MDPs associated with the AFQ-identified CST. This resulted in the identification of 24 unique MDPs from seven white matter ROIs (from a total of 50). The 24 MDPs (12 in each hemisphere) comprised 35.8% of the total set of 67 MDPs (Table 5). These MDPs overlap, are along the same white matter bundle, or are spatially proximal to the CST projections identified in the AFQ analysis.

We conducted two-sample t-tests on a point-by-point basis along each of the identified MDPs. After correcting for multiple comparisons by using FDR independently for each MDP, the MDD and CTL groups exhibited point-wise differences in four MDPs: the left posterior limb of the internal capsule, the right posterior limb of the internal capsule, the right superior *corona radiata*, and the left external capsule (Table 6, Figure 2). Because

Table 1 Participant demographic and clinical characteristics

	CTL ($N = 18$)			MDD ($N = 14$)			p value
Age in years (M | SD | min/max)	30.4	10.2	18.9/52.1	35.6	8.4	22.8/48.5	>0.10[b]
Education level[a] (M | SD | min/max)	6.6	1.5	4/8	7.2	1.1	4/8	>0.10[c]
BDI-II (M | SD | min/max)	2.2	3.2	0/11	31.7	6.6	22/43	<0.001[b]
Global Assessment of Functioning (M | SD | min/max)	87.8	7.0	75/99	53.0	6.6	35/60	<0.001[b]
Age of onset (M | SD | min/max)		NA		16.3	6.8	3/26	NA
Handedness (right | left)	16		2	13		1	>0.10[c]

BDI-II Beck Depression Inventory-II, *GAF* Global Assessment of Functioning, *M* mean, *SD* standard deviation, *MDD* major depressive disorder, *CTL* control.
[a]Level of education was assigned as follows: having finished 1) elementary school, 2) junior high school, 3) high school, 4) some college, 5) technical school, 6) junior college, 7) 4-year college, or 8) graduate or professional education.
[b]Computed using two-sample t-test.
[c]Computed using chi-square test.

Table 2 Current comorbid diagnoses and psychotropic medications of the MDD participants

	Participants	% of total
Comorbidities	7	50
Social phobia	4	28.6
General anxiety disorder	3	21.4
Panic disorder	2	14.3
Post-traumatic stress disorder	2	14.3
Specific phobia	2	14.3
Bulimia nervosa	1	7.1
Psychiatric medications	3	21.4
Aripiprazole	2	14.3
Duloxetine	1	7.1
Gabapentin	1	7.1
Quetiapine	1	7.1
Sertraline	1	7.1
Venlafaxine	1	7.1

MDD major depressive disorder.

each of the four MDPs was located in a unique region, and because each of these regions included two analyzed MDPs, only one of the two MDPs identified for each implicated white matter region yielded point-wise group differences after FDR correction. Of the identified points that differed between groups (27 total across the four MDPs), all except three of the six points of the left external capsule were characterized by greater FA in the MDD than in the CTL group.

Discussion

The literature examining white matter abnormalities in MDD is methodologically varied and sparse and has yielded inconsistent findings. In this context, the current study was designed to capitalize on the improved detection power of tractography, the reduced bias of automated clustering methods, and more systematic and data-driven analysis, to assess abnormalities in white matter in MDD and begin to yield a more systematic and reliable connectomics of depression. Indeed, this is the first study to use automated tractography clustering to characterize white matter in depression. Our analyses

Table 3 AFQ-identified fiber tracts

Laterality	AFQ fiber tracts
L/R	Thalamic radiation
L/R	Corticospinal
L/R	Cingulum cingulate
NA	Callosum forceps major
NA	Callosum forceps minor
L/R	IFOF
L/R	ILF
L/R	SLF
L/R	Uncinate
L/R	Arcuate

AFQ automated fiber quantification, *L* left, *R* right, *IFOF* inferior fronto-occipital fasciculus, *ILF* inferior longitudinal fasciculus, *SLF* superior longitudinal fasciculus.

Table 4 Group differences in FA in AFQ-identified fiber tracts

AFQ fiber group	CTL FA		MDD FA		*p* value
	M	*SD*	*M*	*SD*	
Left corticospinal tract	0.620	0.020	0.644	0.020	<0.002
Right corticospinal tract	0.614	0.021	0.639	0.015	<0.001

p values were computed using two-sample *t*-tests and a false discovery rate (FDR) procedure was used to account for false positives as a result of multiple comparisons. See Figure 1 for corticospinal tract (CST) renderings and graphical display of differences.
AFQ automated fiber quantification, *MDD* major depressive disorder, *CTL* control, *FA* fractional anisotropy, *M* mean, *SD* standard deviation.

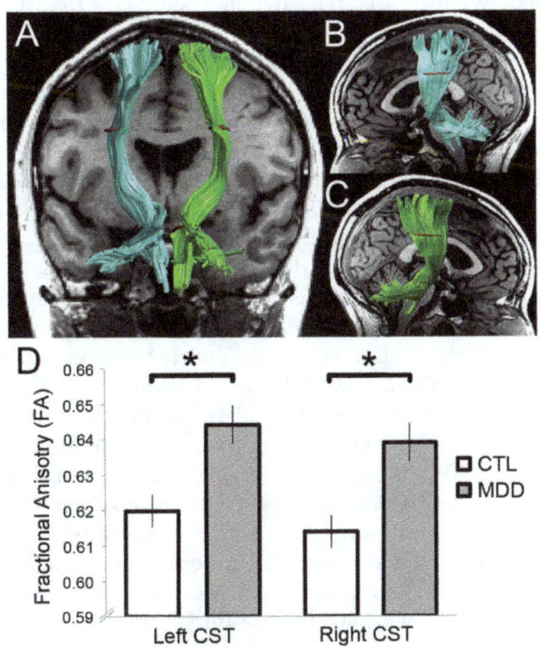

Figure 1 AFQ corticospinal tracts. Corticospinal tracts (CSTs) rendered for an example subject. Three hundred fibers were rendered for each tract. The left CST is colored *teal* and the right CST *green*. Waypoint regions of interest (ROIs) are depicted in *red*. Fractional anisotropy (FA) computed for the fiber tract core, between the waypoint ROIs, was meaned and compared between groups. **(A)** Bilateral CSTs viewed posteriorly with a T1-weighted coronal slice at the anterior commissure. **(B)** Left CST and **(C)** right CST viewed laterally with a mid-sagittal T1-weighted slice. **(D)** Group differences in mean CSTs. *Asterisks* indicate statistical significance from two-sample *t*-tests between groups. *Error bars* represent standard error of the mean (SEM). See Table 4 for group means and standard deviations. *AFQ* automated fiber quantification, *CTL* control group, *MDD* depressed group.

Table 5 MDP locations

White matter region	MDPs per hemisphere
Anterior limb of the internal capsule	2
Posterior limb of the internal capsule	2
External capsule	1
Corticospinal tract	1
Anterior *corona radiata*	2
Superior *corona radiata*	2
Posterior *corona radiata*	2

White matter regions of interest from the Johns Hopkins University Atlas and the number of MDPs per region, per hemisphere. A total of 24 MDPs were assessed.
MDP maximum density path.

included fiber tracts that have been previously studied in this disorder, in addition to several tracts that have not before been examined.

Using AFQ [14], we found that MDD was characterized by abnormalities in FA in the bilateral corticospinal tracts. We then used the MDP procedure [15] to further probe localized abnormalities that were associated with these group differences. This analysis revealed, for the first time, increased FA in the bilateral posterior limbs of the internal capsule, right superior *corona radiata*, and the left external capsule in MDD.

Previous studies have primarily documented reduced FA associated with MDD. In contrast, the current results include almost exclusively *increased* FA in participants diagnosed with this disorder. This discrepancy may be a result of the small number of studies considered in the previous reviews (12 studies [5], 11 studies [4], 7 studies [6]). In addition, Liao et al. only analyzed data indicating increases in FA in MDD [4]; the two quantitative reviews [4,6] excluded tractography studies; and the third review [5] included only one tractography study in the discussion of MDD. Because tractography incorporates directionality information that is used to identify important white matter pathways, it may allow for greater detection power than do whole-brain voxel-wise techniques (e.g., VBA or TBSS) and, thus, may explain why previous research did not report increases in FA in CST in MDD.

Table 6 Group FA differences in MDPs

White matter region	Total points in MDP	Group differences	% of points
Left posterior limb of the internal capsule	16	6	37.5
Right posterior limb of the internal capsule	17	14	82.4
Right superior *corona radiata*	17	1	5.9
Left external capsule	48	6	12.5

Group differences were assessed using two-sample *t*-tests, and a false discovery rate (FDR) procedure was used to account for false positives as a result of multiple comparisons.
FA fractional anisotropy, *MDP* maximum density path.

It is also possible that the automated clustering methods that we implemented yield greater spatial specificity than do earlier methods, and that decreases in FA in MDD that were previously identified using VBA and TBSS were, in fact, inaccurately reported to be localized to major fiber tracts.

It is important to also note that other investigators have reported depression-related increases in FA. For example, Blood et al. found that the ventral tegmental area was associated with greater FA in MDD than in control participants [29]. Moreover, several studies have identified regions of increased FA in bipolar disorder (BD) [5] in areas of the corpus callosum [30] and the frontal lobe [31], including the uncinate fasciculus, optic radiation, and anterior thalamic radiation [32]. Given recent interest in examining transdiagnostic factors in the proposed NIMH RDoC framework, it will be important in future research to investigate how tract-specific FA may correspond to signs and symptoms of disorders of emotion and mood with respect to specific RDoC domains and constructs.

Previous research has suggested that increased FA of the CSTs is related to decreases in FA of the superior longitudinal fasciculi (SLF). Specifically, Douaud et al. reported increases in CST FA in individuals with mild cognitive impairment and Alzheimer's disease compared to healthy controls; moreover, using a method of quantitative crossing fiber tractography, Douaud et al. found that the increases in CST FA were associated with reduced FA of SLF association fibers in a crossing fiber region at the level of the centrum semiovale [33]. Although these findings raise the intriguing possibility that MDD-related increases in FA of the CST are related to selective sparing of this tract with concurrent abnormality in the SLF, we did not find SLF abnormalities in the current study. Future research using imaging and tractography methods that allow for greater resolution of crossing fibers may permit a better assessment of whether increases in CST FA in MDD are related to abnormalities in regions of crossing fibers.

Given the role of the CSTs in motor processes, it is possible that our findings of anomalous FA in these structures are related to psychomotor symptoms that often characterize MDD [34]. More specifically, motor retardation and agitation, criterion symptoms of MDD, may result from aberrations in white matter microstructure connecting the brainstem to motoric regions of cortical gray matter [35]. The current findings offer a foundation from which future research might explore this hypothesis. Importantly, although the white matter of primate CSTs is understood to arise primarily from the primary motor cortex, projections from the somatosensory, cingulate, and insular cortices are also represented [35]. Thus, the CST is likely to be involved in a

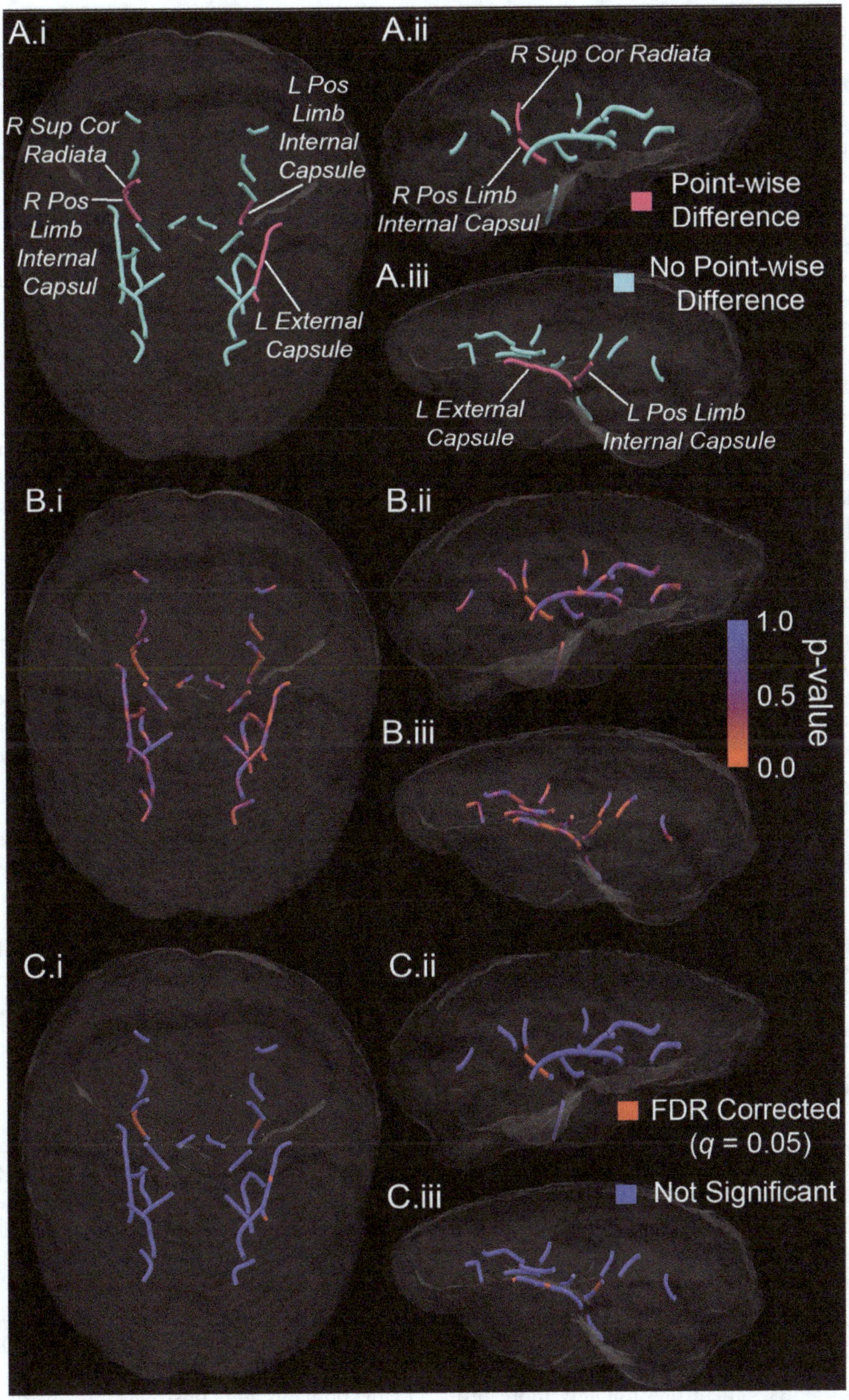

Figure 2 (See legend on next page.)

(See figure on previous page.)

Figure 2 Group differences in MDPs. (A) Rendering of analyzed MDPs associated with the corticospinal tract (CST). A.i Superior view. A.ii Right lateral view. A.iii Left lateral view. MDPs that exhibited point-wise differences (right superior *corona radiata*, right posterior limb of the internal capsule, left posterior limb of the internal capsule, left external capsule) are labeled and colored *magenta*. **(B)** Rendering of analyzed MDPs with point-wise *p* values computed from two-sample *t*-tests. *Red* indicates lower *p* values and greater significance. **(C)** Rendering of analyzed MDPs with FDR-corrected point-wise statistical tests. *Red* indicates significant test. *MDP* maximum density path, *FDR* false discovery rate, *R* right, *L* left, *Sup* superior, *Pos* posterior, *Cor corona*.

variety of functions and thus may be related to a range of depression-related functioning (e.g., somatosensory, affective, and cognitive). Future research, therefore, may profitably assess the relations of these important symptom domains with CST diffusion properties in MDD. Moreover, given the varied projection profile of the CST, future research should assess relations between abnormalities in CST FA and gray matter properties (e.g., volume) in this disorder.

Although controversial, findings of abnormal frontostriatal networks in MDD have led to the formulation that this disorder is a "disconnection syndrome" characterized by reduced connectivity between cortical and subcortical brain regions [4,5,36]. Evidence for this formulation includes observations that frontal white matter FA is reduced in MDD [37] and is correlated with remission from depression [38]. The current findings provide evidence that MDD may be characterized by abnormalities in connectivity between subcortical and brainstem structures and cortical gray matter regions. In future studies, investigators might use the AFQ and MDP procedures to examine the viability of the disconnection syndrome formulation more systematically, given that these procedures yield increased spatial specificity in neuroanatomical abnormalities associated with MDD.

The uncinate fasciculus and thalamic radiation are the most commonly studied fiber tracts in mood disorders [5]; indeed, we had hypothesized that we would find abnormalities of the uncinate fasciculus in MDD. The interest in these white matter tracts is due primarily to their potential involvement in abnormal cognitive control over emotion processing. Specifically, the uncinate fasciculus includes connections between medial temporal lobe regions associated with emotion processing (e.g., the hippocampi and amygdala) and the frontal cortex (involved in cognitive control); similarly, the white matter of the thalamic radiation links the frontal cortex with the thalamus (potentially a key connection in the disconnection syndrome formulation). Notably, we did not find abnormalities in these two tracts. This may be due in part to the location of the default AFQ waypoint ROIs, which are placed to identify the fiber tract cores and, thus, limit the assessment of variability more proximal to cortex.

The current results indicate that AFQ and MDPs are complementary techniques for the quantification and characterization of white matter paths in psychiatric populations and represent an important step towards the automated and efficient characterization of psychopathology, as demonstrated here in MDD. Given the sensitivity and automated nature of these methods, they may prove useful in identifying and characterizing biomarkers that can facilitate efforts to prevent and treat psychiatric disorders.

Despite the strengths of these procedures, we should note three limitations of the present study. First, the sample size in the current study was relatively small; thus, it is possible that the analyses are underpowered to find reductions in FA that have been previously reported, or significant relations between CST FA and age of onset or severity of depression, or level of global functioning. Second, our sample of depressed participants was heterogeneous with respect to the presence of anxiety comorbidities and medication use. We did not find differences in CST FA between the comorbid and non-comorbid participants in the MDD sample, nor did the effects we report appear to be determined by psychotropic medication use in a small subset of our depressed sample. Thus, it seems that these factors did not confound our results. Third, as with all FA-related results, the biological basis of the observed abnormality is unclear, as many factors can influence this metric: the level of orientation dispersion, myelination, numbers of axons, membrane permeability, axonal packing density, geometric properties of the tract, partial volume effects, and influences from branching, merging, or crossing fibers [7].

Conclusions

Using tractography clustering methods, we identified abnormalities in major white matter paths in MDD, specifically in the CSTs and several related pathways, including bilateral posterior limb of the internal capsules, right superior *corona radiata*, and left external capsule. These are the first results to implicate abnormality of the CST and related pathways in MDD. These findings highlight important future research directions, including increasing our understanding of CST abnormalities in the context of depressive symptoms and in relation to RDoC domains and constructs. Finally, the current study demonstrates that tractography clustering techniques can be used to increase our understanding of white matter abnormalities in MDD.

Additional file

Additional file 1: Supplementary information for AFQ and MDP methods. File contains additional information regarding implementations of the AFQ and MDP methods.

Abbreviations

AFQ: Automated fiber quantification; ALE: Activation likelihood estimation; BD: Bipolar disorder; CSPT: Cortico-striatal-pallidal-thalamic; CST: Corticospinal tract; CTL: Control; DSM-IV-TR: Diagnostic and Statistical Manual of Mental Disorders 4th Edition, Text Revision; DTI: Diffusion tensor imaging; FA: Fractional anisotropy; FDR: False discovery rate; MDD: Major depressive disorder; MDP: Maximum density path; MNI: Montreal Neurological Institute; MR: Magnetic resonance; NIMH: National Institute of Mental Health; RDoC: Research domain criteria; ROI: Region of interest; SCID: Structured Clinical Interview for DSM-IV-TR Axis I; SDM: Signed differential mapping; SLF: Superior longitudinal fasciculus; SPGR: Spoiled gradient; TBSS: Tract-based spatial statistics; TE: Echo time; TR: Repetition time; VBA: Voxel-based analysis.

Competing interests

The authors declare that they have no competing interests.

Authors' contributions

MDS conceived of the project, analyzed the data, interpreted the findings, and drafted the manuscript. GP analyzed the data, interpreted the findings, and drafted the manuscript. LCFR coordinated the study, interpreted the findings, and drafted the manuscript. SHJ contributed to the MDP analysis and statistical methods. JPH acquired the data, interpreted the findings, and drafted the manuscript. PMT interpreted the findings and drafted the manuscript. IHG coordinated the study, interpreted the results, and drafted the manuscript. All authors read and approved the final manuscript.

Acknowledgements

We thank Jason Yeatman for technical assistance regarding the implementation of AFQ and Emily Livermore and Meghan Vinograd for help with data collection and organization. This work was supported by grants from the National Institute of Mental Health (MH74849 to IHG and MH090617 to LCFR), the National Alliance for Research in Schizophrenia and Affective Disorders (NARSAD; Distinguished Investigator Award to IHG and Young Investigator Award 19018 to LCFR), and the Hope for Depression Research Foundation (to IHG and LCFR).

Author details

[1]Neurosciences Program, Stanford University, Stanford, CA, USA. [2]Department of Psychology, Stanford University, Jordan Hall, Building 01-420, 450 Serra Mall, Stanford, CA 94305, USA. [3]Imaging Genetics Center, Institute for Neuroimaging and Informatics, Keck School of Medicine of USC, Los Angeles, CA, USA. [4]Ahmanson-Lovelace Brain Mapping Center, Department of Neurology, UCLA, Los Angeles, CA, USA. [5]Laureate Institute for Brain Research, Tulsa, OK, USA.

References

1. Kessler RC, Berglund P, Demler O, Jin R, Koretz D, Merikangas KR, Rush AJ, Walters EE, Wang PS: **The epidemiology of major depressive disorder: results from the National Comorbidity Survey Replication (NCS-R).** *JAMA* 2003, **289:**3095–3105.
2. Whiteford HA, Degenhardt L, Rehm J, Baxter A, Ferrari AJ, Erskine HE, Charlson FJ, Norman RE, Flaxman AD, Johns N, Burstein R, Murray CJL, Vos T: **Global burden of disease attributable to mental and substance use disorders: findings from the Global Burden of Disease Study 2010.** *J Lancet* 2013, **382:**1575–1586.
3. Greenberg PE, Sisitsky T, Kessler RC, Finkelstein SN, Berndt ER, Davidson RT, Ballenger JC, Fyer AJ: **The economic burden of anxiety disorders in the 1990s.** *J Clin Psychiatry* 2003, **60:**427–435.
4. Liao Y, Huang X, Wu Q, Yang C, Kuang W, Du M, Lui S, Yue Q, Chan R, Kemp G, Gong Q: **Is depression a disconnection syndrome? Meta-analysis of diffusion tensor imaging studies in patients with MDD.** *J Psychiatry Neurosci* 2013, **38:**49–56.
5. Sexton CE, Mackay CE, Ebmeier KP: **A systematic review of diffusion tensor imaging studies in affective disorders.** *Biol Psychiatry* 2009, **66:**814–823.
6. Murphy ML, Frodl T: **Meta-analysis of diffusion tensor imaging studies shows altered fractional anisotropy occurring in distinct brain areas in association with depression.** *Biol Mood Anxiety Disord* 2011, **1:**3.
7. Jones DK, Knösche TR, Turner R: **White matter integrity, fiber count, and other fallacies: the do's and don'ts of diffusion MRI.** *Neuroimage* 2013, **73**(C):239–254.
8. van Ewijk H, Heslenfeld DJ, Zwiers MP, Buitelaar JK, Oosterlaan J: **Diffusion tensor imaging in attention deficit/hyperactivity disorder: a systematic review and meta-analysis.** *Neurosci Biobehav Rev* 2012, **36:**1093–1106.
9. Kubicki M, Shenton ME: **Diffusion tensor imaging findings and their implications in schizophrenia.** *Curr Opin Psychiatry* 2014, **27:**179–184.
10. Zhang A, Leow A, Ajilore O, Lamar M, Yang S, Joseph J, Medina J, Zhan L, Kumar A: **Quantitative tract-specific measures of uncinate and cingulum in major depression using diffusion tensor imaging.** *Neuropsychopharmacology* 2011, **37:**959–967.
11. Zhang A, Ajilore O, Zhan L, GadElkarim J, Korthauer L, Yang S, Leow A, Kumar A: **White matter tract integrity of anterior limb of internal capsule in major depression and type 2 diabetes.** *Neuropsychopharmacology* 2013, **38:**1451–1459.
12. Bai F, Shu N, Yuan Y, Shi Y, Yu H, Wu D, Wang J, Xia M, He Y, Zhang Z: **Topologically convergent and divergent structural connectivity patterns between patients with remitted geriatric depression and amnestic mild cognitive impairment.** *J Neurosci* 2012, **32:**4307–4318.
13. Sacchet MD, Prasad G, Foland-Ross LC, Thompson PM, Gotlib IH: **Elucidating brain connectivity networks in major depressive disorder using classification-based scoring.** *Proc IEEE Int Symp Biomed Imaging* 2014, **11:**592–595.
14. Yeatman JD, Dougherty RF, Myall NJ, Wandell BA, Feldman HM: **Tract profiles of white matter properties: automating fiber-tract quantification.** *PLoS One* 2012, **7:**e49790.
15. Prasad G, Joshi SH, Jahanshad N, Villalon-Reina J, Aganj I, Lenglet C, Sapiro G, McMahon KL, de Zubicaray GI, Martin NG, Wright MJ, Toga AW, Thompson PM: **Automatic clustering and population analysis of white matter tracts using maximum density paths.** *Neuroimage* 2014, **97**(C):284–295.
16. Taylor WD, MacFall JR, Gerig G, Krishnan RR: **Structural integrity of the uncinate fasciculus in geriatric depression: relationship with age of onset.** *Neuropsychiatr Dis Treat* 2007, **3:**669.
17. First MB, Dibbon M, Spitzer RL, Williams JB: *Structured Clinical Interview for DSM-IV-TR.* American Psychiatric Association: Washington; 2004.
18. Endicott J, Spitzer RL, Fleiss JL, Cohen J: **The global assessment scale: a procedure for measuring overall severity of psychiatric disturbance.** *Arch Gen Psychiatry* 1976, **33:**766–771.
19. Beck AT, Steer RA, Brown GK: *Manual for the Beck Depression Inventory-II.* San Antonio: Psychological Corporation; 1996.
20. Friston KJ, Ashburner J: **Generative and recognition models for neuroanatomy.** *Neuroimage* 2004, **23:**21–24.
21. Chang L-C, Jones DK, Pierpaoli C: **RESTORE: robust estimation of tensors by outlier rejection.** *Magn Reson Med* 2005, **53:**1088–1095.
22. Mori S, Crain BJ, Chacko VP, Van Zijl P: **Three-dimensional tracking of axonal projections in the brain by magnetic resonance imaging.** *Ann Neurol* 1999, **45:**265–269.
23. Basser PJ, Pajevic S, Pierpaoli C, Duda J, Aldroubi A: **In vivo fiber tractography using DT-MRI data.** *Magn Reson Med* 2000, **44:**625–632.
24. Prasad G, Nir TM, Toga AW, Thompson PM: **Tractography density and network measures in Alzheimer's disease.** In *Proc IEEE Int Symp Biomed Imaging: April 7–11 2013; San Francisco.* Piscataway: IEEE; 2013:692–695.
25. Dijkstra EW: **A note on two problems in connexion with graphs.** *Numer Math* 1959, **1:**269–271.
26. Joshi SH, Klassen E, Srivastava A, Jermyn I: **A novel representation for Riemannian analysis of elastic curves in Rn.** In *Proc IEEE Comput Soc Conf Comput Vis Pattern Recognit: June 17–22 2007; Minneapolis.* Piscataway: IEEE; 2007:1–7.
27. Joshi SH, Klassen E, Srivastava A, Jermyn I: **Removing shape-preserving transformations in square-root elastic (SRE) framework for shape analysis of curves.** In *Proc IEEE Comput Soc Conf Comput Vis Pattern Recognit.* Edited by Yuille A, Zhu S-C, Cremers D, Wang Y. Berlin: Springer; 2007:387–398 [*Lecture Notes in Computer Science*, vol 4679].

28. Benjamini Y, Hochberg Y: **Controlling the false discovery rate: a practical and powerful approach to multiple testing.** *J R Stat Soc Ser A* 1995, **57**:289–300.
29. Blood AJ, Iosifescu DV, Makris N, Perlis RH, Kennedy DN, Dougherty DD, Kim BW, Lee MJ, Wu S, Lee S, Calhoun J, Hodge SM, Fava M, Rosen BR, Smoller JW, Gasic GP, Breiter HC, for the Phenotype Genotype Project on Addiction and Mood Disorders: **Microstructural abnormalities in subcortical reward circuitry of subjects with major depressive disorder.** *PLoS One* 2010, **5**:e13945.
30. Yurgelun-Todd DA, Silveri MM, Gruber SA, Rohan ML, Pimentel PJ: **White matter abnormalities observed in bipolar disorder: a diffusion tensor imaging study.** *Bipolar Disord* 2007, **9**:504–512.
31. Haznedar MM, Roversi F, Pallanti S, Baldini-Rossi N, Schnur DB, LiCalzi EM, Tang C, Hof PR, Hollander E, Buchsbaum MS: **Fronto-thalamo-striatal gray and white matter volumes and anisotropy of their connections in bipolar spectrum illnesses.** *Biol Psychiatry* 2005, **57**:733–742.
32. Versace A, Almeida JR, Hassel S, Walsh ND, Novelli M, Klein CR, Kupfer DJ, Phillips ML: **Elevated left and reduced right orbitomedial prefrontal fractional anisotropy in adults with bipolar disorder revealed by tract-based spatial statistics.** *Arch Gen Psychiatry* 2008, **65**:1041–1052.
33. Douaud G, Jbabdi S, Behrens TEJ, Menke RA, Gass A, Monsch AU, Rao A, Whitcher B, Kindlmann G, Matthews PM, Smith S: **DTI measures in crossing-fibre areas: increased diffusion anisotropy reveals early white matter alteration in MCI and mild Alzheimer's disease.** *Neuroimage* 2011, **55**:880–890.
34. Furman DJ, Hamilton JP, Gotlib IH: **Frontostriatal functional connectivity in major depressive disorder.** *Biol Mood Anxiety Disord* 2011, **1**:11.
35. Galea MP, Darian-Smith I: **Multiple corticospinal neuron populations in the macaque monkey are specified by their unique cortical origins, spinal terminations, and connections.** *Cereb Cortex* 1994, **4**:166–194.
36. Savitz J, Drevets WC: **Bipolar and major depressive disorder: neuroimaging the developmental-degenerative divide.** *Neurosci Biobehav Rev* 2009, **33**:699–771.
37. Li L, Ma N, Li Z, Tan L, Liu J, Gong G, Shu N, He Z: **Prefrontal white matter abnormalities in young adult with major depressive disorder: a diffusion tensor imaging study.** *Brain Res* 2007, **1168**:124–128.
38. Alexopoulos GS, Kiosses DN, Choi SJ, Murphy CF, Lim KO: **Frontal white matter microstructure and treatment response of late-life depression: a preliminary study.** *Am J Psychiatry* 2002, **159**:1929–1932.

13

How research on the meta-structure of psychopathology aids in understanding biological correlates of mood and anxiety disorders

Shani Ofrat* and Robert F Krueger

Abstract

Research on biological correlates of psychopathology stands to benefit from being interwoven with an empirically based, quantitative model of mental disorders. Empirically-based classification approaches help to deal effectively with issues such as comorbidity among diagnoses, which often serve as challenges to interpreting research on biological correlates. With regard to the mood and anxiety disorders specifically, quantitative research shows how mood and anxiety disorders are well conceptualized as elements within a broad internalizing spectrum of psychopathology, such that many putative biological correlates of specific disorders may be better conceptualized as delineating the pathophysiology of the broader mechanisms underlying multiple disorders.

Keywords: Meta-structure, Comorbidity, Biological correlates, DSM-5

Background

The stated goal of the Diagnostic and Statistical Manual for Mental Disorders (DSM) is threefold: to provide a helpful guide to clinical practice, to facilitate research and improve communication among clinicians and researchers, and to serve as an educational tool for teaching psychopathology (DSM-IV-R 4th ed., pp xxiii). Historically, DSM began as a broad set of vignettes that depicted common clinical manifestations of mental disorders, but diagnoses listed in early DSMs were not reliably diagnosed by clinicians, and as a result had little validity [1]. By introducing explicit sets of diagnostic criteria, the DSM-III was instrumental in refining the boundaries of diagnoses so that clinicians were discussing the same clinical entities, supposedly distinct from others. DSM-III also introduced exclusionary criteria that sought to limit overlap between diagnostic sets. DSM-IV did little to change the basic scheme of the DSM-III, which had grown to include hundreds of distinct diagnostic categories. This degree of presumed diagnostic differentiation often contrasts with clinical experiences, where patients typically meet criteria for multiple DSM diagnoses, a phenomenon referred to as comorbidity [2-6], or related experiences where patients present with symptom configurations "not otherwise specified"(NOS), as opposed to symptoms that cohere into a clear DSM-defined focal syndrome [2]. As a result, questions about the validity of DSM-IV's approach to psychodiagnosis are frequently raised [1,7].

Main text

Research focusing on the problem of diagnostic comorbidity has resulted in a literature that has converged on an empirical model of the meta-structure of common mental disorders, or the way in which multiple mental disorders delineate spectrums of interrelated conditions. There is mounting evidence to suggest that common forms of psychopathology are defined by the higher-order groupings or spectrums of *internalizing* and *externalizing*, and that this shared underlying meta-structure contributes to the comorbidity among disorders [8-11]. As shown in Figure 1 [9], internalizing is indicated by unipolar mood disorders and anxiety disorders, like major depressive disorder, generalized anxiety disorder, social and specific phobias, and panic, that load highly on the internalizing factor. Externalizing is indicated by disinhibitory and substance abuse disorders including drug, alcohol, and nicotine dependence, antisocial personality disorder and antisocial traits, pathological gambling, and conduct disorder. Within the higher-order internalizing dimension, some studies have revealed two sub-dimensions: distress, representing unipolar mood

* Correspondence: ofrat001@umn.edu
University of Minnesota, 75 East River Road, Minneapolis, MN, USA

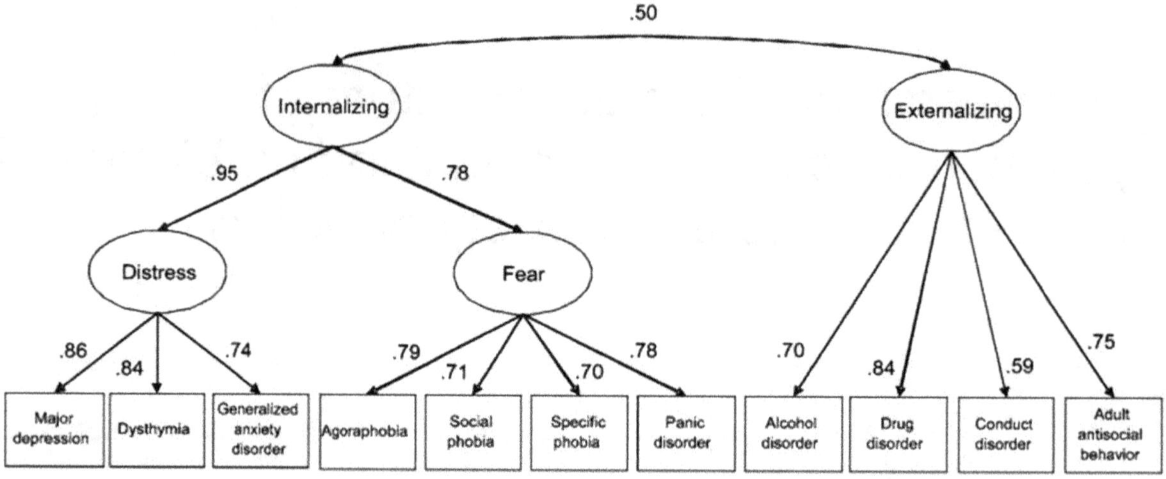

Figure 1 Path diagram for best-fitting meta-analytic model of the structure of common mental disorders. This figure provides parameter estimates from the best-fitting model according to a meta-analytic multiple-groups confirmatory factor analysis [9]. All parameter estimates are standardized and significant, $p < .05$. Reprinted from Krueger and Markon (2006). Copyright 2006 by Annual Review of Clinical Psychology. Reprinted with permission.

disorders and generalized anxiety, and fear, representing panic disorder, social and specific phobia [9], while others have not found evidence of these subfactors [12].

In expanding this work to encompass rarer forms of psychopathology, a recent study in a clinical sample analyzed data on 25 disorders, spanning both rarer and more common disorders, as well as Axes I and II. The best-fitting model consisted of 5 factors: (1) internalizing, which included anxiety and eating disorders, major depressive episodes, as well as cluster C (anxious and inhibited) personality disorders, borderline and paranoid personality disorders; (2) externalizing, including the substance use disorders and antisocial personality disorder; (3) thought disorder, including psychosis, mania, and cluster A personality disorders; (4) somatoform disorders; and (5) antagonism, including cluster B and paranoid personality disorders [13]. This work is important in that it replicates findings from previous work in a clinical sample and demonstrates that the same methods used to establish the existence of the internalizing-externalizing model can be used to extend that model to rarer disorders observed in clinical populations.

Advantages of a quantitative-empirical approach over a case-control approach

As opposed to studies that take a meta-structure approach, studies that use a case–control design in looking for biological correlates of specific disorders are limited both conceptually and empirically in accommodating comorbidity among diagnoses. Searching for biological correlates of one specific disorder often involves designing research to identify cases that have no or few comorbid diagnoses, in order to maintain pure diagnostic categories. This artificial exclusion of cases with comorbidities means that the studies lose ecological validity, inasmuch as a typical clinical case will meet criteria for disorders in addition to the target disorder. Such studies are therefore difficult to extrapolate to actual clinical populations where there is extensive diagnostic comorbidity.

By contrast, in interpreting biological findings through the lens of psychopathological dimensions, research on the underlying biological substrates of disorders becomes more tractable because comorbidity is accommodated in study design and result interpretation. Disorders do not co-occur at random; instead, they group in predictable ways that the meta-structure helps us anticipate, and looking for correlates of these groups of disorders instead of singular diagnoses allows researchers to better reflect the realities of psychiatric diagnoses. Using the meta-structure approach in biological research also allows for a purer and stronger biological 'signal' by allowing disorders to co-vary rather than losing power to artificial distinctions between related diagnoses. The signal of the latent variable, or what is shared between diagnoses, will necessarily be stronger than the signal of each individual diagnosis, and will also reduce noise due to inter-diagnostic similarities that made it difficult to form conclusions about disorder specificity. Conversely, in the case–control designed study if comorbid diagnoses are allowed in the study design, it can be challenging to parse out the relationship between individual diagnoses and results with any sort of specificity, which is supposedly the benefit of conceptualizing disorders as separate entities.

Recent research on biological correlates of the internalizing spectrum illustrates these points. A recent review of studies investigating affect-startle in internalizing disorders found evidence that these particular biological correlates tend to line up with the two subfactors, i.e., fear and distress, that are frequently found to underlie the internalizing factor. Disorders marked by cue-specific fear (specific and social phobia) tend to be associated with one parameter of startle reactivity (potentiation of startle during exposure to aversive stimuli), whereas disorders marked by diffuse negative affectivity or distress tend to be associated with others (heightened general reactivity or increased context-potentiated startle and, possibly, decreased fear-potentiated startle). The authors conclude that there are specific features of fear-based reactivity that map onto the distress and fear sub-factors of internalizing, while the overall concept of pathological fear-based reactivity relates to the overarching internalizing spectrum, implicating fear-potentiated startle as a likely biological indicator of internalizing psychopathology generally [14]. The findings in this study are made more readily interpretable by the metastructure approach, which supports the distinction between fear and distress disorders under the internalizing factor. Additionally, this research demonstrates how research on biological underpinnings can also inform metastructure research itself by providing plausible mechanisms that can further clarify research on the ways in which disorders relate.

Conclusions

The search for biological correlates of psychopathology stands to benefit from being interwoven with the empirical structure of psychopathology. Models of the empirical structure of psychopathology provide a coherent framework through which to interpret biological findings, which can accommodate comorbidity and improve ecological validity. It is important that subsequent versions of the DSM come to reflect the presence of the meta-structure underlying mental disorders if it aims to reflect our current empirical understanding of the data. A DSM-5 study group has proceeded towards the aim of representing the metastructure by developing a group of 11 'validating criteria' that suggest aetiological relatedness between a cluster of disorders. The criteria are (1) genetic factors, (2) familiality, (3) early environmental adversity, (4) temperamental antecedents, (5) neural substrates, (6) biomarkers, (7) cognitive and emotional processing, (8) differences and similarities in symptomatology, (9) comorbidity, (10) course, and (11) treatment. A recent review of the literature has suggested that there is a case for the DSM to unify related disorders under the category of internalizing, also called emotional, disorders [15]. Although the meta-analysis found differences between disorders in the proposed cluster, specifically in the domains of cognitive and emotional processing, neural substrates, and familial studies, there were more similarities than differences in these disorders within the 11 domains studied. The authors suggest that a reorganization of the DSM to reflect this knowledge is possible, and further clarify that the proposed clustering would not remove traditional diagnostic categories, but only reorganize them to better reflect our current understanding. Although our understanding of etiology is still in its nascent stages, to preserve the current classification system with all its flaws until a definitive solution becomes clear would impede biologically and diagnostically-based research [16]. Insofar as the DSM 5 will reflect changes to our understanding of the nature of diagnostic categories, it will be progressing towards a system that will be better suited to research biological underpinnings.

Competing interests
Neither author has any competing interests.

Authors' contributions
SO participated in drafting and editing the manuscript. RF Krueger participated in drafting and editing the manuscript. All authors read and approved the final manuscript.

References

1. Blashfield RK: **Diagnostic models and systems.** In *Clinical Psychology: Assessment, Vol. 4.* Edited by Bellack AS, Herson M, Reynolds CR. New York: Elsevier Science; 1998:57–79.
2. Clark LA, Watson D, Reynolds S: **Diagnostic and classification of psychopathology; challenges to the current system and future directions.** *Annu Rev Psychol* 1995, **46**:121–153.
3. Wittchen HU: **Critical issues in the evaluation of comorbidity of psychiatric disorders.** *Br J Psychiatry Suppl* 1996, **30**:9–16.
4. Angst J, Vollrath M, Merikangas KR, Ernst C: **Comorbidty of anxiety and depression in the Zurich cohort study of young adults.** In *Comorbidity of Mood and Anxiety Disorders.* Edited by Maser JD, Cloninger CR. Washington, DC: American Psychiatric Press; 1990:123–137.
5. Sturt E: **Hierarchical patterns in the distribution of psychiatric symptoms.** *Psychol Med* 1981, **11**:783–794.
6. Boyd JH, Burke JD Jr, Gruenberg E, Holzer CE III, Rae DS, George LK, Karno M, Stoltzman R, McEvoy L, Nestadt G: **Exclusion criteria of DSM-III; a study of co-occurrence of hierarchy-free syndromes.** *Arch Gen Psychiatry* 1984, **41**:983–989.
7. Kirk SA, Kutchins H: **The myth of the reliability of DSM.** *J Mind Behav.* 1994, **15**:71–86.
8. Eaton NR, South SC, Krueger RF: **The meaning of comorbidity among common mental disorders.** In *Contemporary Directions in Psychopathology.* 2nd edition. Edited by Millon T, Krueger R, Simonsen E. New York: Guilford Press; 2010:223–241.
9. Krueger RF, Markon KE: **Reinterpreting comorbidity. A model-based approach to understanding and classifying psychopathology.** *Annu Rev Clin Psychol* 2006, **2**:111–133.
10. Slade T, Watson D: **The structure of common DSM-IV and ICD-10 mental disorders in the Australian general population.** *Psychol Med* 2006, **36**:1593–1600.
11. Vollebergh WAM, Iedema J, Bijl RV, de Graaf R, Smit F, Ormel J: **The structure and stability of common mental disorders: the NEMESIS study.** *Arch Gen Psychiatry* 2001, **58**:597–603.
12. Kessler RC, Ormel J, Petukhova M, McLaughlin KA, Green JG, Russo LJ, Üstün TB: **Development of Lifetime Comorbidity in the World Health Organization World Mental Health Surveys.** *Arch Gen Psychiatry* 2011, **68**(1):90–100. doi:10.1001/archgenpsychiatry.2010.180.

13. Kotov R, Ruggero CJ, Krueger RF, Watson D, Yuan Q, Zimmerman M: **New Dimensions in the Quantitative Classification of Mental Illness.** *Arch Gen Psychiatry* 2011, **68**(10):1003–1011. doi:10.1001/archgenpsychiatry.2011.10.
14. Vaidyanathan U, Patrick CJ, Cuthbert BN: **Linking Dimensional Models of Internalizing Psychopathology to Neurobiological Systems: Affect-Modulated Startle as an Indicator of Fear and Distress Disorders and Affiliated Traits.** *Psych Bull* 2009, **135**:909–942.
15. Goldberg DP, Krueger RF, Andrews G, Hobbs MJ: **Emotional disorders: Cluster 4 of the proposed meta-structure for DSM-V and ICD-11.** *Psych Medicine* 2009, **39**:2043–2059.
16. Hyman SE: **The diagnosis of mental disorders: The problem of reification.** *Annu Rev Clin Psychol* 2010, **6**:155–179.

14

Frontostriatal functional connectivity in major depressive disorder

Daniella J Furman*, J Paul Hamilton and Ian H Gotlib

Abstract

Background: Abnormalities of the striatum and frontal cortex have been reported consistently in studies of neural structure and function in major depressive disorder (MDD). Despite speculation that compromised connectivity between these regions may underlie symptoms of MDD, little work has investigated the integrity of frontostriatal circuits in this disorder.

Methods: Functional magnetic resonance images were acquired from 21 currently depressed and 19 never-disordered women during wakeful rest. Using four predefined striatal regions-of-interest, seed-to-whole brain correlations were computed and compared between groups.

Results: Compared to controls, depressed participants exhibited attenuated functional connectivity between the ventral striatum and both ventromedial prefrontal cortex and subgenual anterior cingulate cortex. Depressed participants also exhibited stronger connectivity between the dorsal caudate and dorsal prefrontal cortex, which was positively correlated with severity of the disorder.

Conclusions: Depressed individuals are characterized by aberrant connectivity in frontostriatal circuits that are posited to support affective and cognitive processing. Further research is required to examine more explicitly the link between patterns of disrupted connectivity and specific symptoms of depression, and the extent to which these patterns precede the onset of depression and normalize with recovery from depressive illness.

Keywords: depression, functional connectivity, striatum, subgenual anterior cingulate cortex, dorsolateral prefrontal cortex, fMRI

Background

Major depressive disorder (MDD) is among the most prevalent and debilitating of all psychiatric illnesses, affecting nearly 20% of the US population, or more than 30 million adults, at some point in their lives [1]. MDD is characterized most commonly by sadness and/or by a marked decrease in the ability to experience reward or pleasure (that is, anhedonia). Individuals diagnosed with MDD also often exhibit psychomotor retardation and deficits in executive function, typically reflected by difficulties concentrating, making decisions, and terminating the processing of negative material [2]. Neuroanatomical models of depression, however, have yet to fully account for the range of symptom domains that characterize this disorder.

* Correspondence: dfurman@stanford.edu
Department of Psychology, Stanford University, 450 Serra Mall, Stanford, CA 94305-2004, USA

Investigators examining neural functioning in depressed individuals have frequently reported anomalies in the structure and function of the frontal lobes. For example, altered regional blood flow [3] and glucose metabolism [4] in the prefrontal cortex (PFC), a region frequently implicated in affect regulation and in a number of cognitive and motor processes, have been linked to both psychomotor retardation and anhedonia in depressed individuals. Interestingly, these studies also implicate anomalous functioning of the striatum in MDD, a revealing co-occurrence given the neuroanatomical linkages between the PFC and striatum. The striatum, composed within each hemisphere of the caudate nucleus, putamen, and core of the nucleus accumbens, comprises the primary input structure to the basal ganglia circuitry, receiving extensive projections from the frontal cortex. Output neurons from the basal ganglia send projections to midbrain structures and the thalamus, which completes a cortico-striatal-pallidal-thalamic (CSPT) circuit by returning projections to the frontal cortices. Whereas the PFC is generally thought to serve central control or goal representation functions, investigators have argued that CSPT circuitry aids in the filtering and focusing of cortical input, selecting among potential cognitive and behavioral representations [5,6]. This formulation has provided a foundation for models of behavior selection [6] and working memory updating [7], and supports the hypothesis that abnormal functioning of frontostriatal pathways contributes to the anhedonic, ruminative, and psychomotor dysfunctions characteristic of MDD.

Importantly, topographical organization within CSPT circuitry is largely preserved, such that corticostriatal neurons from the motor and premotor cortices project most densely to the caudal putamen ('motor' division), whereas input from dorsolateral PFC (DLPFC) innervates the dorsal caudate ('executive' division), and projections from the orbitofrontal cortex (OFC) and anterior cingulate cortex (ACC) tend to populate the ventral striatum ('limbic' or 'affective' division). In general, these divisions along the ventral-dorsal axis of the striatum are posited to be relatively segregated, thereby differentially supporting affective, cognitive, and motor processing [8]. Given that the difficulties experienced in MDD span these domains, it is possible that dysfunction in this system is attributable to global perturbations in microstructure or macrostructure, or in neurotransmission, rather than to abnormalities restricted to a particular CSPT division. Alternatively, the ascending flow of information through the parallel CSPT circuits [9] may enable a circumscribed abnormality in CSPT function to propagate to other subdivisions (for example, disrupting the translation of reward motivation into goal-directed motor behavior). Nonetheless, despite hypotheses that CSPT circuitry, and the frontostriatal connections in particular, may be compromised in MDD [10-12], little empirical work has explicitly examined CSPT circuit function in this disorder.

Over the last decade, there has been a surge in the development and use of methods to investigate network-level brain function [13]. These methods have recently been used to map the correlated activity, or functional connectivity, of normally and abnormally functioning corticostriatal networks in human subjects at rest [14,15]. Using one such method, investigators have documented attenuated functional connectivity between the ACC and a region of interest (ROI) spanning parts of the putamen and globus pallidus in depressed individuals [16]. This finding suggests anomalous frontostriatal connectivity in MDD, but does not permit us to draw conclusions about the subdivisions involved. In the present study, we examined patterns of frontostriatal connectivity in adults diagnosed with MDD, focusing on the dorsal and ventral striatal subdivisions posited to differentially support motor (dorsal putamen), executive (dorsal caudate), and affective (ventral caudate and putamen) functions, all of which have been found to be compromised in MDD. Given previous findings that mood [17] and reward-related behaviors [18] vary with the extent of connectivity between the ventral striatum (VS) and the subgenual anterior cingulate cortex (sACC), we hypothesized that, compared with non-depressed individuals, depressed participants would exhibit abnormal connectivity between the frontal cortex and the striatum, most markedly in this ventral, limbic circuit. Further, given the frequent presentation of cognitive and psychomotor dysfunction in MDD, we hypothesized that depressed persons would also exhibit attenuated frontostriatal connectivity within the executive and motor networks.

Methods

Participants

Twenty-one adults diagnosed with MDD and 19 control (CTL) participants with no history of psychiatric disorder participated in this study. Given the documented gender differences in the prevalence of depression [19], and to reduce possible heterogeneity in neural functioning, we included only female participants in our sample. Participants were recruited from local psychiatric outpatient clinics and through advertisements posted in numerous locations within the community. Participants' responses to a telephone interview provided initial selection information. This phone screen established that participants were fluent in English and were between 18 and 60 years of age. Participants were excluded if they reported severe head trauma, learning disabilities, or bipolar disorder. Participants were also excluded if they met criteria for alcohol or substance dependence or for alcohol or substance abuse within the past 6 months. Trained interviewers administered the Structured Clinical Interview for *Diagnostic and Statistical Manual of Mental Disorders, fourth edition* (DSM-IV) Axis I Disorders (SCID) to eligible individuals; in previous studies, our team of interviewers has demonstrated excellent inter-rater reliability for both the diagnosis of MDD (κ = 0.93) and for the non-psychiatric CTL diagnosis (κ = 0.92). All depressed participants met criteria for a DSM-IV diagnosis of current MDD based on their responses to the SCID. None of the control participants met diagnostic criteria for any current or past Axis-I disorder. In addition, all participants completed the Beck Depression Inventory II (BDI) [20], a self-report measure of the severity of depressive symptoms, and the 22-item Ruminative Responses Scale (RRS) of the Response Styles Questionnaire [21], a self-report measure of ruminative tendencies. Informed consent was obtained from all participants, and all aspects of this study complied with the ethical standards for treatment of human participants from the American Psychiatric Association.

fMRI data acquisition

Blood-oxygen-level dependent (BOLD) signal data were acquired with 3 Tesla General Electric magnetic resonance imaging scanners (General Electric, Milwaukee, WI, USA) using single-channel whole-head coils. Images were acquired used a T2*-weighted, in/out spiral pulse sequence [22]. Scans were acquired as part of three different imaging studies and, therefore, had slightly different parameter specifications (version A: repetition time (TR) = 1,200 ms/frame, echo time (TE) = 30 ms, flip angle = 77, field of view (FOV) = 220 mm, number of temporal frames (NTF) = 250, 18 slices, 3.44 mm^2 in-plane and 5 mm through-plane resolution; version B: TR = 1,300 ms/frame, TE = 30 ms, flip angle = 80, FOV = 220 mm, NTF = 190, 20 slices, 3.44 mm^2 in-plane and 5 mm through-plane resolution; version C: TR = 2,000 ms/frame, TE = 30 ms, flip angle = 77, FOV = 220 mm, NTF = 180, 29 slices, 3.44 mm^2 in-plane and 4 mm through-plane resolution). High-resolution anatomical scans were collected for every participant using a spoiled grass gradient recalled (SPGR) sequence for T1 contrast (TE = 7 ms, flip angle = 15, FOV = 220 mm, 124 axial slices, 0.86 mm^2 in-plane and 1.2 mm through-plane resolution). Participants were instructed to lie still during the scan with their eyes closed.

Data preprocessing

All data preprocessing and analysis were carried out using Analysis of Functional NeuroImages (AFNI; http://afni.nimh.nih.gov/afni/) software. The following procedures were applied to all datasets regardless of data acquisition parameters: (1) removal of first three brain volumes to allow for equilibration of longitudinal magnetization; (2) slice-time correction to the middle axial slice; (3) coregistration to the middle temporal acquisition to correct for head rotation and translation during the scan (Fourier interpolation); (4) temporal band-pass filtering at 0.009 Hz $<f<$ 0.08 Hz, (5) spatial smoothing with a 6 mm Gaussian smoothing kernel; (6) conversion to units of percent signal change; (7) spatial resampling to 27 mm^3 isotropic voxels; and (8) coregistration to high-resolution anatomical images and affine transformation to Talairach space.

Previous investigators have demonstrated the feasibility of pooling data with varying acquisition parameters from multiple studies [23]. Nevertheless, to maximize homogeneity across the three scan types, after preprocessing we took several additional steps to correct for the discrepancy in temporal sampling rate. First, we upsampled all voxel time series data from scan versions A and B using linear interpolation by a factor necessary for subsequent resampling to TR = 2,000 ms/frame (i.e., 6 for version A, 13 for version B). We then downsampled data by the required amount (i.e., selection of every 10th data point for version A and every 20th point for version B). Finally, we resampled head motion data in the same manner as corresponding time-series data. Limiting our analyses to the duration of the shortest scanning session (B), we used only the first 122 time points of each preprocessed dataset, resulting in an effective scan duration of 4 minutes, 4 seconds.

Nuisance signal removal and ROI time series extraction

Consistent with previous studies of basal ganglia functional connectivity [14,24], we regressed participants' preprocessed data on a series of noise predictors, modeling the zero-order through second-order trends in the BOLD time series, and nuisance signals from white matter (WM), cerebrospinal fluid (CSF), global signal, and six motion parameters (three rotational and three translational). Resulting terms were used to generate time series for regressors of no interest, which were then subtracted from the original preprocessed data [25].

For purposes of ROI seed placement, we used eight striatal seeds (four per hemisphere) described by Di Martino *et al.* [14] converted from Montreal Neurological Institute (MNI) space into Talairach coordinates by means of a non-linear transform [26]. In each hemisphere, seed ROIs comprised a spherical mask with 7 mm radius centered in ventral striatum (VS; Talairach x y z: ± 8.9 8.4 -7.1), dorsal caudate (DC; ± 12.9 14.9 7.5), dorsal caudal putamen (DCP; ± 27.7 1.1 2.7), and ventral rostral putamen (VRP, ± 19.8 11.5 -3.1). As detailed by Di Martino *et al.* [14], the locations of these seeds are consistent with identified subdivisions of the striatum. For each participant, the locations of seeds were visually inspected with reference to anatomical images to ensure appropriate placement. BOLD time-series data averaged across all voxels within each of the eight ROIs were then extracted from participants' noise-covariate corrected data. Finally, time-series data from corresponding right and left hemisphere ROIs were averaged to form four bilateral ROIs.

Statistical analyses

We regressed each participant's preprocessed voxel time series data separately for each of the four bilateral seed regions on the spatially averaged ROI time series along with the nuisance covariates (zero-order through second-order trends in the BOLD time series, six motion parameters, and signal from WM, CSF, and whole-brain masks). By regressing the preprocessed data rather than the residuals at this stage, we were able to orthogonalize the basal ganglia seeds with respect to the nuisance covariates, thereby ensuring that the resulting statistical maps reflected the unique contribution of seed mask time series. These analyses yielded subject-level t-statistic maps indexing regional correlations with the ROI time series. Individual statistical maps were Fisher transformed to Z-score maps prior to analysis at the group level. To compare patterns of correlated activity with each bilateral seed region between MDD and CTL samples, we conducted two-sample t-tests on participants' Z-score maps. To elucidate the nature of the group differences, we conducted one-sample t-tests on patterns of striatal functional connectivity within each group. We conducted 2,000 Monte Carlo simulations using AFNI's AlphaSim [27] and determined that an uncorrected single voxel significant threshold of $p < 0.005$ and cluster threshold of $k = 26$ were necessary to hold family-wise type I error at $P < 0.05$.

Exploratory analyses

For each suprathreshold frontal cortical cluster that was identified in the between-groups analyses, connectivity or correlation coefficients (r) were averaged across all voxels falling within the cluster. Within our sample of MDD participants, we then correlated averaged estimates of connectivity strength with measures of disorder severity (BDI) and rumination (RRS). In addition, we conducted two-sample t-tests comparing average correlation coefficients from these clusters between those MDD participants with and without observable psychomotor symptoms (determined on the basis of SCID criteria). Given the exploratory nature of these analyses, we used an uncorrected statistical threshold of $p < 0.05$ for each test.

Results

Demographic and clinical characteristics

The MDD and CTL groups did not differ significantly in age (MDD: mean = 39.2, SD = 11.8; CTL: mean = 33.2, SD = 10.5; $t(38) = 1.7$, $p > 0.1$) or in the distribution of data acquisition protocols from which participants were drawn ($\chi^2(2) = 1.24$, $p > 0.5$). (Age did not moderate levels of functional connectivity for any of the frontal cortical regions reported in the between-group analyses. In addition, we did not observe effects of acquisition protocol, or of an acquisition protocol-by-group interaction, on estimates of frontostriatal connectivity in regions reported here to vary by group.) As expected, scores on the BDI were significantly higher for the MDD (mean = 31.3, SD = 11.7) than for the CTL (mean = 1.5, SD = 2.4) participants, $t(38) = 10.9$, $p < 0.0001$. Fourteen of the participants with MDD were taking at least one of the following psychotropic medications: venlafaxine, bupropion, escitalopram, paroxetine, fluoxetine, duloxetine, atomoxetine, mirtazapine, trazadone, buspirone, temazepam, zoldipem, modafinil, and buprenorphine. (Psychoactive medication status, defined as a dichotomous variable, did not significantly mediate any of the reported frontostriatal connectivity effects [see Additional file 1 for comparisons].) In addition, nine of the MDD participants met diagnostic criteria for at least one comorbid Axis-I disorder: dysthymia (n = 1); panic disorder (n = 2); post-traumatic stress disorder (PTSD) (n = 2); anorexia (n = 1); and social anxiety disorder (n = 5). One CTL participant and two MDD participants reported being regular smokers.

Functional connectivity

The patterns of functional correlations with caudate and putamen identified in the samples of MDD and CTL participants were, in general, consistent with those reported by Di Martino *et al.* [14] (Figure 1 [see Additional files 2 and 3]). Briefly, in CTL participants, activity in the VS was correlated with activity in an extensive region of bilateral caudate, ventromedial prefrontal cortex (vmPFC), OFC, sACC, and posterior cingulate cortex (PCC), as well as with areas of the hippocampal formation, insula, superior temporal gyrus, medial dorsal thalamus, and brainstem. Activity in the DC seed was correlated with activity in regions of dorsal ACC and PFC, medial dorsal thalamus, putamen, inferior frontal gyrus, and the cerebellum.

As in the VS, activity in VRP seeds was correlated with a large region extending through the putamen, ventral caudate, superior temporal gyrus, insula, globus pallidus, and vmPFC. Activity in these seeds was also correlated with activity in the precentral gyrus, cerebellum, and a region of dorsomedial PFC bridging the dorsal aspect of the ACC and supplementary motor area (SMA). The DCP seeds were functionally connected to several cortical and subcortical regions including the globus pallidus, insula, inferior frontal and superior temporal gyri, thalamus, cerebellum, and a region of dorsomedial PFC abutting ACC and SMA. Finally, activity in the right DCP was correlated with activity in the precentral and postcentral gyri.

Given our specific hypotheses of altered frontostriatal connectivity in MDD between striatal seed regions and the frontal cortex, we report significant differences in frontostriatal connectivity between the MDD and CTL participants for each seed region (Figure 1). Detailed results of these analyses, as well as group differences in regions outside of the frontal cortex, are presented in Table 1.

Ventral striatum

Consistent with our hypotheses, we observed attenuated functional connectivity between VS and both vmPFC and sACC in MDD, relative to CTL, participants.

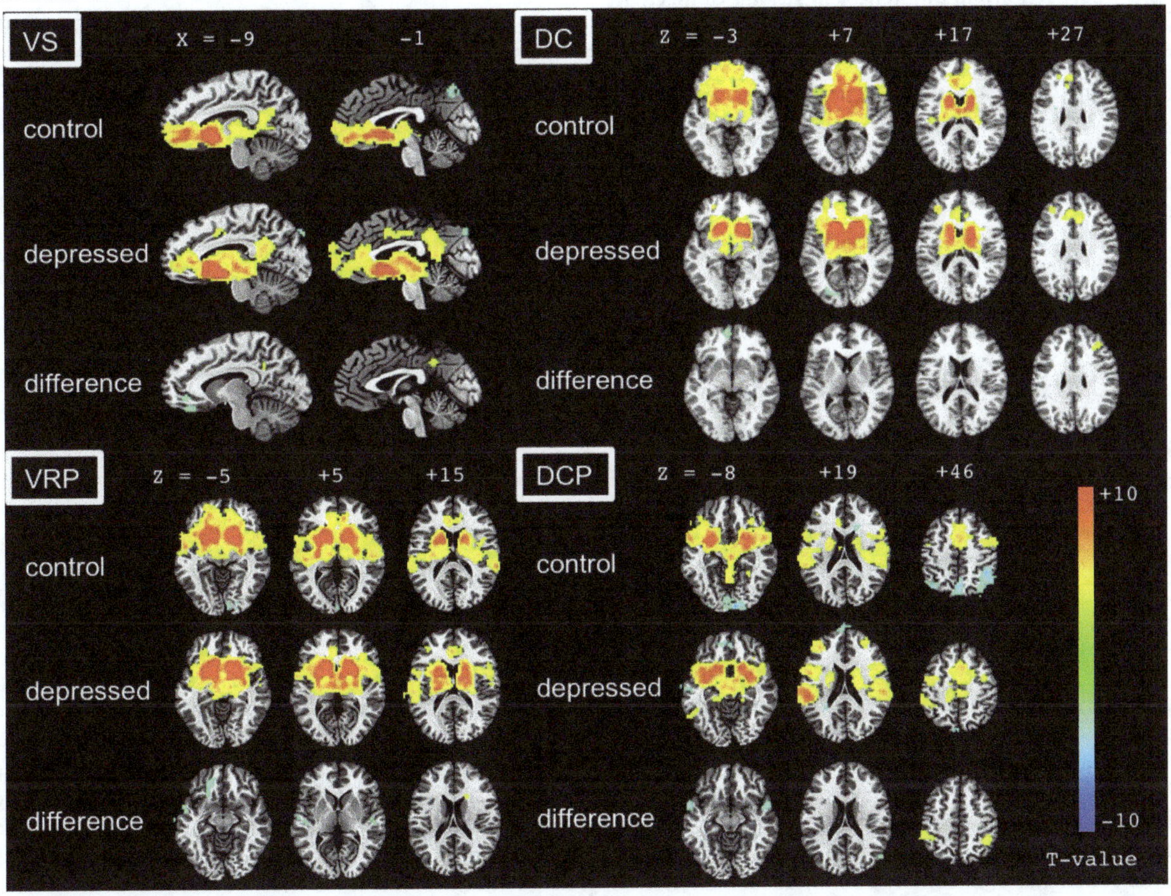

Figure 1 Statistical maps depicting regions of positive and negative functional connectivity with the striatum. Statistical maps depicting regions of positive and negative functional connectivity with the ventral striatum (VS), dorsal caudate (DC), ventral rostral putamen (VRP), and dorsal caudal putamen (DCP) in depressed and control samples, and between-group differences in functional connectivity with these regions (blue = control > depressed; yellow = depressed > control). Voxel-wise $p < 0.005$, minimum cluster size = 26 voxels.

Dorsal caudate

The MDD participants exhibited decreased functional connectivity between the DC seed and the medial frontal gyrus, relative to CTL participants. MDD participants also showed increased positive connectivity between the DC and DLPFC.

Ventral putamen

Compared with CTL participants, individuals with MDD exhibited diminished connectivity between the VRP and ventromedial regions of the frontal lobe.

Dorsal putamen

There were no significant differences between MDD and CTL participants in frontal-DCP connectivity.

Associations with clinical variables

RRS data were collected from all but two participants. BDI and RRS scores were moderately correlated, r = 0.47, $p < 0.05$. Of the four frontostriatal relations examined (VS-sACC, DC-medial frontal gyrus, DC-DLPFC, VRP-vmPFC), only DC-DLPFC connectivity was significantly correlated with depression severity (n = 21, r = 0.52, $p = 0.015$; see Figure 2); for all other correlations with BDI, $|r| < 0.30$, $ps > 0.2$. Although none of the connectivity measures was significantly correlated with RRS score, there was a trend for DC-DLPFC connectivity to correlate with RRS score (n = 19, r = 0.38, $p = 0.105$); for all other correlations with RRS, $|r| < 0.18$, $ps > 0.4$. Depressed participants with observable psychomotor retardation (n = 11) exhibited significantly weaker functional connectivity between the DC and the medial frontal gyrus (mean = 0.003, SD = 0.20) than did depressed participants without this symptom (n = 10; mean = 0.162, SD = 0.14), $t(19) = 2.1$, $p = 0.05$. There was a trend for depressed participants with psychomotor retardation to exhibit weaker VRP-vmPFC connectivity, and stronger DC-DLPFC connectivity, than did

Table 1 Between-group differences in striatal connectivity

Seed	Contrast	Region	Peak voxel (Talairach)			Cluster size	Peak t value
			x	y	z		
VS	CTL > MDD	Left subgenual ACC, medial orbitofrontal cortex	-13	41	-4	40	3.9
	MDD > CTL	Left precuneus, posterior cingulate cortex	-7	-46	32	39	4.1
		Right cerebellum	29	-25	-28	31	4.4
		Right inferior parietal lobule	35	-49	38	30	3.9
DC	CTL > MDD	Left medial frontal gyrus	-7	53	-1	32	3.6
	MDD > CTL	Right middle frontal gyrus	32	32	26	44	4.0
VRP	CTL > MDD	Left superior temporal gyrus	-58	-13	-1	93	4.2
		Left medial frontal gyrus, orbitofrontal cortex	-16	35	-10	78	4.5
		Right posterior insula	44	-13	8	30	4.0
	MDD > CTL	Right caudate body, subgyral	17	14	20	52	4.4
DCP	CTL > MDD	Left superior temporal gyrus	-55	2	-7	50	5.1
		Right superior temporal gyrus	53	5	-10	46	4.6
		Right posterior insula	41	-16	11	44	4.4
		Right middle temporal gyrus	53	-64	14	41	3.8
	MDD > CTL	Left inferior parietal lobule, postcentral gyrus	-46	-37	50	80	4.8
		Right inferior parietal lobule	41	-46	47	54	4.7
		Right lingual gyrus	26	-85	-13	38	4.4

Voxel-wise $p < 0.005$, minimum cluster size = 26 voxels.

ACC = anterior cingulate cortex; CTL = control; DC = dorsal caudate; DCP = dorsal caudal putamen; MDD = major depressive disorder; VRP = ventral rostral putamen; VS = ventral striatum.

depressed participants without psychomotor symptoms, but these differences were not statistically significant, all $t(19) < 1.2$, *ps* > 0.17.

Discussion

The present study was designed to examine alterations in the functional connectivity of frontostriatal networks in MDD. Patterns of connectivity in both control and depressed participants were consistent with the results of previous studies [14]; importantly, however, striking differences between the depressed and non-depressed participants were detected in networks that have been implicated in affective and motivational processing [28]. In particular, we found that, compared with healthy

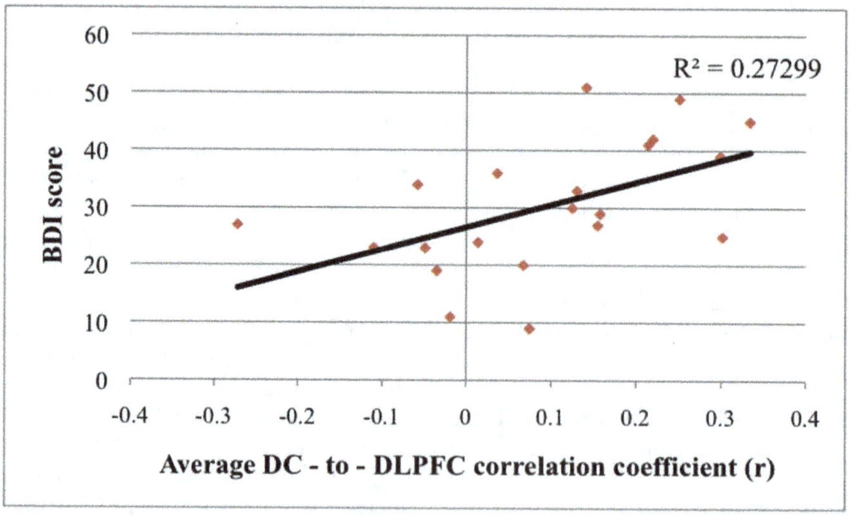

Figure 2 Relation between depression severity and dorsal caudate (DC) to dorsolateral prefrontal cortex (DLPFC) connectivity. Relation between depression severity and dorsal caudate (DC) to dorsolateral prefrontal cortex (DLPFC) functional connectivity in currently depressed participants. BDI = Beck Depression Inventory II.

controls, depressed individuals exhibited attenuated connectivity between seed regions approximating the ventral striatum/nucleus accumbens and ventral rostral putamen, and vmPFC and sACC targets.

It is important to note that these prefrontal target regions fall within the bounds of regions known to have anatomical connectivity with the VS [8,9]. As noted earlier, the pattern of projections from the cortex to the striatum maintains much of its anatomical distinction, such that corticostriatal neurons from the motor and premotor cortices project most densely to the caudal putamen, whereas input from the OFC and vmPFC tends to populate the anteroventral caudate and ventromedial putamen. Indeed, this ventral corticostriatal network is posited to support reward-related processing and affect [8]. Consistent with this framework, several of the ventromedial PFC structures found in this study to correlate differentially with striatal activity in participants with MDD and CTL subjects have previously been implicated in depression and in the processes affected by this disorder [29,30].

Because of its unique interconnectivity with subcortical and limbic structures, the sACC has been hypothesized to be involved in both affective processes and visceromotor integration [31,32], and has specifically been associated with the induction of negative mood [33]. Functional [29], metabolic [34], and volumetric [34,35] anomalies involving the sACC are often reported in studies of MDD. Interestingly, Harrison and colleagues [17] reported a relation between cytokine-induced decrements in mood and the degree of connectivity between the nucleus accumbens and the sACC. Considered in light of our current findings, this body of work suggests that multiple forms of brain pathology, including aberrant structure or functionality of either striatal or frontal regions, ultimately produce a similar, deleterious effect on network-level function. Thus, future research should examine the extent to which volumetric and metabolic anomalies contribute to the pathophysiology of MDD by altering patterns of mesolimbic or corticostriatal connectivity.

Situated just rostral to the sACC, the vmPFC is associated with the production [36] and flexible shifting of emotional states [37] and behavior, as well as with reward processing [38] and reinforcement learning [39]. Interestingly, the integrity of fibers linking the vmPFC, as well as the medial OFC, with the VS appears to mediate individual differences in reward-related behavior. For example, using diffusion tractography, Cohen and colleagues found a positive correlation between the integrity of this tract and reward dependence, a personality trait characterized by learning from reward signals and persistence in repeating actions associated with rewards [18]. Importantly, impaired reinforcement or reward learning is characteristic of MDD, and has been linked to anhedonic symptoms in depressed individuals [30]; the current finding of diminished functional connectivity between the vmPFC and VS in MDD suggests a potential neural correlate of this deficiency. Future work should examine the relation between differences in frontostriatal connectivity and compromised motivational and reward-learning processes in anhedonic depression.

We also observed attenuated connectivity between the dorsal striatum and medial PFC in depressed, relative to control, participants. In contrast to the ventral corticostriatal 'limbic' networks, those networks comprising more dorsal (and caudal) regions of the striatum, along with their respective inputs from the frontal cortices, are thought to support executive function and motor-planning processes, including the initiation of behavior [40]. In addition to detailing associations between MDD and compromised executive and motor function, studies have linked depression to difficulties in the initiation of motor movements [41]. For example, Sabbe *et al.* report that the highest degree of motor slowing in MDD is observed during the early stages of a movement, suggesting a particular difficulty in initiating behaviors [42]. Subsequent work has demonstrated an increased reliance on external cues during the performance of sequential movements in melancholic depressed persons, reminiscent of the deficits of initiative seen in Parkinson's disease (PD) [43]. While preliminary analysis of the relation between psychomotor retardation and dorsal striatal connectivity suggests a plausible mechanism by which psychomotor function is compromised in MDD, future research with larger sample sizes and more detailed assessments of symptom severity will help clarify the extent and specificity of this relation.

We found an unanticipated increase in connectivity between the dorsal caudate and the middle frontal gyrus in MDD. Given the association between dorsal corticostriatal macrocircuitry and both the filtering and manipulation of content in working memory [44,45], it is possible that this result reflects the inability to update the contents of working memory [46] and the maintenance of negative information in MDD [47]. Preliminary support for this formulation comes from our observation that, for depressed participants, increasing tendency to ruminate predicted increasing DC-DLPFC connectivity during rest, though this correlation did not reach statistical significance in the current sample. It is possible that the observed increase in functional connectivity reflects a compensatory mechanism; if output from the basal ganglia circuitry to the frontal cortex (via the thalamus) is compromised in individuals with depression, cortical input to the basal ganglia may be ramped up in an attempt to drive an underactive basal ganglia-thalamus complex.

In addition to differences between depressed and non-depressed participants in the degree or extent of connectivity within corticostriatal networks, alterations observed in this study in the relation between these networks and other known brain systems are noteworthy. Relative to healthy individuals, participants with MDD exhibited enhanced connectivity between the VS and the PCC, a cortical-midline region central to the default mode network (DMN) [48]. The DMN, composed of medial frontal, lateral and medial parietal, as well as temporal lobe regions, has been implicated broadly in self-referential processing [49]. Activity across the various nodes of this network is reduced during periods of non-self-referential processing, such as those that occur during the performance of demanding cognitive tasks [48,49]. Recently, Kelly *et al.* demonstrated that administering L-3,4-dihydroxyphenylalanine (L-DOPA), a precursor to dopamine (DA), to healthy participants diminishes functional connectivity between the PCC and caudate regions [24]; these authors propose that the striatum plays a role in the suppression of the DMN under conditions requiring a shift from self-directed, to externally-directed, processing. In contrast, our finding indicates a *reduction* in the anticorrelation of these two networks in MDD, potentially reflecting the difficulty exhibited by depressed persons shifting attention away from self-referential processing and reducing DMN activity in the face of external demands [50].

Although we did not quantify dopaminergic factors in the present study, there is reason to believe that DA plays an important role in the modulation of these corticostriatal connections. Whereas augmentation of DA levels has been shown to increase functional connectivity between the VS and vmPFC [24], DA depletion has been found to attenuate the functional coupling between VS and both dorsal and ventral PFC [51]. Similarly, connectivity analyses in PD patients have demonstrated attenuated connectivity between the ventromedial caudate (approximating our VS seed) and the vmPFC [52]. The similarity between the connectivity patterns identified in both temporary and disease-related DA-depleted states and those identified in our depressed sample is intriguing, and argues for a more systematic investigation of the relations among DA tone, corticostriatal connectivity, and symptom presentation in MDD.

In closing, we note a number of limitations of this study. First, our sample was composed entirely of females, thereby limiting our ability to generalize the current results to male subjects. Second, our depressed sample was heterogeneous with respect to comorbid DSM-IV diagnoses and psychoactive medication status. Although statistical tests indicated that medication status [see Additional file 1] did not mediate the aberrant patterns of frontostriatal connectivity we found to characterize depressed individuals, we cannot rule out the possibility that certain drug classes might selectively affect these circuits. While previous studies have reported no change in resting state basal ganglia-ACC functional connectivity following selective serotonin reuptake inhibitor (SSRI) treatment [53] and only decreases in DC-frontal lobe connectivity following administration of L-DOPA to healthy controls [24], future research might examine directly the effects of dopaminergic agents on corticostriatal connectivity, particularly in the context of symptom remediation. Third, we may be underpowered in the current study to detect and precisely characterize the associations between clinical variables and frontostriatal abnormalities. It is also possible that certain of the documented abnormalities in frontostriatal connectivity reflect risk factors for the development of depression. In this case, we might not expect to identify correlations with disease or symptom severity. These possibilities highlight the importance of examining corticostriatal connectivity in a larger sample of MDD subjects, in those at elevated risk for the development of MDD, and in individuals who have recovered from the disorder. Finally, the present findings of altered frontostriatal connectivity in MDD may be attributable, in part, to structural changes within the striatum itself [54-56]. Although we assume that the seeds used in this study represent discrete functional divisions of the striatum, it is possible that the boundaries between such divisions are shifted in the brains of depressed persons as a result of structural alteration. Future work directly examining the consequences of gross anatomical, metabolic and/or functional changes on frontostriatal circuitry could advance our understanding of how regional changes in brain function alter system-level function in psychiatric disorders. Despite these limitations, however, the results of the present study provide important empirical support for the hypothesis that MDD is characterized, and even maintained, by compromised frontostriatal function.

Additional material

Additional file 1: Estimates (and standard errors) of functional connectivity between striatal regions-of-interest and frontal cortical regions for control, medicated depressed, and non-medicated depressed participants. Frontal cortical region clusters were identified in the between-groups (control vs depressed) analyses; for each participant, Fisher transformed correlation coefficients were averaged across all voxels falling within a given cluster. In no analysis did medicated and non-medicated depressed participants differ significantly from each other. CTL = control; MDD = major depressive disorder; PFC = prefrontal cortex; sACC = subgenual anterior cingulate cortex.

Additional file 2: Functional connectivity with striatal seeds: control (CTL) group. Voxel-wise $p < 0.005$, minimum cluster size = 26 voxels.

ACC = anterior cingulate cortex; DC = dorsal caudate; DCP = dorsal caudal putamen; PFC = prefrontal cortex; VRP = ventral rostral putamen; VS = ventral striatum.

Additional file 3: Functional connectivity with striatal seeds: major depressive disorder (MDD) group. Voxel-wise $p < 0.005$, minimum cluster size = 26 voxels. ACC = anterior cingulate cortex; DC = dorsal caudate; DCP = dorsal caudal putamen; PFC = prefrontal cortex; VRP = ventral rostral putamen; VS = ventral striatum.

Acknowledgements
This research was supported by National Institute of Mental Health Grant MH59259 awarded to IHG. The authors thank Sarah Victor for her help in data collection.

Authors' contributions
DJF and IHG designed the study, and DJF and JPH conducted the statistical analyses. DJF wrote the first draft of the manuscript. All authors contributed to, and approved, the final manuscript.

Competing interests
The authors declare that they have no competing interests.

References
1. Kessler RC, Wang PS: **Epidemiology of Depression.** In *Handbook of Depression.*. 2 edition. Edited by: Gotlib IH, Hammen CL. New York: The Guilford Press; 2009:5-22.
2. Gotlib IH, Joormann J: **Cognition and depression: current status and future directions.** *Annu Rev Clin Psychol* 2010, **6**:285-312.
3. Videbach P: **PET measurements of brain glucose metabolism and blood flow in major depressive disorder: a critical review.** *Acta Psychiatr Scand* 2000, **101**:11-20.
4. Dunn RT, Kimbrell TA, Ketter TA, Frye MA, Willis MW, Luckenbaugh DA, Post RM: **Principal components of the beck depression inventory and regional cerebral metabolism in unipolar and bipolar depression.** *Biol Psychiatry* 2002, **51**:387-399.
5. Mink JW: **The basal ganglia: focused selection and inhibition of competing motor programs.** *Prog Neurobiol* 1996, **50**:381-425.
6. Grillner S, Hellgren J, Ménard A, Saitoh K, Wilström : **Mechanisms for selection of basic motor programs - roles for the striatum and pallidum.** *Trends Neurosci* 2005, **28**:364-370.
7. Frank MJ, Loughry B, O'Reilly RC: **Interactions between frontal cortex and basal ganglia in working memory: a computational model.** *Cogn Affect Behav Neurosci* 2001, **1**:137-160.
8. Alexander GE, DeLong MR, Strick PL: **Parallel organization of functionally segregated circuits linking basal ganglia and cortex.** *Ann Rev Neurosci* 1986, **9**:357-381.
9. Haber SN, Fudge JL, McFarland NR: **Striatonigrostriatal pathways in primates form an ascending spiral from the shell to the dorsolateral striatum.** *J Neurosci* 2000, **20**:2369-2382.
10. Marchand WR: **Cortico-basal ganglia circuitry: a review of key research and implications for functional connectivity studies of mood and anxiety disorders.** *Brain Struct Funct* 2010, **215**:73-96.
11. Rogers MA, Bradshaw JL, Pantelis C, Phillips JG: **Frontostriatal deficits in unipolar major depression.** *Brain Res Bull* 1998, **47**:297-310.
12. Heller AS, Johnstone T, Shackman AJ, Light SN, Peterson MJ, Kolden GG, Kalin NH, Davidson RJ: **Reduced capacity to sustain positive emotion in major depression reflects diminished maintenance of fronto-striatal brain activation.** *Proc Natl Acad Sci USA* 2009, **106**:22445-22450.
13. Greicius M: **Resting-state functional connectivity in neuropsychiatric disorders.** *Curr Opin Neurol* 2008, **21**:424-430.
14. Di Martino A, Scheres A, Margulies DS, Kelly AM, Uddin LQ, Shehzad Z, Biswal B, Walters JR, Castellanos FX, Milham MP: **Functional connectivity of human striatum: a resting state fMRI study.** *Cereb Cortex* 2008, **18**:2735-2747.
15. Helmich RC, Derikx LC, Bakker M, Scheeringa R, Bloem BR, Toni I: **Spatial remapping of cortiso-striatal connectivity in Parkinson's disease.** *Cereb Cortex* 2010, **20**:1175-1186.
16. Anand A, Li Y, Wang Y, Wu J, Gao S, Bukhari L, Mathews VP, Kalnin A, Lowe MJ: **Activity and connectivity of brain mood rgulating circuit in depression: a functional magnetic resonance study.** *Biol Psychiatry* 2005, **57**:1079-1088.
17. Harrison NA, Brydon L, Walker C, Gray MA, Steptoe A, Critchley HD: **Inflammation causes mood changes through alterations in subgenual cingulate activity and mesolimbic connectivity.** *Biol Psychiatry* 2009, **66**:407-414.
18. Cohen MX, Schoene-Bake J-C, Elger CE, Weber B: **Connectivity-based segregation of the human striatum predicts personality characteristics.** *Nat Neurosci* 2008, **12**:32-34.
19. Nolen-Hoeksema S, Hilt LM: **Gender differences in depression.** In *Handbook of Depression.*. 2 edition. Edited by: Gotlib IH, Hammen CL. New York, NY: Guilford Press; 2009:386-404.
20. Beck AT, Steer RA, Brown GK: *Manual for the Beck Depression Inventory-II* San Antonio, TX: Psychological Corporation; 1996.
21. Nolen-Hoeksema S, Morrow J: **A prospective study of depression and posttraumatic stress symptoms after a natural disaster: the 1989 Loma Prieta earthquake.** *J Pers Soc Psychol* 1991, **61**:115-121.
22. Glover GH, Law CS: **Spiral-in/out BOLD fMRI for increased SNR and reduced susceptibility artifacts.** *Magn Reson Med* 2001, **46**:515-522.
23. Biswal BB, Mennes M, Zuo XN, Gohel S, Kelly C, Smith SM, Beckmann CF, Adelstein JS, Buckner RL, Colcombe S, Dogonowski AM, Ernst M, Fair D, Hampson M, Hoptman MJ, Hyde JS, Kiviniemi VJ, Kötter R, Li SJ, Lin CP, Lowe MJ, Mackay C, Madden DJ, Madsen KH, Margulies DS, Mayberg HS, McMahon K, Monk CS, Mostofsky SH, Nagel BJ, *et al*: **Toward discovery science of human brain function.** *Proc Natl Acad Sci USA* 2010, **107**:4734-4739.
24. Kelly C, de Zubicaray G, Di Martino A, Copland DA, Reiss PT, Klein DF, Castellanos FX, Milham MP, McMahon K: **l-Dopa modulates functional connectivity in striatal cognitive and motor networks: a double-blind placebo-controlled study.** *J Neurosci* 2009, **29**:7364-7378.
25. Chen G: **Simple correlation analysis.**[http://afni.nimh.nih.gov/sscc/gangc/SimCorrAna.html].
26. Brett M: **MRC CBU Imaging Wiki.**[http://imaging.mrc-cbu.cam.ac.uk/imaging/MniTalairach].
27. Ward BD: **Simultaneous inference for fMRI data.**[http://afni.nimh.nih.gov/afni/doc/manual/AlphaSim].
28. Haber SN, Knutson B: **The reward circuit: linking primate anatomy and human imaging.** *Neuropsychopharmacology* 2010, **35**:4-26.
29. Gotlib IH, Sivers H, Gabrieli JDE, Whitfield-Gabrieli S, Goldin P, Minor KL, Canli T: **Subgenual anterior cingulate activation to valenced emotional stimuli in major depression.** *Neuroreport* 2005, **16**:1731-1734.
30. Pizzagalli DA, Iosifescu D, Hallett LA, Ratner KF, Fava M: **Reduced hedonic capacity in major depressive disorder: evidence from a probabilistic reward task.** *J Psychiatr Res* 2008, **43**:76-87.
31. Beckmann M, Johansen-Berg H, Rushworth MFS: **Connectivity-based parcellation of human cingulate cortex and its relation to functional specialization.** *J Neurosci* 2009, **29**:1175-1190.
32. Vogt BA: **Pain and emotion interactions in subregions of the cingulate gyrus.** *Nat Rev Neurosci* 2005, **6**:533-544.
33. Damasio AR, Grabowski TJ, Bechara A, Damasio H, Ponto LLB, Parvizi J, Hichwa RD: **Subcortical and cortical brain activity during the feeling of self-generated emotions.** *Nat Neurosci* 2000, **3**:1049-1056.
34. Drevets WC, Price JL, Simpson JRS Jr, Todd RD, Reich T, Vannier M, Raichle ME: **Subgenual prefrontal cortex abnormalities in mood disorders.** *Nature* 1997, **386**:824-827.
35. Ballmaier M, Toga AW, Blanton RE, Sowell ER, Lavretsky H, Peterson J, Pham D, Kumar A: **Anterior cingulate, gyrus rectus, and orbitofrontal abnormalities in elderly depressed patients: an MRI-based parcellation of the prefrontal cortex.** *Am J Psychiatry* 2004, **161**:99-108.
36. Phillips ML, Drevets WC, Rauch SL, Lane R: **Neurobiology of emotion perception I: the neural basis of normal emotion perception.** *Biol Psychiatry* 2003, **54**:504-514.
37. Fellows LK, Farah MJ: **Ventromedial frontal cortex mediates affective shifting in humans: evidence from a reversal learning paradigm.** *Brain* 2003, **126**:1830-1837.

38. Knutson B, Fong GW, Charles MA, Varner JL, Hommer D: **Dissociation of reward anticipation and outcome with event-related fMRI.** *Neuroreport* 2001, **12**:3683-3687.
39. Wheeler EZ, Fellows LK: **The human ventromedial frontal lobe is critical for learning from negative feedback.** *Brain* 2008, **131**:1323-1331.
40. Boecker H, Jankowski J, Ditter P, Scheef L: **A role of the basal ganglia and midbrain nuclei for initiation of motor sequences.** *Neuroimage* 2008, **39**:1356-1369.
41. Pier MPBI, Hulstijn W, Sabbe BGC: **Differential patterns of psychomotor functioning in unmedicated melancholic and nonmelancholic depressed patients.** *J Psychiatr Res* 2004, **38**:425-435.
42. Sabbe B, Hulstijn W, van Hoof J, Tuynman-Qua HG, Zitman F: **Retardation in depression: assessment by means of simple motor tasks.** *J Affect Disord* 1999, **55**:39-44.
43. Rogers MA, Bradshaw JL, Phillips JG, Chiu E: **Reliance on external cues during serial sequential movement in major depression.** *J Neurol Neurosurg Psychiatry* 2000, **69**:237-239.
44. Lewis SJG, Dove A, Robbins TW, Barker RA, Owen AM: **Striatal contributions to working memory: a functional magnetic resonance imaging study in humans.** *Eur J Neurosci* 2004, **19**:755-760.
45. McNab F, Klingberg T: **Prefrontal cortex and basal ganglia control access to working memory.** *Nat Neurosci* 2008, **11**:103-107.
46. Harvey PO, Le Bastard G, Pochon JB, Levy R, Allilaire JF, Dubois B, Fossati P: **Executive functions and updating of the contents of working memory in unipolar depression.** *J Psychiatr Res* 2004, **38**:567-576.
47. Joormann J, Gotlib IH: **Updating the contents of working memory in depression: interference from irrelevant negative material.** *J Abnorm Psychol* 2008, **117**:182-192.
48. Raichle ME, MacLeod AM, Snyder AZ, Powers WJ, Gusnard DA, Shulman GL: **A default mode of brain function.** *Proc Natl Acad Sci USA* 2001, **98**:676-682.
49. Gusnard DA, Akbudak E, Shulman GL, Raichle ME: **Medial prefrontal cortex and self-referential mental activity: relation to a default mode of brain function.** *Proc Natl Acad Sci USA* 2001, **98**:4259-4264.
50. Sheline YI, Barch DM, Price JL, Rundle MM, Vaishnavi SN, Snyder AZ, Mintun MA, Wang S, Coalson RS, Raichle ME: **The default mode network and self-referential processes in depression.** *Proc Natl Acad Sci USA* 2009, **106**:1942-1947.
51. Nagano-Saito A, Leyton M, Monchi O, Goldberg YK, He Y, Dagher A: **Dopamine depletion impairs frontostriatal functional connectivity during a set-shifting task.** *J Neurosci* 2008, **28**:3697-3706.
52. van Eimeren T, Monchi O, Ballanger B, Strafella AP: **Dysfunction of the default mode network in Parkinson disease: a functional magnetic resonance imaging study.** *Arch Neurol* 2009, **66**:877-883.
53. Anand A, Li Y, Wang Y, Wu J, Gao S, Bukhari L, Mathews VP, Kalnin A, Lowe MJ: **Antidepressant effect on connectivity of the mood-regulating circuit: an fMRI study.** *Neuropsychopharmacology* 2005, **30**:1334-1344.
54. Bora E, Harrison BJ, Davey CG, Yücel M, Pantelis C: **Meta-analysis of volumetric abnormalities in cortico-striatal-pallidal-thalamic circuits in major depressive disorder.** *Psychol Med* .
55. Kim MJ, Hamilton JP, Gotlib IH: **Reduced caudate gray matter volume in women with major depressive disorder.** *Psychiat Res-Neuroim* 2008, **164**:114-122.
56. Parashos IA, Tupler LA, Blitchington T, Krishnan KRR: **Magnetic-resonance morphometry in patients with major depression.** *Psychiat Res-Neuroim* 1998, **84**:7-15.

15

Temporal factors in the extinction of fear in inbred mouse strains differing in extinction efficacy

Kathryn MacPherson[1†], Nigel Whittle[2†], Marguerite Camp[1], Ozge Gunduz-Cinar[1], Nicolas Singewald[2] and Andrew Holmes[1*]

Abstract

Background: Various neuropsychiatric conditions, including posttraumatic stress disorder (PTSD), are characterized by deficient fear extinction, but individuals differ greatly in risk for these. While there is growing evidence that fear extinction is influenced by certain procedural variables, it is unclear how these influences might vary across individuals and subpopulations. To model individual differences in fear extinction, prior studies identified a strain of inbred mouse, 129S1/SvImJ (S1), which exhibits a profound deficit in fear extinction, as compared to other inbred strains, such as C57BL/6J (B6).

Methods: Here, we assessed the effects of procedural variables on the impaired extinction phenotype of the S1 strain and, by comparison, the extinction-intact B6 strain. The variables studied were 1) the interval between conditioning and extinction, 2) the interval between cues during extinction training, 3) single-cue exposure before extinction training, and 4) extinction of a second-order conditioned cue.

Results: Conducting extinction training soon after ('immediately') conditioning attenuated fear retrieval in S1 mice and impaired extinction in B6 mice. Spacing cue presentations with long inter-trial intervals during extinction training augmented fear in S1 and B6 mice. The effect of spacing was lost with one-trial fear conditioning in B6, but not S1 mice. A single exposure to a conditioned cue before extinction training did not alter extinction retrieval, either in B6 or S1 mice. Both the S1 and B6 strains exhibited robust second-order fear conditioning, in which a cue associated with footshock was sufficient to serve as a conditioned exciter to condition a fear association to a second cue. B6 mice extinguished the fear response to the second-order conditioned cue, but S1 mice failed to do so.

Conclusions: These data provide further evidence that fear extinction is strongly influenced by multiple procedural variables and is so in a highly strain-dependent manner. This suggests that the efficacy of extinction-based behavioral interventions, such as exposure therapy, for trauma-related anxiety disorders will be determined by the procedural parameters employed and the degree to which the patient can extinguish.

Keywords: Mouse, Gene, Behavior, Fear, Second order conditioning, PTSD, Prefrontal cortex, Amygdala, Anxiety, Rodent, Exposure-based therapy

* Correspondence: Andrew.Holmes@nih.gov
†Equal contributors
[1]Laboratory of Behavioral and Genomic Neuroscience, National Institute on Alcohol Abuse and Alcoholism, NIH, Bethesda, MD, USA
Full list of author information is available at the end of the article

Background

Fear extinction is a form of learning in which a conditioned fear response is reduced by repeated exposure to the conditioned stimulus (CS) in the absence of the unconditioned stimulus (US) [1]. Various neuropsychiatric conditions, including posttraumatic stress disorder (PTSD) [2] and schizophrenia [3], are characterized by deficient fear extinction. Measuring fear extinction in rodents has emerged as a valuable translational assay for studying both the neural basis of poor extinction [4,5], and identifying novel therapeutic approaches that facilitate extinction [6-8].

Individuals differ greatly in risk for anxiety disorders, including PTSD, in part likely due to the moderating influence of genetic factors [9,10]. With this in mind, recent studies have sought to identify neural mechanisms underlying differences in fear and extinction behaviors between subgroups selected from larger populations [11-13], or identify inbred (isogenic) rodent strains that show reliable trait differences in fear extinction [14]. In this context, we recently identified an inbred strain of mouse, 129S1/SvImJ (S1), that exhibits a profound deficit in fear extinction, as compared to a reference inbred strain, C57BL/6J (B6) [15-19].

Supporting the validity of the S1 inbred mouse strain as a model for the impairment of extinction seen in anxiety disorders, the phenotypic abnormalities in these mice extend to a range of behavioral, autonomic and neuroendocrine disturbances, some of which are characteristic of anxiety disorders including PTSD [18]. Moreover, deficient extinction in these mice can be rescued by chronic treatment with fluoxetine [18], a medication for PTSD and other anxiety disorders, and also by various putative novel therapeutics, including an endocannabinoid-boosting drug [20], histone deacetylase inhibition, and deep brain stimulation [19]. At the neural level, impaired extinction in S1 mice is associated with dendritic hypertrophy in basolateral amygdala (BLA) neurons and a failure to properly recruit corticoamygdala regions mediating extinction [15,17,18]. Importantly, this circuitry can be effectively re-engaged by manipulations that normalize fear extinction in parallel (e.g., dietary zinc restriction) [17]. Taken together, these previous findings suggests that the S1 mouse strain may be a tractable model for studying of the underlying neurobiology and genetics of extinction, and also as a screen for identifying novel interventions that rescue impairments in fear extinction.

There is growing evidence that the efficacy of fear extinction is strongly influenced by the interval between extinction training and the conditioning event and the order and timing of cue presentations during extinction training [21,22]. Such procedural variables could potentially be important considerations when applying extinction-based procedures to clinical settings, in the form of exposure therapy. However, the influence of these variables has not been well studied in the models of impaired extinction despite the fact that the clinical application of exposure therapy typically occurs in extinction impaired patient populations. Therefore, the main aim of the current study was to assess the effects of certain procedural variables on the impaired extinction phenotype of the S1 mouse strain and, by comparison, the good extinguishing B6 mouse strain. The specific variables we studied were 1) the interval between conditioning and extinction [23-25], 2) the interval between cues during extinction training [26-28], 3) single-cue exposure before extinction training [29-32], and 4) extinction of a second-order conditioned cue [33,34].

Methods

Subjects

Subjects were male S1 and B6 mice obtained at ~8-9 weeks of age from The Jackson Laboratory (Bar Harbor, ME) (for experiments at NIAAA) or Charles River (Sulzfeld, Germany) (for experiments at University of Innsbruck). Mice were housed 2–4 per cage in a temperature (~22°C) and humidity (NIAAA = 45 ± 15%, University of Innsbruck = 50-60%) controlled *vivarium* under a 12 hour light/dark cycle (NIAAA = lights on 0600 h, University of Innsbruck = lights on 0700 h). The number of mice used in each experiment is given in the figure legends. Experiments were conducted at the NIAAA with the exception of the second-order conditioning experiment, which was conducted at the University of Innsbruck. All procedures were approved by the NIAAA Animal Care and Use Committee or the Austrian Animal Experimentation Ethics Board (Bundesministerium für Wissenschaft und Verkehr, Kommission für Tierversuchsangelegenheiten), and followed the NIH guidelines outlined in 'Using Animals in Intramural Research.'

General procedures for fear conditioning and extinction

Unless specified differently below, testing consisted of 3 phases: conditioning, extinction training and extinction retrieval. Freezing (no visible movement except that required for breathing) was manually scored every 5 seconds as an index of fear [35], and converted to a percentage [(number of freezing observations/total number of observations) × 100].

Conditioning was conducted in Context A: 27 × 27 × 11 cm (NIAAA) or 25 × 25 × 35 cm (University of Innsbruck) chamber with transparent walls and a metal rod floor, cleaned with a 79.5% water/19.5% ethanol/1% vanilla-extract solution (NIAAA) or water (University of Innsbruck). After a 180-seconds (NIAAA) or 120-second (University of Innsbruck) baseline period, mice received 3 × pairing(s) of a 30-second, 75–80 dB, white noise (NIAAA) or 75 dB 10 kHz pure tone (used as CS1 in second-order conditioning experiments at the University of Innsbruck) conditioned stimulus (CS) and 2 sec, 0.6 mA scrambled footshock [unconditioned stimulus (US)], in which the US was presented during the last 2 seconds of the CS and the inter-trial-interval (ITI) was variable. There was a 120-second no-stimulus period after the final pairing before mice were returned to the home cage.

Extinction training was conducted the day after conditioning, in Context B. At NIAAA, this was a 20 cm-diameter Plexiglas cylinder with black/white-checkered walls, solid-Plexiglas opaque floor, cleaned with a 99% water/ 1% acetic acid solution, located in a different room from Context A. At the University of Innsbruck, Context B was a 25 × 25 × 35 cm cage with a solid grey floor and black walls, cleaned with 100% ethanol. CS presentations began after a 180-second (NIAAA) or 120-second (University of Innsbruck) baseline period. Extinction training data were calculated in 5 × CS trial-blocks. Data were analyzed using the first and last extinction trial-blocks in order to allow for consistent comparison across experiments because fewer than 50 CS presentations were given during extinction training in some experiments (i.e., 10 × CS massed and 10 × CS spaced presentations in the massed vs. spaced experiment).

The following day, **extinction retrieval** was tested in Context B. After a 180-second baseline period, mice received 3 × 30-second non-reinforced CS presentations (5 second inter-stimulus interval). Stimulus presentation was controlled by the Med Associates VideoFreeze system (Med Associates, Burlington, VT, USA) (NIAAA) or a TSE operant system (TSE, Bad Homburg, Germany) (University of Innsbruck).

Effects of varying the interval between conditioning and extinction training

The general procedures for conditioning, extinction training and extinction retrieval were as described above, with the exception that at the time of extinction training, one group had been fear conditioned 24 hour earlier (= 'delayed'), whereas another group had completed conditioning 10 minutes earlier (= 'immediate'), as previously described [23,25]. For a schematic of the experimental design, see Figure 1A.

Effects of varying the interval between cues during extinction training

The general procedures for conditioning, extinction training and extinction retrieval were as described above, with the exception that during extinction training, one group received 10 x CS presentations each separated by 20 minutes (= 'spaced'), whereas the other groups received either 10 × CS (= '10-trial massed') or 50 × CS presentations (= '50-trial massed') separated by 5 seconds, as previously described

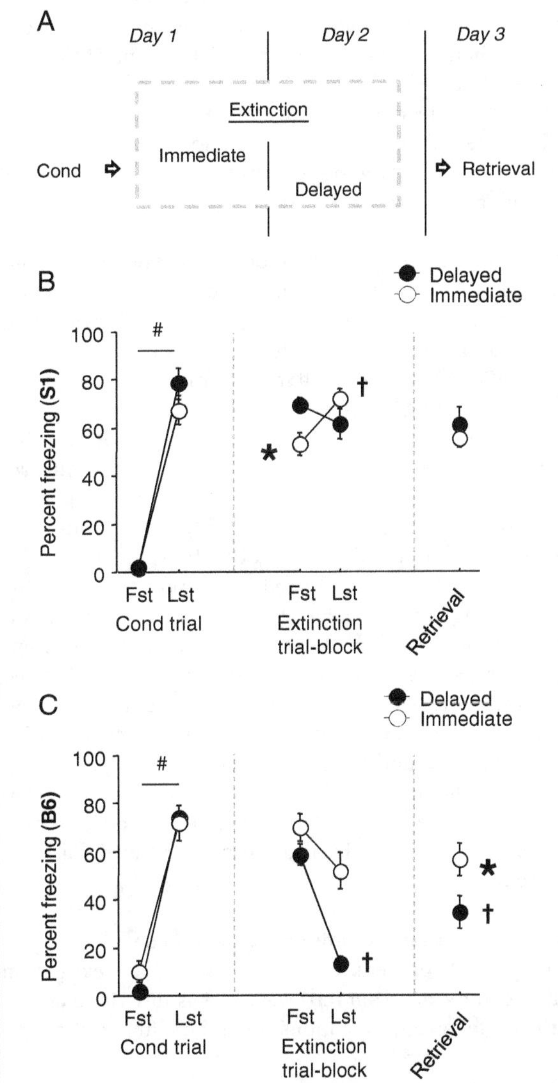

Figure 1 Effects of immediate extinction training. (A) Mice received extinction training 10 minutes (immediate) or 1 day (delayed) after fear conditioning. All mice then received equivalent extinction training and retrieval testing. **(B)** In S1 mice, freezing was significantly lower in the immediate than the delayed group during the first extinction trial-block, and then increased across trial-blocks in the immediate but not delayed group. Freezing was similar between groups during extinction retrieval and neither group showed a decrease in freezing on retrieval as compared to the first extinction trial-block (n = 13-19). **(C)** In B6 mice, freezing significantly decreased across extinction trial-blocks in the delayed but only showed a non-significant trend for a decrease in the immediate group. Freezing was significantly higher in the immediate than delayed group during extinction retrieval, although both groups froze less on retrieval than the first trial-block of extinction training (n = 10). Data are means ± SEM. #$P < .05$ last (Lst) vs. first (Fst) conditioning trial, †$P < .05$ Lst extinction trial-block or retrieval vs. Fst extinction trial-block, *$P < .05$ vs. immediate group at same point in testing.

[26,27]. The massed group was exposed to the extinction training context for the equivalent duration as the spaced group (3 hours, 8 minutes, 30 seconds) to control for context exposure. An additional group of fear 'retention controls' received fear conditioning and no extinction training and were tested for fear on the extinction retrieval test for a comparison with the other groups. For a schematic of the experimental design, see Figure 2A.

Effects of a single-CS exposure prior to extinction training

The general procedures for conditioning and extinction training were the same as above with the exception that 1 hour prior to extinction training, one group received a single (30-second) CS after a 3-minute acclimation period (= '1 × CS'), whereas another group was exposed to the context for the equivalent duration but received no CS presentation (= '0 × CS'). The 1 × CS group received 49 instead of 50 × CS presentations during extinction training to equate total CS presentations with the 0 × CS group. All phases of testing, including CS-pre-exposure, were conducted in Context A (i.e., the conditioning context) for consistency with previous CS-pre-exposure studies [29]. The day after extinction training, fear was reinstated via exposure to unsignaled footshock. After a 180-second baseline period, mice received 5 × USs (0.6 mA) over a 9.5 minute period (ITI = 6–150 seconds) and returned to the home cage 180 seconds after the final US. A fear probe test was conducted the following day via the typical extinction retrieval procedure. For a schematic of the experimental design, see Figure 3A.

Extinction of a second-order conditioned cue

The general procedures for conditioning, extinction training and extinction retrieval were as described above, with the following exceptions. One day after fear conditioning to a pure tone CS (CS1), one group received a second-order conditioning session in which a 75 dB white noise CS (CS2) was presented 5 × immediately prior to presentation of CS1 (without any concomitant US) (= 'CS2×CS1'). Another group received 5 × CS2 presentations in the absence of CS1 during this phase (= 'CS-only'). The following day, after a 120-second baseline, mice were given extinction training involving 16 × CS2 presentations. Fear to the CS2 was tested the following day via 2 × CS2 presentations. For a schematic of the experimental design, see Figure 4A.

Statistical analysis

Data were analyzed using analysis of variance (ANOVA) with repeated measures for conditioning trial and extinction trial-block, followed by Newman Keuls *post hoc* tests where appropriate, or by paired t-tests. The threshold for statistical significance was $P < .05$.

Results and discussion

A short conditioning-extinction training interval reduces fear in S1 and impairs extinction in B6 mice

Previous work in rats has shown that reducing the typical one day interval between conditioning and extinction to less than one hour alters the efficacy of extinction training, as measured by fear levels during an extinction retrieval test. Some studies report a facilitatory effect of 'immediate' extinction [24], while others have observed impaired extinction [23,25,36]. We tested immediate extinction in the extinction impaired S1 and extinction intact B6 mouse strains using a 10 minute conditioning-extinction interval.

Results for S1 mice are shown in Figure 1B. Freezing was negligible at baseline and significantly increased across conditioning trials regardless of group assignment ($F_{1,30} = 219.27$, $P < .01$). During extinction training, baseline freezing trended higher (but not significantly) in the immediate group (as previously reported in rats, [23]), and was significantly lower during the first trial-block in the immediate than the delayed group, and then significantly increased across trial-blocks in the immediate but not delayed group (trial x group interaction: $F_{1,30} = 14.13$, $P < .01$, followed by *post hoc* tests). On the retrieval test, freezing was low at baseline and freezing to the CS was similar between the groups. In addition, in neither group was the level of freezing on retrieval different from that during the first-trial block of extinction training (i.e., prior to training).

Results for B6 mice are shown in Figure 1C. Freezing was negligible at baseline and significantly increased across conditioning trials regardless of group assignment ($F_{1,18} = 277.44$, $P < .01$). During extinction training, baseline freezing was not significantly higher in the immediate group. Freezing during the first trial-block was equivalent between groups and significantly decreased across trial-blocks during extinction training in the delayed but not immediate group, although there was a non-significant trend in the same direction in the immediate group (trial x group interaction: $F_{1,18} = 8.59$, $P < .01$, followed by *post hoc* tests). Moreover, on the extinction retrieval test freezing was similar between groups at baseline but significantly higher in the immediate than delayed group ($t(18) = 2.26$, $P < .05$). Both groups showed less freezing on retrieval relative to the first trial-block of extinction training (immediate: $t(9) = 4.93$, $P < .01$, delayed: ($t(9) = 5.10$, $P < .01$).

Taken together, these results provide a number of confirmatory and novel findings. First, under the typically employed testing procedure, in which there is a delay of one day between conditioning, S1 mice exhibited severely impaired extinction learning and retrieval. This is consistent with previous studies demonstrating an extinction deficient phenotype in this mouse strain, as compared to the B6 strain [15-19]. Prior work has also

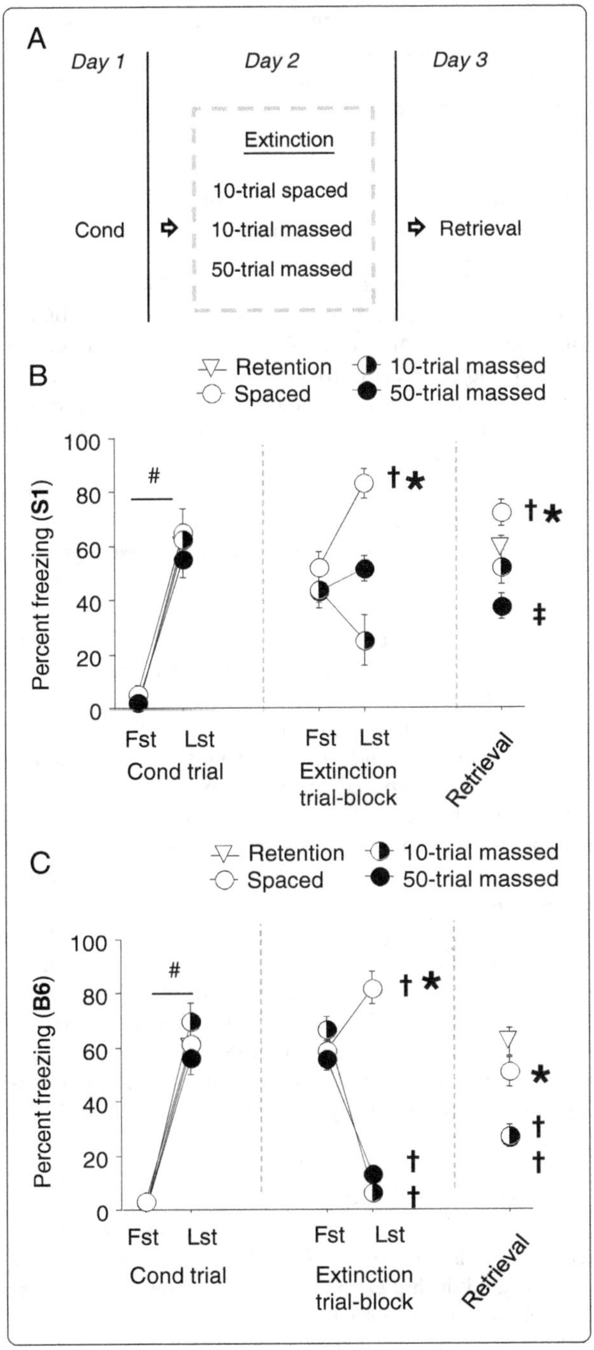

Figure 2 Effects of spaced-CS extinction training. (A) One day after conditioning, mice received 10-trial spaced (20 minute interval), 10-trial massed (5 second interval) or 50-trial massed extinction training. **(B)** In S1 mice, freezing significantly increased across extinction trial-blocks in the spaced group but did not change in the massed groups, such that freezing was significantly higher in the spaced group than the massed groups by the last trial-block. During extinction retrieval, freezing was significantly higher in the spaced group than the massed groups, but was not different from freezing in non-extinguished retention controls. The spaced group showed a significant increase in freezing on extinction retrieval relative to the first-trial block of extinction training (n = 8-26). **(C)** In B6 mice, freezing significantly decreased over extinction trial-blocks in the massed groups, but significantly increased in the spaced group, with higher freezing in the spaced group than in the massed groups by the final trial-block. On extinction retrieval, freezing was higher in the spaced group than the massed groups but no different from retention controls, and the massed groups had lower freezing than retention controls. The massed, but not spaced, groups showed significantly less freezing on retrieval than the first extinction training trial-block (n = 8-26). #$P < .05$ last (Lst) vs. first (Fst) conditioning trial, †$P < .05$ Lst extinction trial-block or retrieval vs. Fst extinction trial-block, *$P < .05$ vs. 10-trial massed group at same point in testing, ‡$P < .05$ vs. retention controls.

shown that this impairment is not an unalterable feature of these mice, but can be rescued by manipulations ranging from antidepressant drug treatment to deep brain simulation [17-19]. However, while studies in rats have found that conducting extinction training soon after conditioning can facilitate extinction [24], the current data found no evidence of a facilitatory effect of 'immediate' extinction in the S1 model. On the contrary, immediate extinction resulted in an extinction impairment in B6 mice, a finding in line with previous findings in rats [23,25,36].

Though immediate extinction did not affect extinction in S1 mice, initial fear levels prior to extinction training were reduced by this procedural manipulation. This could be indicative of a retardation in fear memory consolidation in the strain, such that one hour after conditioning, the memory cannot be fully retrieved. The underlying causes of this deficit are unclear, but could relate to abnormalities in molecular mechanisms underlying the early, protein and RNA synthesis-independent, phase of fear memory formation [37]. This raises interesting questions for future studies on the S1 strain.

Spacing extinction cues increases fear in S1 mice and impairs extinction in B6 mice

Conditioned fear responses can be increased by interposing 1–2 month intervals between conditioning and test [38]. In addition, introducing long (20-minute) intervals between CS presentations during extinction training has been found to impair extinction in the B6 mouse strain [26,27] (c.f. facilitating effect of varying intervals [28]). We tested the effects of long (20-minute)

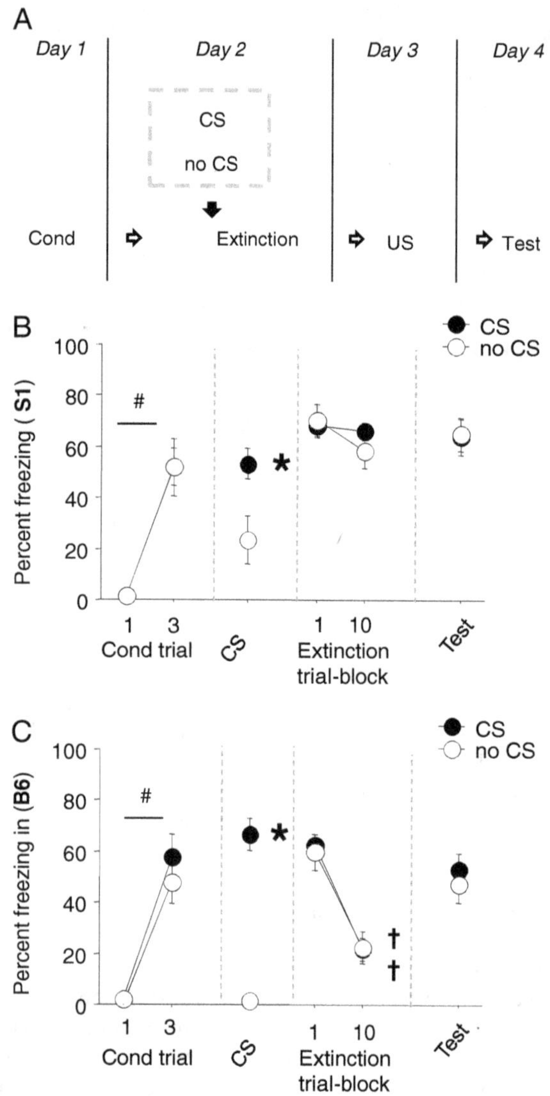

Figure 3 Effects of single-CS exposure prior to extinction training. (A) One day after conditioning, mice received either one CS presentation or no CS/context only 1 hour prior to extinction training. All mice then received equivalent extinction training. One day later, mice received unsignaled US presentations, and we then tested for fear the following day. **(B)** S1 mice significantly increased freezing across conditioning trials. During CS pre-exposure, freezing was higher during the 1xCS presentation than the no CS condition. Freezing did not change during across extinction trial-blocks regardless of CS pre-exposure. Freezing was also no different between groups during the post-reinstatement test (n = 10). **(C)** In B6 mice, freezing significantly increased across conditioning trials. During CS pre-exposure, freezing was higher to the CS presentation relative to the no CS condition. Freezing significantly decreased across extinction trial-blocks regardless of CS pre-exposure. Freezing did not differ between groups during the post-reinstatement test (n = 10). Data are means ± SEM. #$P < .05$ Lst vs. Fst conditioning trial, *$P < .05$ CS vs. no CS at same point in testing.

cue spacing on extinction in S1, and for comparison with previous data, the B6 strain.

Results for S1 mice are shown in Figure 2B. Freezing significantly increased over conditioning trials ($F_{1,39}$ = 120.10, $P < .01$) irrespective of group assignment. During extinction training, the spaced group significantly increased freezing over trial-blocks, whereas there was no significant change in the massed groups (trial-block x group interaction: $F_{2,39} = 6.69$, $P < .01$, followed by *post hoc* tests). The spaced group had significantly higher freezing than the massed group by the last trial-block. On the extinction retrieval test, the spaced group showed higher freezing than the massed group, but not fear retention controls that received no extinction training ($F_{3,50} = 7.56$, $P < .01$, followed by *post hoc* tests). Comparison of freezing during retrieval with the first-trial block of extinction training indicated significantly higher freezing across the test phases in the spaced group ($t(7) = 3.20$, $P < .05$), but neither massed groups. There was minimal baseline freezing across testing phases (Table 1).

Results for B6 mice are shown in Figure 2C. Freezing significantly increased across conditioning trials regardless of group assignment ($F_{1,44} = 171.46$, $P < .01$). During extinction training, freezing significantly decreased over trial-blocks in both massed groups, but significantly increased in the spaced group, such that freezing was significantly higher in the spaced group than the massed groups by the final trial-block (group x trial interaction: $F_{2,44} = 31.60$, $P < .01$, followed by *post hoc* tests). Group differences carried over to the extinction retrieval test, where the spaced group froze significantly more than the 10-trial and 50-trial massed groups, but not more than retention controls ($F_{3,56} = 14.76$, $P < .01$, followed by *post hoc* tests). Finally, the 10-trial massed ($t(7)$ = 6.14, $P < .01$), 50-trial massed ($t(25) = 5.71$, $P < .01$), but not the spaced, group showed significantly lesser freezing during extinction retrieval than the first trial-block of extinction training. There was minimal baseline freezing on any testing phase (Table 1).

Consistent with previous findings [26,27], 10 x 'spacing' cue presentation during extinction training augmented fear over training trials in S1 and B6 mice. Freezing was also elevated during extinction retrieval after spaced training relative to mice that had received either 10 or 50 massed extinction trials, but not relative to mice that had received no extinction training at all. In B6 mice, these group differences on retrieval reflect impaired extinction after spaced training (contrasted with the intact extinction after massing), but not a long-term increase in fear over levels seen with no extinction at all. The retrieval differences in S1 mice reflect a similar pattern of impaired extinction, but no long-term fear increases. However, an interesting footnote to these data was the finding that S1

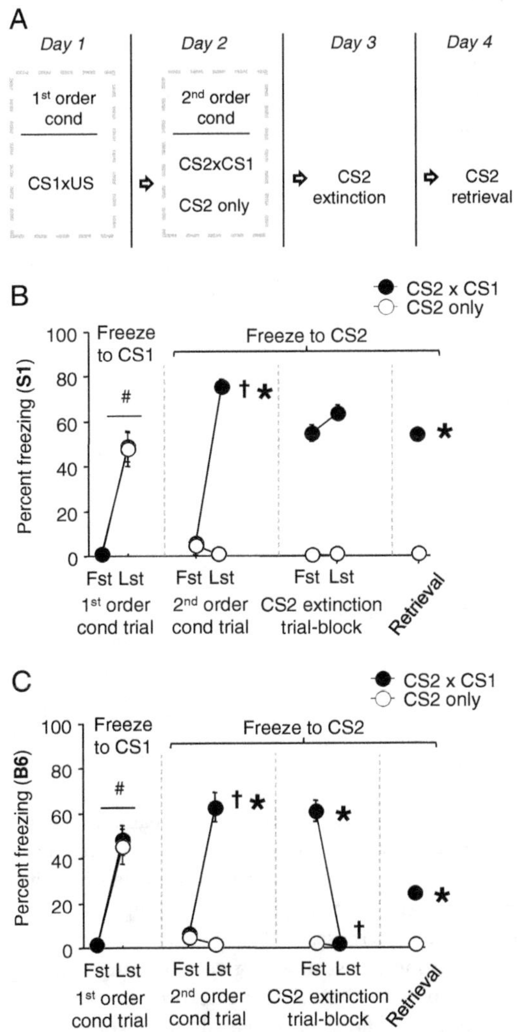

Figure 4 Extinction of a second-order conditioned cue. (A) All mice first received CS1xUS fear conditioning, 1 day prior to exposure to either CS2 paired with CS1 or CS2 exposure alone. All mice then received equivalent extinction training and retrieval testing. **(B).** S1 mice significantly increased freezing across CS1xUS pairings during conditioning. Freezing significantly increased across CS2 trials when the CS2 was paired with the CS1 and not when presented alone. Freezing to the CS2 did not change across extinction trial-blocks in either group and was significantly higher in the CS2-CS1 paired group than the CS2 only group during extinction retrieval (n = 5-10). **(C).** B6 mice significantly increased freezing across CS1xUS pairings during conditioning. Freezing significantly increased across CS2 trials when the CS2 was paired with the CS1 and not when presented alone. Freezing to the CS2 significantly decreased across extinction trial-blocks in the CS2-CS1 paired group. Freezing was significantly higher in the CS2-CS1 paired group than the CS2 only group during extinction retrieval, but was lower relative to the first trial-block of extinction training (n = 5-10). #$P < .05$ last (Lst) vs. first (Fst) conditioning trial, †$P < .05$ Lst vs. Fst trial-block during 2nd order conditioning or extinction, *$P < .05$ vs. CS2-only at same point in testing.

mice given 50 massed extinction trials showed lower freezing on retrieval than non-extinguished controls, which either suggests some, albeit marginal, extinction in this strain, or an augmentation of fear in the interval between conditioning and retrieval of the kind seen with much longer intervals in rats [38].

It should be noted that the design of these experiments does not exclude the possibility that increased freezing at the end of the long extinction training session (> 3 hours) was an artifact of very low levels of exploration, and even sleeping, erroneously detected as freezing. While low exploration could not explain the heightened levels of freezing on the extinction retrieval test, which was the equivalent length in the spaced and massed groups, it is possible that the long spaced training procedure impaired retrieval due to a lack of attention to the later cue presentations during extinction training. To address this caveat, we repeated the spacing procedure in another cohort of B6 mice that was conditioned with a single CS-US pairing. The rationale for this experiment is based on the theory that while a stronger conditioned fear response should be more prone to spacing-induced fear increases, weaker conditioning should be less prone [39].

The results of this experiment showed that B6 mice given either 10 spaced or 10 massed extinction trials showed equivalent freezing on conditioning (trial 1 spaced = 3.3 ± 2.4, trial 1 massed = 6.7 ± 4.2, n = 6-12), extinction training (first trial-block spaced = 50.0 ± 5.0%, first trial-block massed = 52.8 ± 10.0, last trial-block spaced = 27.8 ± 8.8, last massed = 16.8 ± 7.5, effect of trial-block: $F_{1,16} = 16.50$, $P < .01$) and extinction retrieval (spaced = 27.3 ± 5.8, massed = 43.6 ± 6.0). There was minimal baseline freezing across testing phases (Table 1). Thus, B6 mice showed intact fear extinction and no fear increases with spaced training after one-trial conditioning. We repeated the same procedure in S1 mice. Here, freezing on conditioning (trial 1 spaced = 1.3 ± 1.3, trial 1 massed = 0.0 ± 0.0, n = 6-16) was no different between groups, but the spaced, and not massed, group showed increased freezing across extinction trial-blocks during extinction training (first trial-block spaced = 46.8 ± 3.8%, first trial-block massed = 36.0 ± 6.7, last trial-block spaced = 69.8 ± 10.0, last massed = 36.0 ± 11.7, effect of spacing: $F_{1,20} = 6.03$, $P < .05$). Freezing on retrieval was not different between groups (spaced = 48.7 ± 4.4, massed = 44.4 ± 5.9). Again, there was minimal baseline freezing across testing phases (Table 1). These data indicate that, in contrast to B6 mice, fear increases with spacing in the S1 strain occurs even after one-trial conditioning.

These data make three important points. First, they discount the possibility that increased freezing in the spaced group after 3 × CS-US conditioning is an artifact

Table 1 Levels of baseline (pre-CS) percent freezing across testing phases

	S1			B6		
Varying conditioning-extinction training interval						
	Cond	Extinction	Retrieval	Cond	Extinction	Retrieval
Immediate	0.0 ±0.0	15.1 ±22.0	10.2 ±15.7	0.0 ±0.0	16.1 ±23.3	5.0 ±3.1
Delayed	0.0 ±0.0	6.4 ±10.3	10.9 ±13.5	0.0 ±0.0	2.8 ±3.9	2.2 ±3.2
Varying interval between extinction cues (3-shock cond)						
	Cond	Extinction	Retrieval	Cond	Extinction	Retrieval
Spaced	0.0 ±0.0	0.7 ±1.3	2.1 ±2.0	0.2 ±0.8	4.7 ±3.5	3.0 ±2.6
10-trial massed	0.0 ±0.0	4.6 ±3.2	2.6 ±1.9	0.4 ±1.1	5.7 ±3.6	3.2 ±3.8
50-trial massed	0.0 ±0.0	1.7 ±2.5	3.5 ±3.6	0.0 ±0.0	2.4 ±2.3	1.7 ±2.5
Varying interval between extinction cues (1-shock cond)						
	Cond	Extinction	Retrieval	Cond	Extinction	Retrieval
Spaced	0.0 ±0.0	1.2 ±2.9	3.0 ±3.6	0.0 ±0.0	2.3 ±3.3	3.0 ±2.6
Massed	0.0 ±0.0	0.5 ±1.2	2.0 ±2.4	0.0 ±0.0	4.4 ±3.0	1.2 ±3.2
Single-CS exposure prior to extinction training						
	Cond	Extinction	Test	Cond	Extinction	Test
CS	0.0 ±0.0	9.2 ±9.1	29.4 ±18.9	0.0 ±0.0	11.1 ±17.5	33.9 ±22.9
No CS	0.0 ±0.0	19.4 ±18.2	35.6 ±19.9	0.0 ±0.0	5.6 ±13.9	18.6 ±16.9
Extinction of a second-order conditioned cue						
	Cond	Extinction	Retrieval	2nd Cond	Extinction	Retrieval
CS2 x CS1	0.4 ±0.7	0.0 ±0.0	0.0 ±0.0	0.1 ±0.4	0.0 ±0.0	0.0 ±0.0
CS2 only	0.4 ±0.9	0.0 ±0.0	0.0 ±0.0	0.0 ±0.0	0.0 ±0.0	0.0 ±0.0

of low exploration because the extinction training session duration is the same after 1 × CS-US experiment, and no increase in freezing is evident with this procedure. Second, and by extension, these data demonstrate that increased fear with spaced extinction training is determined in part by the intensity of the initial conditioning. This is consistent with the notion that the outcome of extinction training will be dependent upon the strength of the excitatory fear memory [40], and also agrees with the predictions of certain conceptual models of excessive fear in humans [39]. Third, the finding that S1 mice showed elevated fear even with one-trial conditioning suggests extinction-impaired populations may be more liable to this effect. This is consistent with the recent finding that extinction-impaired CB1 knockout mice displayed fear augmentation with massed training after being conditioned to a high intensity (0.8 mA) US, but not standard (0.6 mA) US [41].

The precise nature of the fear increases seen with spacing is unclear. Some authors have proposed that under some circumstances, the conditioned fear response to the CS can itself serve as a reinforcer to maintain fear and counter the effects of the CS-no-US association formed during extinction [39]. Alternatively, Cain and colleagues have suggested that spacing the presentation of CSs could promote fear by favoring the rehearsal of the original CS-US association with each presentation [26]. In a similar vein, it has been shown that there is more fear reconsolidation when conditioned fear stimuli are more widely spaced [42]. Our finding that spacing-induced fear increases, at least in B6 mice, was dependent upon the strength of conditioning would generally concur with these latter interpretations, assuming that stronger fear favored rehearsal/ reconsolidation over weaker conditioning. Aside from these interpretative questions, to our knowledge there is still no clear evidence of fear elevations with spaced extinction training in humans, and until such evidence is obtained, the relevance of these data in mice to clinical contexts should be viewed with caution.

A single pre-extinction cue presentation is insufficient to prevent fear reinstatement

Presenting a conditioned cue one hour prior to extinction training has been found to facilitate extinction memory formation in humans [30,43], rats [29] (but see, [31]) and the B6 mouse strain [32,44], possibly by reactivating the fear memory to render it more labile and thereby sensitive to extinction training. Here we tested whether impaired extinction in the S1 strain could be rescued by pre-extinction cue exposure. B6 mice were also tested to ascertain the efficacy of this manipulation in a reference population.

Results for S1 mice are shown in Figure 3B. Freezing was negligible at baseline and significantly increased in freezing across conditioning trials regardless of group assignment ($F_{1,18} = 59.64$, $P < .01$). Baseline freezing prior to single CS presentation was slightly but not significantly elevated in the no CS group (Table 1). Cue presentation prior to extinction training elicited significant freezing, as compared to no-CS/context only exposure ($t(18) = 2.70$, $P < .05$). During extinction training, freezing did not significantly differ across trial-blocks, regardless of pre-training CS presentation. Following US-reinstatement, freezing was similar between groups during baseline, as well as during CS presentation, on the fear probe test. It was notable that baseline freezing on the fear probe test was higher than in other experiments (Table 1), reflecting contextual fear acquired during reinstatement (conducted in the same context). Strong contextual fear could potentially have affected (e.g., summed with) fear to the CS during the fear probe test and mitigated possibly fear-reducing effect of the pre-extinction CS exposure. This issue could be explored further by using a design involving multiple contexts.

Results for B6 mice are shown in Figure 3C. Freezing was negligible at baseline and significantly increased across conditioning trials irrespective of group assignment ($F_{1,18} = 81.12$, $P < .01$). Baseline freezing prior to the single CS trended higher in the CS group (Table 1). Freezing was elicited by CS presentation, and significantly more than no-CS/context only exposure ($t(18) = 10.30$, $P < .01$). Both the CS and no-CS groups showed a significant, and equivalent, decrease in freezing across extinction trial-blocks ($F_{1,18} = 63.59$, $P < .01$). Finally, freezing on the fear probe test after US-induced reinstatement was not different between the CS and no CS groups. As in S1 mice, baseline freezing was relatively high on this test and slightly higher in the CS than US group.

In contrast to recent findings in humans, rats and B6 mice [29,30,32,43,44] we did not find that exposure to the CS before extinction training facilitated extinction memory formation, either in B6 or S1 mice. One reason for this apparent discrepancy may be that we tested for extinction facilitation after unsignaled-US reinstatement, which is a strong fear-promoting procedure relative to other probes for facilitation such as spontaneous recovery and context-driven renewal. In other words, an extinction facilitation effect of CS presentation may have been overcome by such strong fear reinstatement. On the other hand, Monfils and colleagues were able to see a significant effect of pre-extinction CS presentation, in rats, under conditions of reinstatement [29]. Thus, there appear to be additional factors involved in determining the effects of CS presentation. Indeed, this is borne by a recent study in rats which found that pre-extinction CS exposure can actually *increase* fear following reinstatement (or renewal) [31]. Clearly, further studies will be necessary to elucidate the critical variables modulating this effect (for further discussion, see [45]).

Impaired extinction of a second-order conditioned cue in S1 mice

Some authors have posited that anxiety disorders such as PTSD can be maintained by a process of second-order conditioning, in which previously neutral stimuli acquire associative strength after pairing with trauma reminders and then act as additional stimuli maintaining fear [46]. It is not known, however, whether individuals or populations differ in the ability to acquire and extinguish second-order conditioned fear memories. We therefore tested for this in the S1 and B6 mouse strains, using procedures previously described in rats [33,34].

Results for S1 mice are shown in Figure 4B. During conditioning to CS1, there was a significant increase in freezing across trials regardless of group assignment ($F_{1,13} = 76.29$, $P < .01$). On the second-order conditioning sessions, freezing to CS2 increased in the CS2-CS1 paired group across trials, but was negligible in the group presented with the CS2 alone (group x trial interaction: $F_{1,13} = 163.23$, $P < .01$, followed by *post hoc* tests). During extinction training, freezing to CS2 was significantly higher in the CS2-CS1 than CS2-only group ($F_{1,13} = 203.55$, $P < .01$), and did not change across trials in either group. Freezing was significantly higher to CS2 in the CS2-CS1 group than the CS2-only group on the extinction retrieval test ($t(13) = 18.61$, $P < .01$). There was minimal baseline freezing across testing phases (Table 1).

Results for B6 mice are shown in Figure 4C. Freezing significantly increased across CS1 conditioning trials regardless of group assignment ($F_{1,13} = 74.76$, $P < .01$). With second-order conditioning, freezing to CS2 increased across trials in the CS2-CS1 group but not the CS2-only group (group x trial interaction: $F_{1,13} = 30.02$, $P < .01$, followed by *post hoc* tests). During extinction training, freezing significantly decreased across trials in the CS2-CS1 group, whereas there was virtually no freezing in the CS2-only group (group x trial interaction: $F_{1,13} = 72.53$, $P < .01$, followed by *post hoc* tests). Freezing was significantly higher to CS2 in the CS2-CS1 than CS2-only group on the extinction retrieval test ($t(13) = 10.62$, $P < .01$). There was minimal baseline freezing across testing phases (Table 1).

These data show that both the S1 and B6 strains exhibit robust second-order fear conditioning under a procedure similar to those previously reported in rats [34]. This demonstrates that the CS1 served as a sufficient US ('conditioned exciter') to condition a new association with the CS2 that had no direct connection with footshock [33]. The conditioned response to CS2 successfully underwent extinction in B6 mice but, remarkably, could not be extinguished in S1 mice. As far as we are aware, this is some of the first evidence that an extinction-impaired population that also has a major deficit in extinguishing fear to stimuli only indirectly associated with the initial conditioning event. From a clinical perspective, these results suggest that post-trauma anxiety in certain at-risk individuals may be maintained by impaired extinction of second-order conditioned stimuli, and that it may be important to extinguish these stimuli in order to produce a fully effective therapeutic effect of extinction-based procedures such as exposure therapy. As such, it will be of great interest to elucidate the neurobiological basis of this form of extinction, and to determine to what degree it shares or differs from extinction of first-order conditioned stimuli. Studies are planned to investigate this further.

Further work is also needed to establish what abnormal learning processes underlie failed extinction of second-order conditioned stimuli. In one scheme, conditioning to CS1 might render S1 mice more attentive to the CS2-CS1 pairing during second-order conditioning, resulting in stronger learning of a CS2-CS1 association and subsequently poor extinction. One way to probe over-attention to the CS2 could be to test S1 mice for a deficit in the ability of prior conditioning to one CS to block conditioning to a second CS that is paired with the same US [47,48]. Alternatively, the S1 strain may have had a deficit in learning the conditioned inhibitor properties of the CS2 - i.e., learning that this stimulus is associated with the absence of an aversive outcome. This could also be more formally tested, for example by demonstrating that the presentation of the CS2 in the presence of the CS1 would inhibit fear to CS1 in B6 mice, but fail to do so in S1 mice. In lieu of such an analysis, however, a prior study found that, in contrast to B6, S1 mice fail to learn to reduce fear to a CS that had previously been explicitly unpaired with US [18] – consistent with a disruption of conditioned inhibition. This suggests that the S1 strain may have a fundamental problem with learning to suppress fear that manifests under various conditions, that includes but is not limited to the severe deficit in fear extinction that was initially found to characterize these mice [15,19].

Conclusions

The current study examined the effects of manipulating the interval between conditioning and extinction training, the interval between CS presentations during training and exposure to a CS prior to training on fear extinction. It also examined extinction of a second-order conditioned fear response. Results provide further evidence that fear extinction is an ostensibly simple behavioral assay that is strongly influenced by multiple procedural variables and, importantly, is so in a strain-dependent manner. These findings in mice could have important implications for the application of extinction-based behavioral interventions, such as exposure therapy, for trauma-related anxiety disorders because it suggests that the efficacy of such interventions will be determined both by the procedural parameters employed and the clinical profile of the patient.

Competing interests

The authors declare that they have no competing interests.

Authors' contributions

KM, NW, MC, and OG-C performed experiments. NW, NS and AH designed experiments. All authors read and approved the final manuscript.

Acknowledgements

We are very grateful to Dr. Charles Pickens for valuable comments. Research supported by the National Institute on Alcohol Abuse and Alcoholism Intramural Research Program and the Austrian Science Fund (SFB F4410-B19).

Author details

[1]Laboratory of Behavioral and Genomic Neuroscience, National Institute on Alcohol Abuse and Alcoholism, NIH, Bethesda, MD, USA. [2]Department of Pharmacology & Toxicology, Institute of Pharmacy and CMBI, University of Innsbruck, Innsbruck, Austria.

References

1. Pavlov IP: *Conditioned reflexes.* London: Oxford University Press; 1927.
2. Milad MR, Pitman RK, Ellis CB, Gold AL, Shin LM, Lasko NB, Zeidan MA, Handwerger K, Orr SP, Rauch SL: **Neurobiological basis of failure to recall extinction memory in posttraumatic stress disorder.** *Biol Psychiatry* 2009, **66:**1075–1082.
3. Holt DJ, Lebron-Milad K, Milad MR, Rauch SL, Pitman RK, Orr SP, Cassidy BS, Walsh JP, Goff DC: **Extinction memory is impaired in schizophrenia.** *Biol Psychiatry* 2009, **65:**455–463.
4. Quirk GJ, Mueller D: **Neural mechanisms of extinction learning and retrieval.** *Neuropsychopharmacology* 2008, **33:**56–72.
5. Herry C, Ferraguti F, Singewald N, Letzkus JJ, Ehrlich I, Luthi A: **Neuronal circuits of fear extinction.** *Eur J Neurosci* 2010, **31:**599–612.
6. Myers KM, Davis M: **Mechanisms of fear extinction.** *Mol Psychiatry* 2007, **12:**120–150.
7. Holmes A, Quirk GJ: **Pharmacological facilitation of fear extinction and the search for adjunct treatments for anxiety disorders–the case of yohimbine.** *Trends Pharmacol Sci* 2010, **31:**2–7.
8. Graham BM, Langton JM, Richardson R: **Pharmacological enhancement of fear reduction: preclinical models.** *Br J Pharmacol* 2011, **164:**1230–1247.
9. Caspi A, Hariri AR, Holmes A, Uher R, Moffitt TE: **Genetic sensitivity to the environment: the case of the serotonin transporter gene and its implications for studying complex diseases and traits.** *Am J Psychiatry* 2010, **167:**509–527.
10. Skelton K, Ressler KJ, Norrholm SD, Jovanovic T, Bradley-Davino B: **PTSD and gene variants: new pathways and new thinking.** *Neuropharmacology* 2012, **62:**628–637.
11. Muigg P, Hetzenauer A, Hauer G, Hauschild M, Gaburro S, Frank E, Landgraf R, Singewald N: **Impaired extinction of learned fear in rats selectively bred for high anxiety–evidence of altered neuronal processing in prefrontal-amygdala pathways.** *Eur J Neurosci* 2008, **28:**2299–2309.
12. Burgos-Robles A, Vidal-Gonzalez I, Quirk GJ: **Sustained conditioned responses in prelimbic prefrontal neurons are correlated with fear expression and extinction failure.** *J Neurosci* 2009, **29:**8474–8482.

13. Duvarci S, Bauer EP, Pare D: **The bed nucleus of the stria terminalis mediates inter-individual variations in anxiety and fear.** *J Neurosci* 2009, **29:**10357–10361.
14. Holmes A, Singewald N: **Individual differences in recovery from traumatic fear.** *Trends Neurosci* 2013, **36:**23–31.
15. Hefner K, Whittle N, Juhasz J, Norcross M, Karlsson R, Saksida LM, Bussey TJ, Singewald N, Holmes A: **Impaired fear extinction learning and cortico-amygdala circuit abnormalities in a common genetic mouse strain.** *J Neurosci* 2008, **28:**8074–8085.
16. Camp M, Norcross M, Whittle N, Feyder M, D'Hanis W, Yilmazer-Hanke D, Singewald N, Holmes A: **Impaired Pavlovian fear extinction is a common phenotype across genetic lineages of the 129 inbred mouse strain.** *Genes Brain Behav* 2009, **8:**744–752.
17. Whittle N, Hauschild M, Lubec G, Holmes A, Singewald N: **Rescue of impaired fear extinction and normalization of cortico-amygdala circuit dysfunction in a genetic mouse model by dietary zinc restriction.** *J Neurosci* 2010, **30:**13586–13596.
18. Camp MC, Macpherson KP, Lederle L, Graybeal C, Gaburro S, Debrouse LM, Ihne JL, Bravo JA, O'Connor RM, Ciocchi S, Wellman CL, Luthi A, Cryan JF, Singewald N, Holmes A: **Genetic strain differences in learned fear inhibition associated with variation in neuroendocrine, autonomic, and amygdala dendritic phenotypes.** *Neuropsychopharmacology* 2012, **37:**1534–1547.
19. Whittle N, Schmuckermair C, Gunduz Cinar O, Hauschild M, Ferraguti F, Holmes A, Singewald N: **Deep brain stimulation, histone deacetylase inhibitors and glutamatergic drugs rescue resistance to fear extinction in a genetic mouse model.** *Neuropharmacology* 2013, **64:**414–423.
20. Gunduz-Cinar O, Macpherson KP, Cinar R, Gamble-George J, Sugden K, Williams B, Godlewski G, Ramikie TS, Gorka AX, Alapafuja SO, Nikas SP, Makriyannis A, Poulton R, Patel S, Hariri AR, Caspi A, Moffitt TE, Kunos G, Holmes A: **Convergent translational evidence of a role for anandamide in amygdala-mediated fear extinction, threat processing and stress-reactivity.** *Mol Psychiatry* 2013, **8:**813–823.
21. Quirk GJ, Pare D, Richardson R, Herry C, Monfils MH, Schiller D, Vicentic A: **Erasing fear memories with extinction training.** *J Neurosci* 2010, **30:**14993–14997.
22. Orsini CA, Maren S: **Neural and cellular mechanisms of fear and extinction memory formation.** *Neurosci Biobehav Rev* 2012, **36:**1773–1802.
23. Maren S, Chang CH: **Recent fear is resistant to extinction.** *Proc Natl Acad Sci U S A* 2006, **103:**18020–18025.
24. Myers KM, Ressler KJ, Davis M: **Different mechanisms of fear extinction dependent on length of time since fear acquisition.** *Learn Mem* 2006, **13:**216–223.
25. Chang CH, Maren S: **Early extinction after fear conditioning yields a context-independent and short-term suppression of conditional freezing in rats.** *Learn Mem* 2009, **16:**62–68.
26. Cain CK, Blouin AM, Barad M: **Temporally massed CS presentations generate more fear extinction than spaced presentations.** *J Exp Psychol Anim Behav Process* 2003, **29:**323–333.
27. Cain CK, Blouin AM, Barad M: **Adrenergic transmission facilitates extinction of conditional fear in mice.** *Learn Mem* 2004, **11:**179–187.
28. Plendl W, Wotjak CT: **Dissociation of within- and between-session extinction of conditioned fear.** *J Neurosci* 2010, **30:**4990–4998.
29. Monfils MH, Cowansage KK, Klann E, LeDoux JE: **Extinction-reconsolidation boundaries: key to persistent attenuation of fear memories.** *Science* 2009, **324:**951–955.
30. Schiller D, Monfils MH, Raio CM, Johnson DC, Ledoux JE, Phelps EA: **Preventing the return of fear in humans using reconsolidation update mechanisms.** *Nature* 2009, **463:**49–53.
31. Chan WY, Leung HT, Westbrook RF, McNally GP: **Effects of recent exposure to a conditioned stimulus on extinction of Pavlovian fear conditioning.** *Learn Mem* 2010, **17:**512–521.
32. Clem RL, Huganir RL: **Calcium-permeable AMPA receptor dynamics mediate fear memory erasure.** *Science* 2010, **330:**1108–1112.
33. Gewirtz JC, Davis M: **Using pavlovian higher-order conditioning paradigms to investigate the neural substrates of emotional learning and memory.** *Learn Mem* 2000, **7:**257–266.
34. Parkes SL, Westbrook RF: **The basolateral amygdala is critical for the acquisition and extinction of associations between a neutral stimulus and a learned danger signal but not between two neutral stimuli.** *J Neurosci* 2010, **30:**12608–12618.
35. Blanchard RJ, Blanchard DC: **Passive and active reactions to fear-eliciting stimuli.** *J Comp Physiol Psychol* 1969, **68**(1):129–135.
36. Stafford JM, Maughan DK, Ilioi EC, Lattal KM: **Exposure to a fearful context during periods of memory plasticity impairs extinction via hyperactivation of frontal-amygdalar circuits.** *Learn Mem* 2013, **20:**156–163.
37. Hutton-Bedbrook K, McNally GP: **The promises and pitfalls of retrieval-extinction procedures in preventing relapse to drug seeking.** *Front Psychiatry* 2013, **4:**14.
38. Izquierdo I, Bevilaqua LR, Rossato JI, Bonini JS, Medina JH, Cammarota M: **Different molecular cascades in different sites of the brain control memory consolidation.** *Trends Neurosci* 2006, **29:**496–505.
39. Pickens CL, Golden SA, Adams-Deutsch T, Nair SG, Shaham Y: **Long-lasting incubation of conditioned fear in rats.** *Biol Psychiatry* 2009, **65:**881–886.
40. Eysenck HJ: **A theory of the incubation of anxiety-fear responses.** *Behav Res Ther* 1968, **6:**309–321.
41. Eisenberg M, Kobilo T, Berman DE, Dudai Y: **Stability of retrieved memory: inverse correlation with trace dominance.** *Science* 2003, **301:**1102–1104.
42. Jacob W, Marsch R, Marsicano G, Lutz B, Wotjak CT: **Cannabinoid CB1 receptor deficiency increases contextual fear memory under highly aversive conditions and long-term potentiation in vivo.** *Neurobiol Learn Mem* 2012, **98:**47–55.
43. Kindt M, Soeter M: **Reconsolidation in a human fear conditioning study: a test of extinction as updating mechanism.** *Biol Psychol* 2013, **92:**43–50.
44. Costanzi M, Cannas S, Saraulli D, Rossi-Arnaud C, Cestari V: **Extinction after retrieval: effects on the associative and nonassociative components of remote contextual fear memory.** *Learn Mem* 2013, **18:**508–518.
45. Jarome TJ, Kwapis JL, Werner CT, Parsons RG, Gafford GM, Helmstetter FJ: **The timing of multiple retrieval events can alter GluR1 phosphorylation and the requirement for protein synthesis in fear memory reconsolidation.** *Learn Mem* 2012, **19:**300–306.
46. Wessa M, Flor H: **Failure of extinction of fear responses in posttraumatic stress disorder: evidence from second-order conditioning.** *Am J Psychiatry* 2007, **164:**1684–1692.
47. Rescorla RA, Wagner AR: **A theory of Pavlovian conditioning: Variations in the effectiveness of reinforcement and nonreinforcement.** In *Classical conditioning II.* Edited by Black AH, Prokasy WF. New York: Appleton-Century-Crofts; 1972:64–99.
48. Pearce JM, Hall G: **A model for Pavlovian learning: variations in the effectiveness of conditioned but not of unconditioned stimuli.** *Psychol Rev* 1980, **87:**532–552.

16

Rumination in bipolar disorder: evidence for an unquiet mind

Sharmin Ghaznavi* and Thilo Deckersbach

Abstract

Depression in bipolar disorder has long been thought to be a state characterized by mental inactivity. However, recent research demonstrates that patients with bipolar disorder engage in rumination, a form of self-focused repetitive cognitive activity, in depressed as well as in manic states. While rumination has long been associated with depressed states in major depressive disorder, the finding that patients with bipolar disorder ruminate in manic states is unique to bipolar disorder and challenges explanations put forward for why people ruminate. We review the research on rumination in bipolar disorder and propose that rumination in bipolar disorder, in both manic and depressed states, reflects executive dysfunction. We also review the neurobiology of bipolar disorder and recent neuroimaging studies of rumination, which is consistent with our hypothesis that the tendency to ruminate reflects executive dysfunction in bipolar disorder. Finally, we relate the neurobiology of rumination to the neurobiology of emotion regulation, which is disrupted in bipolar disorder.

Keywords: bipolar disorder, rumination, executive functioning, emotion regulation

Introduction

Bipolar disorder is characterized by episodes of mania or hypomania, with or without one or more episode(s) of depression. By recent estimates, it affects between 1 and 2.5% of the general population in the United States [1]. Although mania/hypomania is the distinguishing feature of bipolar disorder, recurrent depressive episodes constitute the most frequent and functionally debilitating, unresolved aspect of the illness for individuals with bipolar disorder [2,3]. For example, over their lifetime, patients with bipolar disorder experience many more depressive episodes than manic or hypomanic episodes and spend longer amounts of time depressed than manic or hypomanic [4,5]. They are also more likely to consult a physician or psychiatrist for depression rather than for mania [6]. Likewise, depressive episodes are associated with comparatively greater occupational and psychosocial disruption then manic/hypomanic episodes. This includes impairments at work [6,7] as well as disruptions of patients' family and social life [6]. Unfortunately, despite the advancements in pharmacotherapy and the emergence of adjunctive psychosocial treatments, the diagnosis and management of bipolar depression remain significant challenges [8,9].

Melancholic depression in bipolar disorder

One of the earliest observations about bipolar depression is that it is more likely to be a *melancholic* depression. According to DSM-IV, the *melancholic* subtype is a depressed state characterized by anhedonia, excessive weight loss, psychomotor agitation or retardation, insomnia, worsening of symptoms in the morning, early morning awakening and excessive guilt. Although operational definitions of *melancholia* have varied over the years and across diagnostic systems (DSM III [10], DSMIII-R [11], Research Diagnostic Criteria [12], the World Health Organization Depression Scale [13], the Newcastle Scale - Versions I and II [13,14], Hamilton Depression Rating Scale [15]; see [16] for a review), the one consistent feature across the various definitions has been that of psychomotor retardation [16], described as a slowed or decreased rate of movement and/or speech.

In one of the early studies of the phenomenology of depressed states, Dunner and colleagues [17] found that in the midst of a depressive phase, inpatients with bipolar I disorder showed significantly less attention to personal appearance and exhibited greater psychomotor

* Correspondence: sghaznavi@partners.org
Massachusetts General Hospital, Boston, MA, USA

slowing than inpatients with major depressive disorder (MDD). Similarly, in a study looking at melancholic depression in patients who met criteria for melancholic depression based on three different definitions, including DSM-III, the rate of bipolar disorder was significantly higher than unipolar depression, regardless of the definition of melancholia employed [18]. They also found that melancholia was most clearly distinguished by psychomotor disturbance. Likewise, in a study by Mitchell and colleagues [19] that compared bipolar I disorder patients with patients with MDD, patients with bipolar disorder were found to be more likely to have psychomotor retardation and atypical features (such as hypersomnia and leaden paralysis) than depressed patients with MDD.

The generally held belief that patients with bipolar disorder (in particular bipolar I disorder) are more likely to experience a melancholic depression characterized by psychomotor retardation than patients with MDD, as well as the research showing that melancholic depression is more common in bipolar I disorder, has led to the notion, among clinicians, that there is a corresponding mental slowing as well [20,21]. However, there have been no studies to suggest that patients with bipolar disorder are less mentally active. The notion that there is mental slowing in bipolar depression may also be, in part, a contrast to the large body of evidence that points to an active mind in major depressive disorder, in the form of rumination.

Rumination in major depressive disorder

Major depressive disorder (MDD), sometimes referred to as unipolar depression, is characterized by one or more episodes of depression, without any episodes of mania or hypomania. Thus, it is nosologically distinguished from bipolar disorder by the absence of hypomanic or manic episodes. One feature of MDD which has received considerable attention is the tendency to ruminate [22], that is responding to negative affect or depressed mood by focusing on self and symptoms of distress, without actively engaging in active problem solving [23].

Rumination represents a behavioral and attentional style of responding to negative affect or depressed mood. Thus, rumination is distinguished from such problems as indecisiveness, as well as a set of recurrent thoughts about death and suicide. Similarly, rumination is distinguished from dysfunctional attitudes, which are a set of general beliefs about the self, world and future which are negatively biased, as opposed to a means of responding to a negative affective state. In fact, dysfunctional attitudes are thought to be present in individuals at risk for depression when they are euthymic (that is, not in a negative affective state).

By the same token, rumination is also distinguished from negative automatic thoughts, which refers to a set of thoughts with distorted negative content. As Nolen-Hoeksema originally pointed out, patient's ruminative thoughts may often in fact be realistic rather than distorted (for example, "I can't complete my work on time.") These distinct features of rumination were demonstrated in early studies of rumination in which participants were asked to state their responses to prompts in a rumination induction paradigm developed by Nolen-Hoeksema and colleagues [24]. While it might be argued that yet another difference between rumination and automatic thoughts is that there seems to be a volitional component to a ruminative response style, whereas negative automatic thoughts seem less volitional, such a characterization is oversimplified. As discussed later, the cognitive underpinnings of rumination suggest that while a ruminative response style may start off as seemingly volitional, its perpetuation may not be volitional.

The tendency to ruminate is highly correlated to depressed mood (see [22] for a review). To date, much of the research on rumination has been carried out on individuals with dysphoria and patients with MDD [22]. Early studies on rumination found that rumination can maintain or even worsen depressed mood [25,26]. Additionally, the tendency to ruminate predicts the likelihood to go on to develop a first major depressive episode following a stressor [23], as well as a worse prognosis in patients with major depression. The tendency to ruminate was found to be predictive of higher levels of depressed mood at discharge and follow-up after hospitalization in a group of inpatients with MDD [27]. Studies on the phenomenology of rumination reveal that it is a repetitive and persistent phenomenon that is difficult to stop and maladaptive [28-30]. To date, there are no studies examining whether rumination is more prevalent in certain types of depression (for example, excited depression or melancholic depression); however, such research might illuminate differences in the phenomenology of mood states in different types of depression.

Rumination is related to a negative self-concept in individuals with major depression. In fact, in the course of their research on rumination, Nolen-Hoeksema and Morrow [31] developed a rumination induction task, which consists of self-focused but neutral statements, (for example, "think about the sensations in your body"). When healthy normal controls are asked to engage in the task, they do not show any changes in mood. However, when depressed individuals are asked to perform the same task, they report maintenance or even worsening of depressed mood [31]. Presumably, self-focus promoting statements activate negative self-schemata, which trigger corresponding negative thoughts associated with maintenance or worsening of mood in depressed patients, thereby creating a vicious cycle of increased self-focus, negative thoughts and depressed mood.

Studies of negative thoughts and beliefs as assessed by two widely used and well validated measures, the Automatic Thoughts Questionnaire (ATQ)[32] and Dysfunctional Attitudes Scale (DAS) [33], show that negative automatic thoughts and dysfunctional attitudes, often related to the self, are elevated in depressed states (ATQ: [32,34-37]; DAS: [33,37-40]). This does not appear to be the case when patients are euthymic (ATQ: [34,37,38]; DAS: [37-40]). A few studies have also found that dysfunctional attitudes interact with negative life events, or stress, to predict depressive symptoms [41,42]. Thus, latent negative self-concepts, when activated, as in rumination, may trigger depressed mood and relapse into depression.

Negative self-concept in bipolar disorder

There is an emerging literature documenting persistent negative self-concepts (schemata) in individuals with bipolar disorder as well. In one study, using the ATQ and DAS, Hollon *et al.* [37] found that regardless of nosology (MDD, bipolar disorder, substance induced depression), among patients who were currently depressed, scores on both the ATQ and DAS were higher than in other clinical and control groups. Additionally, the ATQ covaried directly with levels of depression as measured by the Beck Depression Inventory (BDI). In a study directly comparing scores on the DAS between patients with bipolar disorder and patients with MDD, Jones and colleagues [43] found that, when current levels of depression were taken into account, there was no difference on scores on the DAS between the two groups. More recently Scott and Pope [44] also found that patients with MDD and bipolar disorder did not differ significantly on overall scores on the DAS. The finding that scores on the DAS and ATQ do not differ between patients with MDD and bipolar disorder suggests that self-concept in depressed states in both disorders is equally negative.

Consistent with this, Reilly-Harrington *et al.* [45] found patients with bipolar disorder and MDD performed similarly on a Self-Referent Information Processing Task [46] that consisted of a battery of four tasks which tap into self-attributes. Both groups performed the tasks in a manner consistent with a negative self-concept.

Additionally, research on self-esteem suggests that patients with bipolar disorder and major depression demonstrate similar low levels of self-esteem. In their study comparing patients with bipolar disorder and MDD on the DAS, Scott and Pope [44] also used the Rosenberg Self-Esteem Questionnaire (SEQ; [47]). The SEQ is a measure of trait self-esteem consisting of five negative and five positive statements (corresponding to negative and positive self-esteem respectively), which participants rate on a 1 to 4 scale. They found that patients with bipolar disorder and MDD did not differ significantly on overall scores on the SEQ. Similarly, in the Jones and colleagues study [43], when current levels of depression were taken into account; there was no difference on scores on the SEQ between depressed patients with bipolar disorder and depressed patients with MDD, and both patient groups had significantly lower scores on the SEQ than control participants.

Unique to bipolar disorder, scores on the DAS are elevated in patients with bipolar disorder during the manic phase as well as the depressed phase. Goldberg and colleagues [48] compared scores on the DAS in patients with bipolar disorder who were manic, patients with MDD who were depressed, and controls. They found that while patients with MDD, who were currently depressed, had the highest scores on the DAS, patients with bipolar disorder who were manic, had significantly higher scores on the DAS than healthy controls.

As in MDD, scores on the ATQ and DAS do not appear elevated when patients with bipolar disorder are in remission. For example, in the study by Hollon and colleagues [37], they found that scores on the ATQ and DAS were not elevated compared to controls, in patients with bipolar disorder who were in remission. Likewise, in a study by Lex and colleagues [49] investigating cognitive styles in patients with bipolar disorder in full remission, there were no significant differences on scores on the DAS and ATQ between patients with bipolar disorder who were in remission and normal controls.

Finally, similar to patients with MDD, negative self-concept or schemata seem to predict relapse into mania and depression in patients with bipolar disorder. In the study by Reilly-Harrington and colleagues [45], scores on the DAS interacted with the number of negative life events to predict increases in depressive, as well as manic, symptoms. Depressed patients with bipolar disorder, who possessed greater dysfunctional attitudes and experienced more negative life events, showed worsening in their mood symptoms, both depressive and manic symptoms.

Rumination in bipolar disorder

While the bulk of the research on rumination has been conducted in individuals with major depression, given the research showing negative self-concept/schemata in bipolar disorder and the role of rumination or self-focus in sustaining depressed mood one might expect that depressed patients with bipolar disorder engage in ruminative thinking, similar to patients with MDD. Indeed, this is what Johnson *et al.* [50] found in a recent study looking at the tendency to ruminate in individuals with bipolar disorder, MDD and normal controls. They used the Response Styles Questionnaire (RSQ; [51]), which is a measure of the tendency to engage in ruminative responses when feeling depressed, and found that both individuals with MDD and bipolar disorder endorsed heightened rumination in response to negative affect, compared to normal controls.

Consistent with this, van der Gucht *et al.* [52] found that the tendency to ruminate was highly correlated with depressive symptoms, (as assessed by the Hamilton Depression Rating Scale; HDRS), in patients with bipolar disorder. In a recent study, in our group with patients with bipolar disorder, using the RSQ, we also found that patients with bipolar disorder, who are depressed, show a greater tendency to ruminate, when compared to levels previously reported in normal controls [53].

Given the repetitive and persistent nature of ruminative thinking, its presence in depressed states in patients with bipolar disorder is contrary to the widely held belief that depression in bipolar disorder is characterized by mental slowing, decreased mental activity, or a relative dearth of thought. Early studies of rumination in unipolar depressed states, in which participants were asked to state their thoughts in response to the prompts on the rumination task developed by Nolen-Hoeksema and colleagues, demonstrate that individuals who ruminate are mentally quite active, with numerous thoughts, albeit with a negative bias [24]. Patients with bipolar disorder in depressed states ruminate and, as such, are mentally quite active, suggesting an unquiet mind in depressed states in bipolar disorder as well.

Notably, melancholia and rumination are not necessarily contrasting phenomena. As reviewed above, various definitions of melancholia exist, but generally these definitions, including the current DSM-IV definition, encompass primarily physical symptoms (for example, psychomotor disturbance). Thus, cognitive states in melancholia are not well characterized. It is possible, given the greater depressive symptom load in melancholic depression and the correlation between rumination and depressive symptom load, that rumination is prevalent among individuals afflicted with melancholia. Thus, rumination and melancholia are not necessarily contrasting phenomena, and, in fact, it is likely that rumination is a key feature of melancholia, not previously described.

What appears to be unique to bipolar disorder is that studies of rumination in bipolar disorder reveal that not only do individuals with bipolar disorder ruminate in response to negative affect in depressed states, they ruminate in response to positive affect as well. In the study by Johnson *et al.* [50], individuals with bipolar disorder endorsed ruminating in response to positive affect as well as negative affect, albeit with a more positive focus. Using the Response to Positive Affect Questionnaire [54] which assesses tendencies in responses to positive affect, Johnson and colleagues found that individuals with bipolar disorder, who were hypomanic, endorsed a tendency to focus on positive affective experiences and positive self-qualities. Thus, patients with bipolar disorder engage in a positive ruminative style in response to positive affect in a hypomanic state, as well as a negative ruminative style in response to negative affect, in a depressed state. Notably, positive rumination is conceptually different from grandiosity, which is defined as an inflated sense of self-esteem or believing that one has special powers, spiritual connections or religious relationships. Ruminative thoughts of a positive nature may often be realistic (for example, "I did a good job on a project at work last week", which describes a positive affective experience that is reality based). Additionally, positive rumination is distinguished from flight of ideas by the fact that the content of positive ruminations is organized around positive affective experiences and qualities, and not random associations. Studies which record the content of positive ruminations, as Nolen-Hoeksema and colleagues have done with negative rumination [24], are needed to provide empirical support for these distinctions.

Surprisingly, the tendency to engage in rumination to negative affect may also be associated with hypomania. In studies of college sample students [55,56], scores on the RSQ are found to be positively correlated with hypomanic traits (as assessed by the Eckblad and Chapman's Hypomanic Personality Scale; HPS [57]). Individuals who have a tendency to focus on their symptoms of distress and negative self-qualities also possess more hypomanic traits. Notably, in another study, van der Gucht *et al.* [52] did not find a correlation between rumination (as assessed by the RSQ) and manic traits (as assessed by the Bech-Rafaelson mania scale [58]) in patients with bipolar disorder.

Psychological accounts of why patients with bipolar disorder ruminate

Given the role of rumination in persistence of negative mood, the question arises, why do depressed patients ruminate? One account that has been put forward to explain rumination in unipolar depression by Papageorgiou and Wells [28] is that rumination is a coping strategy. Papageorgiou and Wells found that patients identified advantages as well as disadvantages to rumination, suggesting that they engage in rumination in part because of a perceived benefit from rumination. The advantages cited by patients included a sense of improved understanding of their depression and the causes of their depression, and a sense of control over their symptoms and problem solving.

This account is likely applicable to patients with bipolar disorder who are depressed. They may engage in rumination for reasons similar to their MDD counterparts. However, such an account does not explain why rumination has been associated with hypomania in patients with bipolar disorder as well. One possibility that has been put forward to account for this finding [55] invokes the age old idea of the manic defense to depression. On this account, the hypomania/mania is a coping strategy just like rumination, so the correlation between hypomania and rumination reflects that they are both coping strategies used by patients with bipolar disorder who are struggling with depression. Support for this account comes from a recent study by Goldberg and colleagues [48] showing that patients with bipolar disorder in a manic phase endorse negative core beliefs, suggesting that the mania may be a means of coping with the negative core beliefs. Another account is based on research that patients with bipolar disorder generally have higher expectations [59] and are goal attainment focused [60], but when depressed, have greater difficulty realizing those expectations and goals. The account proposes that this difficulty leads to a failure to achieve those expectations and goals in depressed states, which in turn may lead to negative self-appraisal and rumination. A final related hypothesis explaining the link between the tendency to ruminate and mania in bipolar disorder is rooted in the possibility that individuals with mania may have experienced more failures, as well as destructive complications, as a result of their mania (as opposed to failures due to their depression). According to this account [61], hypomania/mania may have led to more failures and in turn may lead to a greater likelihood to resort to self-blame, negative self-appraisal and rumination.

One problem with these three psychological accounts is the finding from Johnson and colleagues (2008) that patients with bipolar disorder engage in positive rumination (that is, positive self-appraisal) in response to positive affect in a hypomanic state. Similarly, Eisner and colleagues [62] found that there is a tendency to engage in positive generalization, similar to positive rumination, in response to successes. An account of why patients with bipolar disorder ruminate must take into account why they ruminate in response to both negative and positive affect.

The tendency to ruminate in bipolar disorder and executive dysfunction

We propose that the link between the tendency to ruminate in manic and depressed states in bipolar disorder reflects executive dysfunction in bipolar disorder. Research on neuropsychological functioning in bipolar disorder reveals deficits in several cognitive domains, including attention, learning and memory, and executive functioning [63-66]. The executive dysfunction seen in bipolar disorder is present in euthymic, depressed and manic states, suggesting that the executive dysfunction is not state specific, but rather trait-like. In one study, investigating neuropsychological functioning in bipolar patients in manic, depressed and euthymic mood states, Martinez-Aran *et al.* [66] found that regardless of mood state, all patients with bipolar disorder showed impaired functioning on tests of executive functioning, including the Wisconsin Card Sort Task (WCST) and Stroop Color and Word Interference task. While a more recent study calls into question the presence of executive dysfunction in euthymic states in bipolar disorder, they nonetheless found a trend towards executive dysfunction in patients with bipolar disorder who are euthymic [67]. It is possible that the executive dysfunction present in patients with bipolar disorder in euthymic states is exacerbated in mania and depression.

In fact, in studies using tests of executive functioning, including attentional set-shifting [68,69], planning ability [70] and decision making [69,70], researchers consistently find deficits in executive functioning in mania. And the finding by Martinez-Aran *et al.* [66] of executive dysfunction in depressed states in bipolar disorder is consistent with the literature showing executive dysfunction in depressed states in MDD (see [71] for a review). Of note, many of the tasks used to assess executive functioning are tasks which incorporate multiple executive processes (for example, the WCST incorporates shifting attention as well as inhibition), so a fine grain approach to executive functioning as suggested by Miyake *et al.* [72] is not currently possible. However, such an approach would be invaluable at more precisely identifying particular executive deficits in bipolar disorder. This highlights the need for research into specific executive processes in bipolar disorder.

There is some initial evidence that the tendency to ruminate is associated with executive dysfunction. In a study by Davis and Nolen-Hoeksema [73], individuals with a tendency to ruminate were found to demonstrate perseverative tendencies and failures to maintain adaptive cognitive sets on the WCST. Similarly, Watkins and Brown [74] found that depressed patients who underwent a rumination induction and were asked to perform a random number generation task showed failures of inhibitory executive control compared to depressed participants who underwent distraction, and non-depressed participants. More recently, Whitmer and Banich [75] found that individuals with a tendency to ruminate have trouble inhibiting mental representations of previous task demands when they switch their attention to new task demands. Thus, rumination seems to be associated with executive dysfunction, particularly inhibitory executive control. Of course, given the dearth of studies, further research into executive functioning and rumination is much needed.

Taken together, the evidence for executive dysfunction in bipolar disorder and the relationship between rumination and executive dysfunction suggests that the tendency to ruminate may be symptomatic of executive dysfunction in bipolar disorder, specifically inhibitory executive dysfunction. Patients with bipolar disorder may experience an exacerbation in executive dysfunction when manic or depressed, which may lead to a tendency to ruminate because of a failure to inhibit self-focused thoughts of a positive or negative nature. This possibility invites investigation into the effects of mood states on executive functioning and rumination in bipolar disorder.

Neural correlates of bipolar disorder and rumination

Research into neural correlates of bipolar disorder has increased dramatically in the last few decades with advances in structural and functional neuroimaging. The data for structural differences are somewhat mixed, with a few studies showing no differences between individuals with bipolar disorder and healthy controls in prefrontal regions [76-78] and amygdala [79], and other studies reporting differences in both prefrontal regions [80-83] as well as amygdala [84-87]. Two recent meta-analyses using region of interest analyses found no evidence of gray matter abnormalities [88,89], but more recently one meta-analysis study using voxel based morphometry (VBM), which uses a whole brain technique, found reductions in grey matter in the rostral anterior cingulate cortex and the right fronto insular cortex [90], while another meta-analysis study, also using VBM, found reductions in grey matter in the anterior cingulate and insula [91].

Functional neuroimaging studies comparing patients with bipolar disorder and healthy controls consistently report differences in prefrontal cortices, with early studies showing blood flow and/or metabolic abnormalities in overall frontal metabolism in patients with bipolar disorder compared to healthy subjects [92-96], and later studies suggesting more fine-tuned differences in activation in subgenual prefrontal cortex in patients with bipolar disorder compared to healthy controls [97].

More recently, studies using functional Magnetic Resonance Imaging (fMRI) while performing various tasks, such as presentation of emotional stimuli, the Stroop task and the Go/No-Go, and memory encoding tasks, consistently find differences in activation in prefrontal regions in patients with bipolar disorder across all mood states. Studies have found differences in activation in dorsolateral prefrontal cortex (DLPFC; BA9/46) [98,99], left ventral prefrontal cortex (VLPFC; BA47) [100], rostral ventral prefrontal cortex (VLPFC; BA10/47) [101], and orbital and medial prefrontal (BA 8/9) cortices in patients with bipolar disorder who are euthymic [100]. One study found differences in activation in left ventral prefrontal cortex (BA 10/47) in patients with bipolar disorder who were manic as well as those who were depressed [101]. Functional neuroimaging studies also consistently report differences in amygdalar activitation in response to negative stimuli relative to healthy controls in patients with bipolar disorder who are euthymic [98], depressed [102] and manic [103].

Additionally, there are two studies that suggest a link between activity in prefrontal cortices and amygdala in bipolar disorder. Yuerglen-Todd *et al.* [98] found that patients with bipolar disorder who are euthymic demonstrate a reduction in DLPFC (BA 9/46) activation and an increase in amygdalar activation in response to fear faces, relative to healthy controls. Ketter *et al.* [102] found that patients with bipolar disorder who were depressed had decreased global prefrontal and paralimbic cortical metabolism and increased metabolism in right amygdala, ventral striatum and thalamus. Taken together, these two studies suggest that decreased functional activation in prefrontal areas may reflect a loss of cognitive control or executive dysfunction, and a failure of emotion regulation, which may in turn lead to increased amygdala activation. Consistent with this, a recent meta-analysis of 65 fMRI studies in bipolar disorder by Chen and colleagues [104] found evidence for fronto-limbic activation in bipolar disorder, which was characterized by attenuated ventrolateral prefrontal cortex activation across emotional and cognitive tasks and enhanced limbic activation with emotional tasks.

In a recent review on the neurophysiology of emotion regulation, Phillips *et al.* [105] conceptualized a model of emotion regulation consisting of a voluntary emotion regulation system involving lateral prefrontal cortices (DLPFC and VLPFC) and an automatic emotion regulation system involving medial prefrontal cortices (OFC, subgenual ACC and medial dorsal PFC). The model is based on research in healthy controls which demonstrates increased activity in lateral prefrontal cortices in tasks of voluntary behavioral control to positive and negative stimuli (for example, suppressing facial reactions to emotional stimuli), voluntary attentional control (in which participants are directed to selectively attend to task-relevant emotional stimuli/inhibit distraction from task-irrelevant emotional stimuli, for example) and voluntary reappraisal (for example, decreasing negative affect from a negative stimulus); and increased activity in medial prefrontal cortices in tasks of automatic behavioral control (for example, decreased affect to emotional stimuli), automatic attentional control (implicit direction of attention to or away from emotional stimuli, for example, the Stroop task), and automatic reappraisal (for example, implicit appraisal of novel contexts).

Phillips *et al.* [105] show that there is an overlap with the above findings in bipolar disorder. They report mixed findings with regards to voluntary emotion regulation: studies of voluntary attentional control show reduced activation in lateral PFC and DLPFC regions, while studies of voluntary emotion regulation show greater activation in those same areas. The literature on automatic emotion regulation in patients with bipolar disorder is more consistent with studies of automatic attentional control showing reduced activitation in ventromedial PFC in bipolar disorder compared to healthy controls and studies of emotion regulation showing reduced activation within ventromedial PFC. Thus, overall, while it is clear that more research on emotion regulation in bipolar disorder is much needed, it is nonetheless apparent that there are differences in bipolar disorder in brain regions that are involved in emotion regulation.

Compared to the research on neural substrates of bipolar disorder, the research on neural substrates of rumination is relatively new. In fact, there have been less than a handful of studies, most of them in the last few years. These studies suggest overlap with brain regions implicated in affective dysregulation in bipolar disorder, including anterior cingulate, DLPFC, OFC, as well as amygdala, suggesting a common neural substrate for rumination and affective dysregulation in bipolar disorder. In one of the first studies, which investigated the relationship between the tendency to ruminate and amygdalar response to word stimuli, Siegle and colleages [106] found that in depressed individuals, the tendency to ruminate was moderately correlated with sustained amygdala activity following presentation of negative items.

Ray *et al.* [107] investigated the relationship between the tendency to ruminate and cognitive reappraisal after emotional responses in a non-clinical sample. They found that the tendency to ruminate was correlated with increases in amygdala response, when participants were instructed to increase negative affect, and with decreases in prefrontal regions, including anterior cingulate cortex and medial prefrontal cortex, when participants were instructed to decrease negative affect. More recently, Cooney *et al.* [108] looked at neural activity during a brief rumination induction, a concrete distraction induction, and an abstract distraction induction in depressed individuals and normal controls. They found that depressed individuals showed greater activation in the OFC (BA 11), subegenual cingulate (BA25), and DLPFC (BA 9) than normal controls during rumination compared to concrete distraction. Additionally, depressed participants showed greater activity than healthy controls in the rumination condition compared to abstract distraction in the amygdala, dorsal anterior cingulate (BA 24), rostral anterior cingulate (BA 32), DLPFC (BA 46), posterior cingulate (BA 31), and parahippocampus. More recently, Hamilton *et al.* found a correlation between the depressive rumination in depressed patients correlated with resting state activity in posterior cingulate and medial prefrontal cortices [109].

Notably, many of the brain regions implicated in bipolar disorder overlap with regions implicated in rumination, namely prefrontal cortical areas, including the anterior cingulate, DLPFC, and OFC, as well as the amygdala. The evidence for common neural substrates in bipolar disorder and rumination, particularly in prefrontal cortical regions, which are believed to be involved in executive functioning, is consistent with our hypothesis that executive dysfunction may underlie the tendency to ruminate in bipolar disorder. Patients with bipolar disorder may ruminate because they experience difficulty inhibiting their persistent self-focus, once it has been initiated. The fact that prefrontal brain regions implicated in bipolar disorder and rumination include regions involved in automatic emotion regulation (ACC, OFC) and voluntary emotion regulation (DLPFC) point to a common neural substrate for affective dysregulation as well. Thus, patients with bipolar disorder, due to differences in functioning in prefrontal cortical regions may experience difficulty inhibiting and regulating emotion, just as they have difficulty inhibiting their persistent self-focus in response to positive or negative affect (that is, rumination). In fact, rumination, more generally speaking, might be explained by differences in functioning in prefrontal cortical regions and a deficit in inhibiting self-focus. These hypotheses provide interesting lines of investigation that might be pursued in future neuroimaging studies.

Conclusions and future directions

The mind in bipolar disorder, whether manic or depressed, is never quiet. Patients with bipolar disorder struggle and tend to ruminate in depressed states, just like their MDD counterparts. Unique to bipolar disorder is the finding that patients with bipolar disorder ruminate about positive things in hypomanic and possibly manic states, which raises several questions.

One question that arises is whether rumination contributes to worsening in hypomanic or manic states [50]. Research on rumination in depressed states [22] demonstrates that rumination maintains and even worsens depressed mood. However, it is unclear whether rumination plays a role in exacerbating or maintaining hypomanic or manic mood. On this point, Johnson *et al.* [50] not only found that patients with bipolar disorder ruminate in response to positive affect, but that it was explained by hypomanic symptoms. Also, Johnson and Tran [110] found that individuals with bipolar disorder show an increased focus on goals and increased confidence during manic states. Research is needed on the relationship between rumination in response to positive affect and future hypomanic or manic episodes.

Another question which arises is why do patients with bipolar disorder ruminate in response to positive affect? We know that in major depression, rumination begins with a desire to problem solve [28], but then evolves into a vicious cycle of repetitively focusing on one's symptoms of distress and how they came to be. One possibility is that rumination in response to positive affect is intended to maintain the positive mood. Johnson *et al.* [111] assessed the tendency to ruminate in response to positive affect using a measure which assesses the tendency to think about positive qualities of the self, positive affective experiences, and favorable life circumstances that might amplify the positive affect, and found that patients with bipolar disorder endorsed a greater tendency to ruminate to positive affect. It seems possible that such thinking might be geared towards maintaining a positive mood. However, research on the effects of positive rumination on mood is needed. Additionally, research on the reasons why people engage in positive rumination is also needed. It is also possible that patients with bipolar disorder ruminate in response to positive affect because the prospect of reward initiates a cycle of thinking which might maximize reward. Perhaps the positive affect serves as a sort of reward, and sets in cycle a desire for additional reward.

Finally, related to our hypothesis that the tendency to ruminate reflects executive dysfunction, there are several questions which warrant investigation. Is intact executive functioning protective? Are patients with bipolar disorder with little or no executive dysfunction less likely to ruminate in response to positive or negative affect? What are the neural mechanisms underlying the failure to inhibit rumination? It may be that the failure to inhibit rumination is simply a product of prefrontal dysfunction and an inability to inhibit certain cognitive processes as needed. Alternatively, it is possible that deficits in automatic and voluntary emotion regulation as posited by Phillips [105] perpetuates the cycle of rumination by affecting prefrontal functioning. Thus, there are several avenues of research related to rumination and bipolar disorder that have the potential to inform our understanding of what contributes to and maintains mood states in bipolar disorder.

Abbreviations

ATQ: Automatic Thoughts Questionnaire; BDI: Beck Depression Inventory; DAS: Dysfunctional Attitudes Scale; DLPFC: dorsolateral prefrontal cortex; HDRS: Hamilton Depression Rating Scale; HPS: Eckblad and Chapman's Hypomanic Personality Scale; MDD: major depressive disorder; RSQ: Response Styles Questionnaire; SEQ: Rosenberg Self-Esteem Questionnaire; VBM: voxel based morphometry; VLPFC: left ventral prefrontal cortex; WCST: Wisconsin Card Sort Task

Authors' contributions

SG and TD were involved in research for this manuscript and drafted the manuscript. Both authors read and approved the final manuscript.

Competing interests

SG and TD have no competing interests.

References

1. Merikangas KR, Akiskal HS, Angst J, Greenberg PE, Hirschfeld RM, Petukhova M, Kessler RC: **Lifetime and 12-month prevalence of bipolar spectrum disorder in the National Comorbidity Survey replication.** *Arch Gen Psychiatry* 2007, **64**:543-552.
2. Dion GL, Tohen M, Anthony WA, Waternaux CS: **Symptoms and functioning of patients with bipolar disorder six months after hospitalization.** *Hosp Community Psychiatry* 1988, **39**:652-657.
3. Coryell W, Andreasen NC, Endicott J, Keller M: **The significance of past mania or hypomania in the course and outcome of major depression.** *Am J Psychiatry* 1987, **144**:309-315.
4. Judd LL, Akiskal HS, Schettler PJ, Endicott J, Maser J, Solomon DA, Leon AC, Rice JA, Keller MB: **The long-term natural history of the weekly symptomatic status of bipolar I disorder.** *Arch Gen Psychiatry* 2002, **59**:530-537.
5. Judd LL, Akiskal HS, Schettler PJ, Coryell W, Endicott J, Maser JD, Solomon DA, Leon AC, Keller MB: **A prospective investigation of the natural history of the long-term weekly symptomatic status of bipolar II disorder.** *Arch Gen Psychiatry* 2003, **60**:261-269.
6. Calabrese JR, Hirschfeld RM, Frye MA, Reed ML: **Impact of depressive symptoms compared with manic symptoms in bipolar disorder: results of a U.S. community-based sample.** *J Clin Psychiatry* 2004, **65**:1499-1504.
7. Kessler RC, Akiskal HS, Ames M, Birnbaum H, Greenberg P, Hirschfeld RM, Jin R, Merikangas KR, Simon GE, Wang PS: **Prevalence and effects of mood disorders on work performance in a nationally representative sample of U.S. workers.** *Am J Psychiatry* 2006, **163**:1561-1568.
8. Thase ME, Sachs GS: **Bipolar depression: pharmacotherapy and related therapeutic strategies.** *Biol Psychiatry* 2000, **48**:558-572.
9. Gijsman HJ, Geddes JR, Rendell JM, Nolen WA, Goodwin GM: **Antidepressants for bipolar depression: a systematic review of randomized, controlled trials.** *Am J Psychiatry* 2004, **161**:1537-1547.
10. American Psychiatric Association. Task Force on Nomenclature and Statistics., American Psychiatric Association.Committee on Nomenclature and Statistics: *Diagnostic and statistical manual of mental disorders.* 3 edition. Washington, D.C.: American Psychiatric Association; 1980.
11. American Psychiatric Association., American Psychiatric Association. Work Group to Revise DSM-III: *Diagnostic and statistical manual of mental disorders: DSM-III-R.* 3 edition. Washington, DC: American Psychiatric Association; 1987.
12. Spitzer RL, Endicott J, Robins E: **Research diagnostic criteria: rationale and reliability.** *Arch Gen Psychiatry* 1978, **35**:773-782.
13. Bech P, Gram LF, Reisby N, Rafaelsen OJ: **The WHO Depression Scale. Relationship to the Newcastle Scales.** *Acta Psychiatr Scand* 1980, **62**:140-153.
14. Roth M, Gurney C, Mountjoy CQ: **The Newcastle rating scales.** *Acta Psychiatr Scand Suppl* 1983, **310**:42-54.

15. Hamilton M: **A rating scale for depression.** *J Neurol Neurosurg Psychiatry* 1960, **23**:56-62.
16. Rush AJ, Weissenburger JE: **Melancholic symptom features and DSM-IV.** *Am J Psychiatry* 1994, **151**:489-498.
17. Dunner DL, Dwyer T, Fieve RR: **Depressive symptoms in patients with unipolar and bipolar affective disorder.** *Compr Psychiatry* 1976, **17**:447-451.
18. Parker G, Roy K, Wilhelm K, Mitchell P, Hadzi-Pavlovic D: **The nature of bipolar depression: implications for the definition of melancholia.** *Journal of Affective Disorders* 2000, **59**:217-224.
19. Mitchell PB, Wilhelm K, Parker G, Austin MP, Rutgers P, Malhi GS: **The clinical features of bipolar depression: a comparison with matched major depressive disorder patients.** *J Clin Psychiatry* 2001, **62**:212-216, quiz 217.
20. Potter WZ: **Bipolar depression: specific treatments.** *J Clin Psychiatry* 1998, **59(Suppl 18)**:30-36.
21. Goodwin FK, Jamison KR, Ghaemi SN: *Manic-depressive illness: Bipolar disorders and recurrent depression.* 2 edition. New York, N.Y.: Oxford University Press; 2007.
22. Nolen-Hoeksema S, Wisco BE, Lyubomirsky S: **Rethinking rumination.** *Perspectives on Psychological Science* 2008, **3**:400-424.
23. Nolen-Hoeksema S: **The role of rumination in depressive disorders and mixed anxiety/depressive symptoms.** *J Abnorm Psychol* 2000, **109**:504-511.
24. Lyubomirsky S, Tucker KL, Caldwell ND, Berg K: **Why ruminators are poor problem solvers: clues from the phenomenology of dysphoric rumination.** *J Pers Soc Psychol* 1999, **77**:1041-1060.
25. Morrow J, Nolen-Hoeksema S: **Effects of responses to depression on the remediation of depressive affect.** *J Pers Soc Psychol* 1990, **58**:519-527.
26. Nolen-Hoeksema S: **Responses to depression and their effects on the duration of depressive episodes.** *Journal of Abnormal Psychology* 1991, **100**:569-582.
27. Kuehner C, Weber I: **Responses to depression in unipolar depressed patients: an investigation of Nolen-Hoeksema's response styles theory.** *Psychol Med* 1999, **29**:1323-1333.
28. Papageorgiou C, Wells A: **Metacognitive beliefs about rumination in recurrent major depression.** *Cognitive and Behavioral Practice* 2001, **8**:160-164.
29. Watkins E, Baracaia S: **Why do people ruminate in dysphoric moods?** *Personality and Individual Differences* 2001, **30**:723-734.
30. Watkins E, Moulds M: **Positive beliefs about rumination in depression–a replication and extension.** *Personality and Individual Differences* 2005, **39**:73-82.
31. Nolen-Hoeksema S, Morrow J: **Effects of rumination and distraction on naturally occurring depressed mood.** *Cognition and Emotion* 1993, **7**:561-570.
32. Hollon SD, Kendall PC: **Cognitive self-statements in depression: Development of an automatic thoughts questionnaire.** *Cognitive Therapy and Research* 1980, **4**:383-395.
33. Weissman AN, Beck AT: **Development and validation of the Dysfunctional Attitude Scale.** *Paper presented at the Association for the Advancement of Behavior Therapy, Chicago* 1978.
34. Blackburn IM, Jones S, Lewin RJ: **Cognitive style in depression.** *Br J Clin Psychol* 1986, **25(Pt 4)**:241-251.
35. Crandell CJ, Chambless DL: **The validation of an inventory for measuring depressive thoughts: the Crandell Cognitions Inventory.** *Behav Res Ther* 1986, **24**:403-411.
36. Eaves G, Rush AJ: **Cognitive patterns in symptomatic and remitted unipolar major depression.** *J Abnorm Psychol* 1984, **93**:31-40.
37. Hollon SD, Kendall PC, Lumry A: **Specificity of Depressotypic Cognitions in Clinical Depression.** *Journal of Abnormal Psychology* 1986, **95**:52-59.
38. Dohr KB, Rush AJ, Bernstein IH: **Cognitive biases and depression.** *Journal of Abnormal Psychology* 1989, **98**:263-267.
39. Hamilton EW, Abramson LY: **Cognitive patterns and major depressive disorder: A longitudinal study in a hospital setting.** *Journal of Abnormal Psychology* 1983, **92**:173-184.
40. Reda MA, Carpiniello B, Secchiaroli L, Blanco S: **Thinking, depression, and antidepressants: Modified and unmodified depressive beliefs during treatment with amitriptyline.** *Cognitive Therapy and Research* 1985, **9**:135-143.
41. Olinger LJ, Kuiper NA, Shaw BF: **Dysfunctional attitudes and stressful life events: An interactive model of depression.** *Cognitive Therapy and Research* 1987, **11**:25-40.
42. Wise EH, Barnes DR: **The relationship among life events, dysfunctional attitudes, and depression.** *Cognitive Therapy and Research* 1986, **10**:257-266.
43. Jones L: **Cognitive style in bipolar disorder.** *The British Journal of Psychiatry* 2005, **187**:431-437.
44. Scott J, Pope M: **Cognitive styles in individuals with bipolar disorders.** *Psychological Medicine* 2003, **33**:1081-1088.
45. Reilly-Harrington NA, Alloy LB, Fresco DM, Whitehouse WG: **Cognitive styles and life events interact to predict bipolar and unipolar symptomatology.** *J Abnorm Psychol* 1999, **108**:567-578.
46. Alloy LB, Abramson LY, Whitehouse WG, Hogan ME, Tashman NA, Steinberg DL, Rose DT, Donovan P: **Depressogenic cognitive styles: predictive validity, information processing and personality characteristics, and developmental origins.** *Behav Res Ther* 1999, **37**:503-531.
47. Rosenberg M: *Society and the adolescent self-image* Princeton, N.J.,: Princeton University Press; 1965.
48. Goldberg JF, Gerstein RK, Wenze SJ, Welker TM, Beck AT: **Dysfunctional Attitudes and Cognitive Schemas in Bipolar Manic and Unipolar Depressed Outpatients.** *The Journal of Nervous and Mental Disease* 2008, **196**:207-210.
49. Lex C, Meyer TD, Marquart B, Thau K: **No strong evidence for abnormal levels of dysfunctional attitudes, automatic thoughts, and emotional information-processing biases in remitted bipolar I affective disorder.** *Psychology and Psychotherapy: Theory, Research and Practice* 2008, **81**:1-13.
50. Johnson S, McKenzie G, McMurrich S: **Ruminative Responses to Negative and Positive Affect Among Students Diagnosed with Bipolar Disorder and Major Depressive Disorder.** *Cognitive Therapy and Research* 2008, **32**:702-713.
51. Nolen-Hoeksema S, Morrow J: **A prospective study of depression and posttraumatic stress symptoms after a natural disaster: The 1989 Loma Prieta earthquake.** *Journal of Personality and Social Psychology* 1991, **61**:115-121.
52. Van der Gucht E, Morriss R, Lancaster G, Kinderman P, Bentall RP: **Psychological processes in bipolar affective disorder: negative cognitive style and reward processing.** *The British Journal of Psychiatry* 2009, **194**:146-151.
53. Deckersbach T, Hölzel BK, Eisner LR, Stange JP, Peckham AD, Dougherty DD, Rauch SL, Lazar S, Nierenberg AA: **Mindfulness-based Cognitive Therapy for Nonremitted Patients with Bipolar Disorder.** *CNS Neuroscience & Therapeutics* 2011.
54. Feldman GC, Joormann J, Johnson SL: **Responses to Positive Affect: A Self-Report Measure of Rumination and Dampening.** *Cognit Ther Res* 2008, **32**:507-525.
55. Thomas J, Bentall RP: **Hypomanic traits and response styles to depression.** *Br J Clin Psychol* 2002, **41**:309-313.
56. Knowles R, Tai S, Christensen I, Bentall R: **Coping with depression and vulnerability to mania: A factor analytic study of the Nolen-Hoeksema (1991) Response Styles Questionnaire.** *British Journal of Clinical Psychology* 2005, **44**:99-112.
57. Eckblad M, Chapman LJ: **Development and validation of a scale for hypomanic personality.** *J Abnorm Psychol* 1986, **95**:214-222.
58. Bech P, Rafaelsen OJ, Kramp P, Bolwig TG: **The mania rating scale: scale construction and inter-observer agreement.** *Neuropharmacology* 1978, **17**:430-431.
59. Johnson SL, Eisner LR, Carver CS: **Elevated expectancies among persons diagnosed with bipolar disorder.** *British Journal of Clinical Psychology* 2009, **48**:217-222.
60. Lam D: **Dysfunctional assumptions in bipolar disorder.** *Journal of Affective Disorders* 2004, **79**:193-199.
61. Mansell W, Colom F, Scott J: **The nature and treatment of depression in bipolar disorder: A review and implications for future psychological investigation.** *Clinical Psychology Review* 2005, **25**:1076-1100.
62. Eisner LR, Johnson SL, Carver CS: **Cognitive responses to failure and success relate uniquely to bipolar depression versus mania.** *Journal of Abnormal Psychology* 2008, **117**:154-163.
63. Martinez-Aran A, Vieta E, Colom F, Reinares M, Benabarre A, Gasto C, Salamero M: **Cognitive dysfunctions in bipolar disorder: evidence of neuropsychological disturbances.** *Psychother Psychosom* 2000, **69**:2-18.

64. Bearden CE, Hoffman KM, Cannon TD: **The neuropsychology and neuroanatomy of bipolar affective disorder: a critical review.** *Bipolar Disord* 2001, **3**:106-150, discussion 151-103.
65. Quraishi S, Frangou S: **Neuropsychology of bipolar disorder: a review.** *J Affect Disord* 2002, **72**:209-226.
66. Martinez-Aran A, Vieta E, Reinares M, Colom F, Torrent C, Sanchez-Moreno J, Benabarre A, Goikolea JM, Comes M, Salamero M: **Cognitive function across manic or hypomanic, depressed, and euthymic states in bipolar disorder.** *Am J Psychiatry* 2004, **161**:262-270.
67. Olley AL, Malhi GS, Bachelor J, Cahill CM, Mitchell PB, Berk M: **Executive functioning and theory of mind in euthymic bipolar disorder.** *Bipolar Disord* 2005, **7(Suppl 5)**:43-52.
68. Morice R: **Cognitive inflexibility and pre-frontal dysfunction in schizophrenia and mania.** *British Journal of Psychiatry* 1990, **157**:50-54.
69. Clark L, Iversen SD, Goodwin GM: **A neuropsychological investigation of prefrontal cortex involvement in acute mania.** *The American Journal of Psychiatry* 2001, **158**:1605-1611.
70. Murphy FC: **Neuropsychology of bipolar disorder.** *The British Journal of Psychiatry* 2001, **178**:120s-127.
71. Gotlib IH, Joormann J: **Cognition and depression: current status and future directions.** *Annu Rev Clin Psychol* 2010, **6**:285-312.
72. Miyake A, Friedman NP, Emerson MJ, Witzki AH, Howerter A, Wager TD: **The unity and diversity of executive functions and their contributions to complex "Frontal Lobe" tasks: a latent variable analysis.** *Cogn Psychol* 2000, **41**:49-100.
73. Davis RN, Nolen-Hoeksema S: **Cognitive Inflexibility Among Ruminators and Nonruminators.** *Cognitive Therapy and Research* 2000, **24**:699-711.
74. Watkins E, Brown RG: **Rumination and executive function in depression: An experimental study.** *Journal of Neurology, Neurosurgery & Psychiatry* 2002, **72**:400-402.
75. Whitmer AJ, Banich MT: **Inhibition versus switching deficits in different forms of rumination.** *Psychol Sci* 2007, **18**:546-553.
76. Hoge EA, Friedman L, Schulz SC: **Meta-analysis of brain size in bipolar disorder.** *Schizophr Res* 1999, **37**:177-181.
77. Strakowski SM, DelBello MP, Adler C, Cecil DM, Sax KW: **Neuroimaging in bipolar disorder.** *Bipolar Disord* 2000, **2**:148-164.
78. Strakowski SM, Adler CM, DelBello MP: **Volumetric MRI studies of mood disorders: do they distinguish unipolar and bipolar disorder?** *Bipolar Disord* 2002, **4**:80-88.
79. Swayze VW, Andreasen NC, Alliger RJ, Yuh WT, Ehrhardt JC: **Subcortical and temporal structures in affective disorder and schizophrenia: a magnetic resonance imaging study.** *Biol Psychiatry* 1992, **31**:221-240.
80. Sax KW, Strakowski SM, Zimmerman ME, DelBello MP, Keck PE Jr, Hawkins JM: **Frontosubcortical neuroanatomy and the continuous performance test in mania.** *Am J Psychiatry* 1999, **156**:139-141.
81. Lopez-Larson MP, DelBello MP, Zimmerman ME, Schwiers ML, Strakowski SM: **Regional prefrontal gray and white matter abnormalities in bipolar disorder.** *Biol Psychiatry* 2002, **52**:93-100.
82. Lochhead RA, Parsey RV, Oquendo MA, Mann JJ: **Regional brain gray matter volume differences in patients with bipolar disorder as assessed by optimized voxel-based morphometry.** *Biol Psychiatry* 2004, **55**:1154-1162.
83. Rimol LM, Hartberg CB, Nesvag R, Fennema-Notestine C, Hagler DJ Jr, Pung CJ, Jennings RG, Haukvik UK, Lange E, Nakstad PH, *et al*: **Cortical thickness and subcortical volumes in schizophrenia and bipolar disorder.** *Biol Psychiatry* 2010, **68**:41-50.
84. Pearlson GD, Barta PE, Powers RE, Menon RR, Richards SS, Aylward EH, Federman EB, Chase GA, Petty RG, Tien AY: **Ziskind-Somerfeld Research Award 1996. Medial and superior temporal gyral volumes and cerebral asymmetry in schizophrenia versus bipolar disorder.** *Biol Psychiatry* 1997, **41**:1-14.
85. Strakowski SM, DelBello MP, Sax KW, Zimmerman ME, Shear PK, Hawkins JM, Larson ER: **Brain magnetic resonance imaging of structural abnormalities in bipolar disorder.** *Arch Gen Psychiatry* 1999, **56**:254-260.
86. Altshuler LL, Bartzokis G, Grieder T, Curran J, Jimenez T, Leight K, Wilkins J, Gerner R, Mintz J: **An MRI study of temporal lobe structures in men with bipolar disorder or schizophrenia.** *Biol Psychiatry* 2000, **48**:147-162.
87. Brambilla P, Harenski K, Nicoletti M, Sassi RB, Mallinger AG, Frank E, Kupfer DJ, Keshavan MS, Soares JC: **MRI investigation of temporal lobe structures in bipolar patients.** *J Psychiatr Res* 2003, **37**:287-295.
88. Kempton MJ, Geddes JR, Ettinger U, Williams SC, Grasby PM: **Meta-analysis, database, and meta-regression of 98 structural imaging studies in bipolar disorder.** *Arch Gen Psychiatry* 2008, **65**:1017-1032.
89. McDonald C, Zanelli J, Rabe-Hesketh S, Ellison-Wright I, Sham P, Kalidindi S, Murray RM, Kennedy N: **Meta-analysis of magnetic resonance imaging brain morphometry studies in bipolar disorder.** *Biol Psychiatry* 2004, **56**:411-417.
90. Bora E, Fornito A, Yucel M, Pantelis C: **Voxelwise meta-analysis of gray matter abnormalities in bipolar disorder.** *Biol Psychiatry* 2010, **67**:1097-1105.
91. Ellison-Wright I, Bullmore E: **Anatomy of bipolar disorder and schizophrenia: a meta-analysis.** *Schizophr Res* 2010, **117**:1-12.
92. Buchsbaum MS, DeLisi LE, Holcomb HH, Cappelletti J, King AC, Johnson J, Hazlett E, Dowling-Zimmerman S, Post RM, Morihisa J, *et al*: **Anteroposterior gradients in cerebral glucose use in schizophrenia and affective disorders.** *Arch Gen Psychiatry* 1984, **41**:1159-1166.
93. Baxter LR Jr, Phelps ME, Mazziotta JC, Schwartz JM, Gerner RH, Selin CE, Sumida RM: **Cerebral metabolic rates for glucose in mood disorders. Studies with positron emission tomography and fluorodeoxyglucose F 18.** *Arch Gen Psychiatry* 1985, **42**:441-447.
94. Buchsbaum MS: **Brain imaging in the search for biological markers in affective disorder.** *J Clin Psychiatry* 1986, **47(Suppl)**:7-12.
95. Buchsbaum MS, Wu J, DeLisi LE, Holcomb H, Kessler R, Johnson J, King AC, Hazlett E, Langston K, Post RM: **Frontal cortex and basal ganglia metabolic rates assessed by positron emission tomography with [18F]2-deoxyglucose in affective illness.** *J Affect Disord* 1986, **10**:137-152.
96. Baxter LR Jr, Schwartz JM, Phelps ME, Mazziotta JC, Guze BH, Selin CE, Gerner RH, Sumida RM: **Reduction of prefrontal cortex glucose metabolism common to three types of depression.** *Arch Gen Psychiatry* 1989, **46**:243-250.
97. Drevets WC, Price JL, Simpson JR Jr, Todd RD, Reich T, Vannier M, Raichle ME: **Subgenual prefrontal cortex abnormalities in mood disorders.** *Nature* 1997, **386**:824-827.
98. Yurgelun-Todd DA, Gruber SA, Kanayama G, Killgore WD, Baird AA, Young AD: **fMRI during affect discrimination in bipolar affective disorder.** *Bipolar Disord* 2000, **2**:237-248.
99. Deckersbach T, Dougherty D, Savage C, McMurrich S, Fischman A, Nierenberg A, Sachs G, Rauch S: **Impaired Recruitment of the Dorsolateral Prefrontal Cortex and Hippocampus During Encoding in Bipolar Disorder.** *Biological Psychiatry* 2006, **59**:138-146.
100. Malhi GS, Lagopoulos J, Sachdev PS, Ivanovski B, Shnier R: **An emotional Stroop functional MRI study of euthymic bipolar disorder.** *Bipolar Disorders* 2005, **7**:58-69.
101. Blumberg HP, Leung HC, Skudlarski P, Lacadie CM, Fredericks CA, Harris BC, Charney DS, Gore JC, Krystal JH, Peterson BS: **A functional magnetic resonance imaging study of bipolar disorder: state- and trait-related dysfunction in ventral prefrontal cortices.** *Arch Gen Psychiatry* 2003, **60**:601-609.
102. Ketter TA, Kimbrell TA, George MS, Dunn RT, Speer AM, Benson BE, Willis MW, Danielson A, Frye MA, Herscovitch P, Post RM: **Effects of mood and subtype on cerebral glucose metabolism in treatment-resistant bipolar disorder.** *Biological Psychiatry* 2001, **49**:97-109.
103. Altshuler L, Bookheimer S, Townsend J, Proenza M, Eisenberger N, Sabb F, Mintz J, Cohen M: **Blunted Activation in Orbitofrontal Cortex During Mania: A Functional Magnetic Resonance Imaging Study.** *Biological Psychiatry* 2005, **58**:763-769.
104. Chen CH, Suckling J, Lennox BR, Ooi C, Bullmore ET: **A quantitative meta-analysis of fMRI studies in bipolar disorder.** *Bipolar Disord* 2011, **13**:1-15.
105. Phillips ML, Ladouceur CD, Drevets WC: **A neural model of voluntary and automatic emotion regulation: implications for understanding the pathophysiology and neurodevelopment of bipolar disorder.** *Molecular Psychiatry* 2008, **13**:833-857.
106. Siegle GJ, Steinhauer SR, Thase ME, Stenger VA, Carter CS: **Can't shake that feeling: event-related fMRI assessment of sustained amygdala activity in response to emotional information in depressed individuals.** *Biol Psychiatry* 2002, **51**:693-707.
107. Ray RD, Ochsner KN, Cooper JC, Robertson ER, Gabrieli JD, Gross JJ: **Individual differences in trait rumination and the neural systems supporting cognitive reappraisal.** *Cogn Affect Behav Neurosci* 2005, **5**:156-168.

108. Cooney RE, Joormann J, Eugène F, Dennis EL, Gotlib IH: **Neural correlates of rumination in depression.** *Cognitive, Affective, & Behavioral Neuroscience* 2010, **10**:470-478.
109. Hamilton JP, Furman DJ, Chang C, Thomason ME, Dennis E, Gotlib IH: **Default-mode and task-positive network activity in major depressive disorder: implications for adaptive and maladaptive rumination.** *Biol Psychiatry* 2011, **70**:327-333.
110. Johnson S, Tran T: **Bipolar disorder: What can psychotherapists learn from the cognitive research?** *Journal of Clinical Psychology* 2007, **63**:425-432.
111. Johnson SL, McKenzie G, McMurrich S: **Ruminative Responses to Negative and Positive Affect Among Students Diagnosed with Bipolar Disorder and Major Depressive Disorder.** *Cognitive Therapy and Research* 2007, **32**:702-713.

17

Botulinum toxin-induced facial muscle paralysis affects amygdala responses to the perception of emotional expressions: preliminary findings from an A-B-A design

M Justin Kim[1], Maital Neta[2], F Caroline Davis[3,4], Erika J Ruberry[5], Diana Dinescu[6], Todd F Heatherton[1], Mitchell A Stotland[7,8] and Paul J Whalen[1*]

Abstract

Background: It has long been suggested that feedback signals from facial muscles influence emotional experience. The recent surge in use of botulinum toxin (BTX) to induce temporary muscle paralysis offers a unique opportunity to directly test this "facial feedback hypothesis." Previous research shows that the lack of facial muscle feedback due to BTX-induced paralysis influences subjective reports of emotional experience, as well as brain activity associated with the imitation of emotional facial expressions. However, it remains to be seen whether facial muscle paralysis affects brain activity, especially the amygdala, which is known to be responsive to the perception of emotion in others. Further, it is unknown whether these neural changes are permanent or whether they revert to their original state after the effects of BTX have subsided. The present study sought to address these questions by using functional magnetic resonance imaging to measure neural responses to angry and happy facial expressions in the presence or absence of facial paralysis.

Results: Consistent with previous research, amygdala activity was greater in response to angry compared to happy faces before BTX treatment. As predicted, amygdala activity in response to angry faces was attenuated when the corrugator/procerus muscles were paralyzed via BTX injection but then returned to its original state after the effects of BTX subsided. This preliminary study comprises a small sample size and no placebo condition; however, the A-B-A design affords the present sample to serve as its own control.

Conclusions: The current demonstration that amygdala responses to facial expressions were influenced by facial muscle paralysis offers direct neural support for the facial feedback hypothesis. Specifically, the present findings offer preliminary causal evidence that amygdala activity is sensitive to facial feedback during the perception of the facial expressions of others. More broadly, these data confirm the utility of using BTX to address the effect of facial feedback on neural responses associated with the *perception*, in addition to the experience or expression of emotion.

Keywords: Amygdala, Botulinum toxin, Corrugator supercilii, Facial feedback hypothesis

* Correspondence: paul.j.whalen@dartmouth.edu
[1]Department of Psychological and Brain Sciences, Dartmouth College, 6207 Moore Hall, Hanover, NH 03755, USA
Full list of author information is available at the end of the article

Background

It has long been suggested that feedback signals from facial muscle activity associated with forming facial expressions are critical to emotional experience [1,2]. This notion has developed into what we now know as the facial feedback hypothesis [3]. According to this hypothesis, our brain receives afferent feedback signals from facial muscles that significantly influence how we process and experience emotion [4]. Importantly, a number of psychological experiments have shown support for the facial feedback hypothesis [5-9].

In a classic demonstration by Strack and colleagues, participants judged the funniness of cartoons while unknowingly contracting their zygomaticus (the facial muscle used during smiling) by holding a pen in their mouths [9]. This subtle manipulation influenced their perception of the cartoons; such that they found the cartoons to be funnier when contracting the zygomaticus muscles compared to a control condition where the zygomaticus muscles were not contracted. This study offered clear behavioral evidence that feedback signals from the facial muscles influence our emotional experiences.

Seminal studies such as this would be strengthened by additional work seeking to establish a direct causal relationship between facial feedback and emotional phenomena. Though Strack and colleagues convincingly employed methods that protected against demand characteristics (i.e., participants ostensibly were not aware of the fact that they were being asked to smile) [9], there are additional considerations when asking participants to actively alter their facial muscle contractions. Specifically, intentional alteration of facial muscle activity calls for novel efferent signals to be sent to the facial muscles, which might influence how we experience emotion independent of any change in the afferent facial feedback signals to the brain. To put it another way, this method does not allow us to distinguish between whether the observed outcomes are due to a change in brain activity that is responsible for producing the emotional facial expression (efferent) or a change in facial feedback signals to the brain (afferent) [10,11]. Thus, it would be ideal to leave the efferent brain signals intact while selectively shutting down the afferent facial muscle signals.

Recent widespread cosmetic use of botulinum toxin (BTX) type-A has allowed researchers to perform exactly this separation of afferent and efferent signals, making it possible to directly test causal factors related to facial feedback. BTX induces a temporary paralysis of the muscles at the injection site by inhibiting the release of the neurotransmitter acetylcholine at the muscle nerves [12]. By injecting BTX into the muscles that we use to make emotional facial expressions, a "reversible lesion" of target facial muscles can be temporarily created. This effectively "severs" afferent feedback signals from these muscles while leaving the efferent signals intact, thus allowing us to study emotional experience and processing devoid of facial muscle feedback.

The corrugator supercilii—an important component of the glabellar muscles (the "frown muscles" between the eyebrows) along with the procerus [13]—has been implicated in the experience and processing of negative emotions. One prototypical feature of an angry facial expression is that the medial portions of the eyebrows are pulled down using the corrugator supercilii muscles [14]. Using facial electromyography (EMG), researchers have shown that corrugator activity is selectively potentiated when viewing photos of angry facial expressions [15-17]. A similar pattern of corrugator activity is found in response to negative affective pictures [18-20] and sounds [20].

Based on this established link between corrugator activity and negative emotion, a number of recent studies have used BTX to directly test the facial feedback hypothesis and found that feedback from facial muscles influenced subjective experience of emotion and emotional language processing [10,21]. Other studies suggest that BTX injections mitigate depression symptoms and help elevate mood in major depressive disorder patients [22,23]. Functional neuroimaging studies are also beginning to explore the relationship between facial feedback and responses to emotional stimuli. The first such study assessed the effect of BTX on the ability to imitate emotional expressions [24]. Amygdala activity, and its coupling with brain stem activity, was diminished when the corrugator muscle was paralyzed with BTX as participants attempted to imitate angry facial expressions. Taken together, these data suggest that our emotional experiences as well as brain activity to emotional stimuli can be influenced by feedback signals from the facial muscles.

The present study sought to determine whether the activity of the amygdala—a brain region within the medial temporal lobe that is known to be sensitive to facial expressions of emotion, including anger [25]—in response to angry facial expressions could be manipulated by BTX-induced glabellar (i.e., corrugator/procerus) muscle paralysis. Critically, when the effect of BTX injection subsides, would amygdala activity in response to angry facial expressions be restored? If so, this would provide strong evidence in favor of the facial feedback hypothesis and shed further light on its underlying neural mechanism. To this end, we used functional magnetic resonance imaging (fMRI) in an A-B-A design to assess neural responses to facial expressions a total of three times: prior to BTX treatment, shortly after BTX treatment (i.e., during corrugator/procerus paralysis), and after the effects of BTX had subsided. We hypothesized that amygdala activity would be greater to angry compared to happy facial expressions prior to BTX administration, that these signal increases to angry expressions would be mitigated by BTX, and that they would return to their pre-injection state (i.e., relatively enhanced amygdala responses to angry vs. happy faces) after BTX had subsided.

Methods

Participants

Initially, ten female volunteers were recruited through the Department of Plastic Surgery at Dartmouth Hitchcock Medical Center. Our study sample was limited to women for two reasons. First, reliable dosing is best obtained in females, as men have a larger glabellar muscle mass and require variable dosing. Second, the vast majority of BTX patients are women—for example, in 2013, women received 94% of 6.3 million BTX treatments in the United States [26]. Thus, we chose to focus on a female study sample. Of the ten volunteers, three did not return for at least one of the subsequent sessions, and thus, data reported here are from seven volunteers between the ages of 35–44 (mean age 40.43 ± 3.69 years). All participants had corrected-to-normal vision and were right handed. The current study was approved by the Committee for the Protection of Human Subjects at Dartmouth College, and written informed consent was obtained from each subject prior to the experiment.

BTX injection

None of the participants had received BTX treatments prior to the current study. All participants were injected with botulinum toxin type-A a total of five times during a single visit; twice in the corrugator supercilii on each side and once in the procerus (a vertically oriented, midline muscle which pulls the medial ends of the eyebrows downward). The BTX was diluted as 100 units botulinum toxin/2 ccs non-preserved injectable saline. The volume per injection was 0.1 cc/5 units, for a total dose of 25 units. All participants received the injection 2–5 weeks after the first experimental session and then returned to the lab 3–6 weeks after the first session for a second experimental session. Finally, participants were instructed to return at least 9 months after the injection, a time known to be sufficient for the effect of BTX to dissipate [13,27]. Our participants returned for their third session an average of 54 (range 37–63) weeks after their initial BTX injection.

Experimental paradigm

Participants were asked to participate in an fMRI scanning session at each of the three time points. During fMRI, each subject viewed a series of angry, happy, and surprised facial expressions consisting of 18 identities (9 males and 9 females), which were selected from a standardized set (NimStim) [28]. The order of presentation of all faces was randomized for each run. All of the stimuli were back-projected (Panasonic PT-D4000U DLP) onto the center of a screen, which the participants viewed using a mirror that was mounted on the head coil.

During each trial, photos of faces with angry, happy, and surprised expressions were presented for 17, 50, and 1,000 ms, followed by a black-and-white pattern that was presented for 250 ms, which served as a retinal wipe. The length of intertrial intervals was jittered between 750 and 6,750 ms (average = 3,750 ms). Each run consisted of 54 trials (18 trials for each emotion type, presented in a pseudorandom order) lasting 4.5 total minutes, and the participants underwent three runs per scanning session. During each trial, participants were asked to report using a button box whether they thought each of the faces they saw was positive or negative in emotional valence (i.e., two-alternative forced choice paradigm). We note that all trials (correct and error in ratings) were included in the subsequent fMRI analysis independent of their responses. For our purposes here, we have collapsed the data across stimulus presentation durations because our main focus was to elicit amygdala activity to angry and happy faces, regardless of the differences in duration. Surprised faces and variable stimulus durations were included as a part of a larger study, and our goal was to have the participants work on the same tasks as our previous investigation of surprise [17]. Here, we report our preliminary findings on the effects of BTX injections into the corrugator muscle on amygdala responses to angry and happy expressions.

Image acquisition

All participants were scanned at the Dartmouth Brain Imaging Center, using a 3.0 Tesla Philips Intera Achieva Scanner (Philips Medical Systems, Bothell, WA) equipped with a SENSE birdcage head coil. Following our standard imaging protocol that is known to maximize signal to noise ratio in the amygdala in our scanner, functional images were acquired using echo-planar T2*-weighted imaging sequence. Each volume consisted of 36 interleaved 3-mm-thick axial slices with 0.5-mm interslice gap (echo time [TE] = 35 ms, repetition time [TR] = 2,000 ms, field of view [FOV] = 240 mm, flip angle = 90°, voxel size = 3 × 3 × 3.5 mm). Anatomical T1-weighted images were collected using a high-resolution 3D magnetization-prepared rapid gradient echo sequence, with 160 contiguous 1-mm-thick sagittal slices (TE = 4.6 ms, TR =9.8 ms, FOV = 240 mm, flip angle = 8°, voxel size = 1 × 0.94 × 0.94 mm).

fMRI data analysis

All fMRI images were processed using Statistical Parametric Mapping software (SPM5, Wellcome Department of Imaging Neuroscience, London, UK). First, functional blood-oxygen-level dependent (BOLD) data were preprocessed using slice-time correction. Then, data were preprocessed to accommodate each subject's head movement for all six directions. We note here that none of the participants showed head movement exceeding 2.5 mm or 2.5 degrees in any direction. Spatial normalization of the functional images was performed by warping our data to fit into standard space, using the Montreal Neurological Institute (MNI)-152 template. In our final preprocessing step, normalized functional images were smoothed using a Gaussian kernel of 6-mm full width at half maximum.

At each voxel, the parameter estimates of event-related activity were fit to a general linear model. Three types of events were entered in the model—angry, happy, and surprised faces. Covariates of no interest (a session mean, a linear trend for each run, and six motion parameters derived from realignment corrections) were also accounted for in the general linear model. For the purposes of the current study, we used angry and happy faces in further analysis of variance (ANOVA) investigations. Surprised faces were also included in the experimental design for another experimental hypothesis. Since surprised faces have ambiguous valence (i.e., they can be interpreted as having either positive or negative valence), understanding of these data will require further data collection in a greater number of participants. Here, we present a 3 (Session: pre-BTX, BTX, post-BTX) × 2 (Emotion: angry, happy) voxelwise ANOVA model of the data for the negative (angry) and positive (happy) expressions, since even seven participants can offer consensus on the valence of these expressions. To accommodate the 3 × 2 design (Session × Emotion), a voxelwise ANOVA model was constructed for each subject, using linear contrasts (angry vs. baseline, happy vs. baseline) generated for the three time points (pre-BTX, BTX, and post-BTX). An implicit baseline was derived from all unmodeled events in SPM—that is, all events other than angry, happy, and surprised faces. They were subsequently entered into a random effects model, which allows population-based inferences to be made from our data [29]. Given our specific hypothesis that amygdala activity would follow an A-B-A pattern in response to angry vs. happy faces, we searched for voxels that tracked this pattern by entering a quadratic contrast vector in our ANOVA model.

Since our aim was to investigate the impact of BTX on amygdala activity specifically, we selected a significance threshold of $p < 0.05$ corrected for multiple comparisons over the amygdala volume (~4,500 mm^3), which was defined using the Automated Anatomical Labeling atlas [30]. The significance threshold was calculated through Monte Carlo simulations, using the AlphaSim tool included with the AFNI software [31]. For all other brain regions about which we did not have *a priori* hypotheses, we imposed a statistical threshold of $p < 0.001$ (uncorrected for multiple comparisons, k = 10 voxels) for exploratory purposes.

Results

Behavioral data

A Session (pre-BTX, BTX, post-BTX) × Emotion (angry, happy) ANOVA revealed a significant main effect of Emotion ($F_{(1,6)}$ = 496.73, p <0.001; Figure 1). As expected, post hoc pairwise comparisons revealed that across all three time points, angry faces were consistently rated more negatively than happy faces (all p's < 0.001, Bonferroni corrected). We note here that accuracy was calculated by combining 50 and 1,000 ms data. Behavioral data from 17 ms were not included because past research has shown that accuracy ratings from 17 ms were not significantly different from chance [17]. Angry faces were rated as negative on 86.5% of the trials, and happy faces were rated as positive on 85.7% of the trials. The main effect of Session and the Session × Emotion interaction were not significant (all p's > 0.05).

fMRI data

Voxelwise ANOVA results showed a significant Session × Emotion interaction characterized by a quadratic pattern of activity in the right amygdala (MNI 21, 3, −24; $t_{(36)}$ = 3.28, p <0.05 corrected, cluster size = 432 mm^3) in response to angry vs. happy faces (Figure 2). Specifically, this quadratic pattern was characterized by significantly increased right amygdala activity to angry vs. happy faces in pre-BTX (p = 0.03, one-tailed) and post-BTX (p = 0.04, one-tailed) conditions but no significant activity in the BTX condition. No significant main effects of Session or Emotion, as well as linear interaction effects were observed in the amygdala. No other brain regions showed this quadratic pattern of activity in response to angry vs. happy faces at the pre-determined statistical threshold.

In an attempt to examine the possibility that the observed quadratic effect was driven by amygdala activity to angry faces or happy faces compared to baseline, we further probed the right amygdala voxel cluster defined by the voxelwise ANOVA (see Figure 2A) and analyzed angry vs. baseline and happy vs. baseline separately. An ANOVA with a planned quadratic contrast revealed that right amygdala activity to angry vs. baseline ($F_{(1,6)}$ = 6.08, p = 0.049) and happy vs. baseline ($F_{(1,6)}$ =10.9, p = 0.016) had significant quadratic effects across sessions, showing that the aforementioned voxelwise ANOVA results were not driven by angry faces or happy faces alone (Figure 2). In fact, the quadratic pattern of amygdala activity to angry faces had a U-shaped curve, which matched the pattern observed in response to angry vs. happy faces, whereas amygdala activity to happy faces demonstrated an inverted U-shaped curve. There were no significant linear effects across sessions for either angry vs. baseline or happy vs. baseline comparisons (all p's > 0.05).

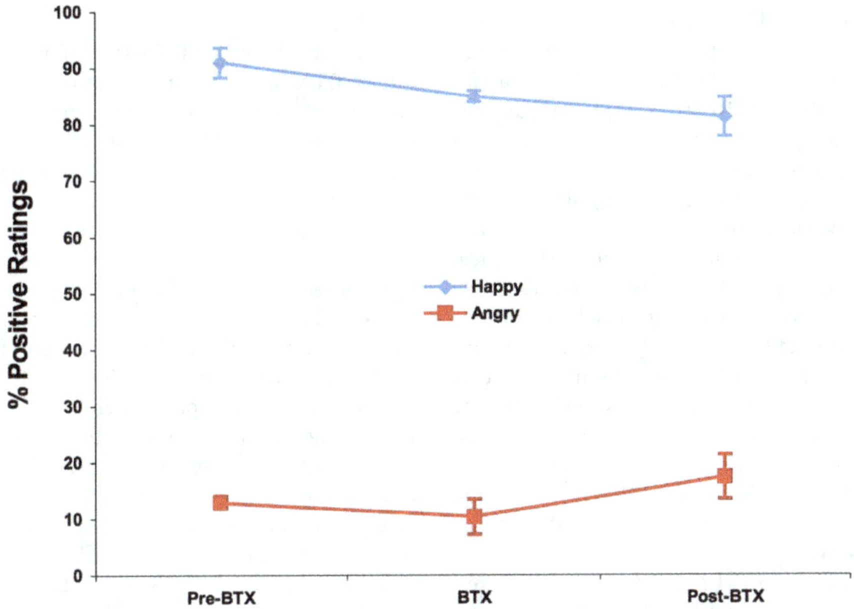

Figure 1 Behavioral performance. Behavioral data showing that angry faces are consistently rated as negative (86.5%), and happy faces are consistently rated as positive (85.7%), regardless of BTX injection. *Error bars* indicate standard error of the mean, which was computed by removing between subject-variability to account for the within-subject design [32].

Discussion

The aim of the current study was to investigate the effects of BTX-induced corrugator/procerus paralysis on amygdala activity to angry faces by adapting an A-B-A experimental design, a powerful method that allowed us to determine the neural consequence of BTX treatment. Consistent with our hypothesis, we observed diminished amygdala activity to angry vs. happy faces when the facial muscles used to produce angry facial expressions were paralyzed. Importantly, amygdala activity was restored to its pre-BTX injection state after the effects of BTX subsided. In other words, amygdala activity in response to angry vs. happy faces was modulated in parallel with the activity state of the corrugator supercilii and the procerus. When the corrugator and procerus muscles were unaffected by BTX, greater amygdala activity to angry vs. happy faces was observed. However, when the corrugator and procerus muscles were paralyzed via BTX injection, amygdala activity in response to angry vs. happy faces was attenuated. Our finding implies that feedback signals from the corrugator supercilii and the procerus to the brain are modulating amygdala activity.

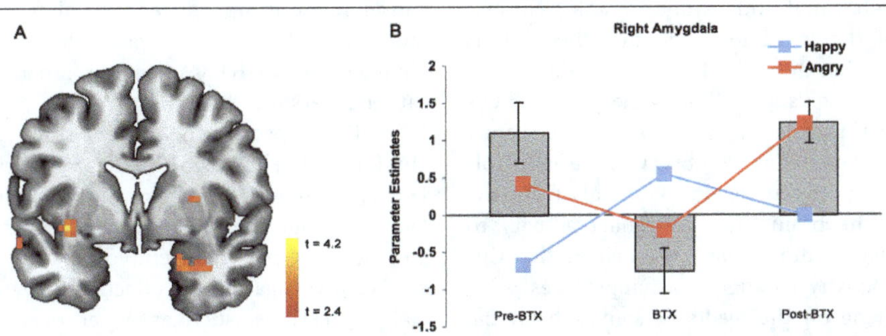

Figure 2 Right amygdala activity tracks BTX-induced corrugator/procerus paralysis. (A) Statistical map (coronal plane, $Y = 3$, $p < 0.01$, $k = 7$ voxels) depicting the right amygdala (MNI 21, 3, −24; $t_{(36)} = 3.28$, $p < 0.05$ corrected, cluster size = 432 mm^3) that corresponded to the effects of BTX. **(B)** Bar graph showing right amygdala activity to angry vs. happy faces, showing a distinctive quadratic pattern of activity (parameter estimates for angry vs. happy faces were calculated by subtracting happy vs. baseline from angry vs. baseline). *Red lines* indicate right amygdala activity to angry faces vs. baseline, and *blue lines* indicate right amygdala activity to happy faces. *Error bars* indicate standard error of the mean.

According to the facial feedback hypothesis, our emotional experience is modulated by feedback signals from the facial muscles that we use to create expressions, and this argument is supported, at least in part, by a number of psychological studies [6,8-10,21]. Temporary paralysis of facial muscles using BTX essentially cuts off all afferent feedback signals from the injection site while leaving the efferent signals untouched [12], providing researchers with an ideal setup to directly test the facial feedback hypothesis. Behavioral and psychophysiological studies utilizing these unique properties of BTX have also partially supported the facial feedback hypothesis [10,21]. Here, we use the term "partially" because the reports from the existing literature make it quite clear that not all of our emotional experience can be accounted for by afferent facial feedback signals [6,9,10,33]. At the same time, however, these studies do show evidence supporting the facial feedback hypothesis; that at least some of our emotional experience is influenced by afferent signals from facial muscles.

Our data add further support to the facial feedback hypothesis by offering direct neural evidence. We chose to focus on the amygdala, which is known to be responsive to biologically relevant and socially salient stimuli, including facial expressions [34]. We specifically selected angry faces to probe the amygdala, since the BTX treatment in our study targeted the corrugator supercilii and the procerus – the glabellar muscles that we use when we frown and make angry faces. Prior to BTX treatment, our participants demonstrated greater amygdala activity to angry faces compared to happy faces. Similar activity of the amygdala was observed when effects of BTX wore off at least 9 months after its injection to the corrugator supercilii and the procerus. It was only during the period when BTX was active and the corrugator and procerus muscles were paralyzed that we did not see greater amygdala activity to angry vs. happy faces. This quadratic pattern of amygdala activity is consistent with the aforementioned behavioral and psychophysiological evidence in favor of the facial feedback hypothesis. It is clear from the data that the lack of afferent feedback signals from the corrugator supercilii and the procerus has impacted how the amygdala responds to angry vs. happy faces. The causal relationship we observe here is as follows: if there are no afferent feedback signals from the facial muscles to the brain, then amygdala activity to angry vs. happy faces is diminished. We believe that this means amygdala activity to angry vs. happy faces is, at least partially, relying on the feedback signals from the corrugator supercilii and the procerus. This implies that when we see an angry face, we detect and experience negatively valenced emotion by contracting and flexing the relevant muscles—the corrugator supercilii being the most prominent one in this case—and our amygdala uses these afferent signals to properly process the information.

Our data showing diminished activity of the amygdala due to BTX-induced paralysis of the corrugator/procerus are consistent with the findings reported by Hennenlotter and colleagues [24]. In their fMRI investigation, they also observed attenuated amygdala activity to angry faces when the participants were treated with BTX and had their corrugator paralyzed, compared to their placebo-injected controls [24]. There were slight differences as well—for instance, they found BTX-induced attenuation of amygdala activity only when the participants were asked to imitate the facial expressions that were shown on the screen, as opposed to just viewing them passively. In our study, participants were not explicitly asked to imitate the facial expressions they were viewing on the screen, but we observed diminished amygdala activity nonetheless. This discrepancy could stem from many factors, among which include differences in the experimental paradigm that was used to probe the amygdala. Since we did not explicitly instruct the participants to either imitate or not imitate the facial expressions, they might have been less aware of their facial muscular movements and thus less resistant to spontaneous elicitations of their own facial expressions when viewing other people's faces. This may have also influenced the difference in the observed laterality of the amygdala—that is, whereas Hennenlotter and colleagues report that BTX affected the left amygdala [24], we found the right amygdala to be modulated by BTX-induced paralysis of the corrugator supercilii. Despite these relatively minor differences, we believe our data are in the same vein as the findings by Hennenlotter and colleagues, in the sense that both provide neural evidence supporting the facial feedback hypothesis [24]. Furthermore, an important contribution of the current study is the addition of a third post-BTX condition. As the last 'A' in the A-B-A design, this third condition allows us to directly test a causal relationship between facial feedback signals and amygdala activity and suggests that amygdala activation changes due to BTX injections are not permanent but rather reversible.

Another aspect of the current study that warrants discussion is the inclusion of happy faces in the analysis. Happy faces were used as a direct comparison to angry faces to gauge the level of amygdala activity—a common strategy that has been employed in a number of fMRI studies investigating the effects of negatively valenced facial expressions, such as anger or fear [35-37]. Upon closer examination of the data, our observations revealed that amygdala activity to happy faces actually showed an opposite quadratic pattern compared to angry faces. By subtracting amygdala activity to happy faces from angry faces and thus calculating amygdala activity to angry vs.

happy faces, the U-shaped quadratic pattern became more prominent in our data. This inverted U-shaped pattern of activity to happy faces emerges as a topic of future inquiry, as BTX only had an effect on the corrugator supercilii and the procerus, not the zygomaticus major—the facial muscle we use to smile—but nevertheless had an impact on amygdala activity.

BTX-induced corrugator/procerus paralysis did not alter the participants' perception of the valence of angry or happy faces. Regardless of BTX treatment, angry faces were consistently rated as being negatively valenced, and happy faces were consistently rated as being positively valenced. This was expected, as judging such clearly valenced facial expressions would not necessarily require feedback signals from the corrugator, given that the participants have prior experience and knowledge of the meaning of angry and happy faces. It is important to note that these behavioral data do not imply that afferent signals from the corrugator/procerus are not being used during processing of emotional facial expressions. Rather, these results hint at our ability to utilize multiple sources of information when making decisions on a given clearly valenced face, such that the lack of corrugator feedback signal is compensated by other factors including past experience and learned responses. Taking into account the EMG findings that show increased corrugator activity to angry facial expressions [15-17], negative pictures [18-20] and sounds [20], as well as other BTX-induced corrugator paralysis studies demonstrating behavioral effects such as impaired negative emotional language processing (i.e., significantly delayed reading times for sentences describing angry and sad situations) [21] and diminished subjective emotional experience in response to mildly positive video clips [10], it is clear that the feedback signals from the corrugator impact our emotional experiences, and it is beneficial to interpret our data within this context.

Limitations of the current study include the relatively small sample size. While within subject repeated measures (i.e., A-B-A design) mitigates this limitation to an extent, having a larger sample size, as well as a control group that is also cosmetically treated but without paralysis (see [10]) would strengthen the study. In addition, the present results might generalize only to females who would voluntarily report for BTX treatment. Next, it should be noted that the participants were exposed to surprised faces along with angry and happy faces during the experiment, and so the results reported here for happy and angry expressions could depend on the presence of surprised expressions in the experimental context. Finally, the current A-B-A design comprised uneven time intervals between each repeated measure, raising the possibility that the decrement in responses between pre-BTX and BTX (3–6 weeks) might be due to response habituation alone compared to the longer BTX and post-BTX interval (9 months). However, previous studies examining the test-retest reliability of amygdala BOLD activity to angry and fearful faces report reliable responsivity for both short (2 weeks; [38]) and long (1 year; [39]) time intervals.

Conclusions

To summarize, our data support the facial feedback hypothesis by offering neural evidence concerning the causal relationship between activity in the corrugator/procerus muscles and in the amygdala. Using BTX to temporarily paralyze facial muscles, we have found that the amygdala closely tracks the state of the corrugator/procerus by displaying a quadratic pattern of activity. Specifically, amygdala responses to angry faces were diminished by BTX-induced corrugator/procerus paralysis but reverted to pre-BTX injections levels once the effect of the drug wore off. These findings offer preliminary causal evidence that amygdala activity is sensitive to facial feedback during the perception of the facial expressions of others.

Abbreviations

BTX: botulinum toxin; fMRI: functional magnetic resonance imaging; EMG: electromyography; BOLD: blood-oxygen-level dependent; MNI: Montreal Neurological Institute; ANOVA: analysis of variance.

Competing interests

The authors declare that they have no competing interests.

Authors' contributions

MJK, MN, FCD, EJR, and DD participated in the collection of the fMRI data and analyzed the data. MJK, PJW, TFH, and MAS conceived of the study, directed its design and coordination. MJK, PJW and MAS drafted the manuscript. All authors read and approved the manuscript.

Acknowledgements

Brain scans were provided by the Dartmouth Brain Imaging Center. Manuscript preparation was supported by the National Institute of Mental Health grants to MJK (F31 MH090672), PJW (R01 MH080716) and TFH (R01 MH059282).

Author details

[1]Department of Psychological and Brain Sciences, Dartmouth College, 6207 Moore Hall, Hanover, NH 03755, USA. [2]Department of Psychology, B84 East Stadium, University of Nebraska-Lincoln, Lincoln, NE 68588-0156, USA. [3]US Army Natick Soldier Research Development and Engineering Center, Cognitive Science Research Team, 10 Kansas St., Natick, MA 01760, USA. [4]Department of Psychology, Tufts University, 490 Boston Avenue, Medford, MA 02155, USA. [5]Department of Psychology, University of Washington, 119A Guthrie Hall, Seattle, WA 98195, USA. [6]Department of Psychology, University of Virginia, 102 Gilmer Hall, Charlottesville, VA 22904, USA. [7]Department of Surgery (Plastic) and Pediatrics, Geisel School of Medicine at Dartmouth, Dartmouth-Hitchcock Medical Center, Lebanon, NH 03756, USA. [8]Department of Surgery (Plastic and Craniofacial), Sidra Research and Medical Center, Doha, Qatar.

References

1. Darwin CR: *The Expression of the Emotions in Man and Animals.* London: Murray; 1872.
2. James W: *The Principles of Psychology.* New York: Holt; 1890.
3. Tomkins S: *Affect, Imagery, and Consciousness: The Positive Affects.* New York: Springer; 1962.

4. Buck R: **Nonverbal behavior and the theory of emotion: the facial feedback hypothesis.** *J Pers Soc Psychol* 1980, **38:**811–824.
5. Adelmann PK, Zajonc RB: **Facial efference and the experience of emotion.** *Annu Rev Psychol* 1989, **40:**249–280.
6. Keillor JM, Barrett AM, Crucian GP, Kortenkamp S, Heilman KM: **Emotional experience and perception in the absence of facial feedback.** *J Int Neuropsychol Soc* 2002, **8:**130–135.
7. McIntosh DN: **Facial feedback hypotheses: evidence, implications, and directions.** *Motiv Emot* 1996, **20:**121–147.
8. Soussignan R: **Duchenne smile, emotional experience, and autonomic reactivity: a test of the facial feedback hypothesis.** *Emotion* 2002, **2:**52–74.
9. Strack F, Martin LL, Stepper S: **Inhibiting and facilitating conditions of the human smile: a nonobtrusive test of the facial feedback hypothesis.** *J Pers Soc Psychol* 1988, **54:**768–777.
10. Davis JI, Senghas A, Brandt F, Ochsner KN: **The effects of BOTOX injections on emotional experience.** *Emotion* 2010, **10:**433–440.
11. Davis JI, Senghas A, Ochsner KN: **How does facial feedback modulate emotional experience?** *J Res Pers* 2009, **43:**822–829.
12. Hambleton P: **Clostridium botulinum toxins: a general review of involvement in disease, structure, mode of action and preparation for clinical use.** *J Neurol* 1992, **239:**16–20.
13. Olver JM: **Botulinum toxin A treatment of overactive corrugator supercilii in thyroid eye disease.** *Br J Ophthalmol* 1998, **82:**528–533.
14. Jancke L: **Facial EMG in an anger-provoking situation: individual differences in directing anger outwards or inwards.** *Int J Psychophysiol* 1996, **23:**207–214.
15. Dimberg U: **Facial reactions to facial expressions.** *Psychophysiology* 1982, **19:**643–647.
16. Dimberg U, Thunberg M, Elmehed K: **Unconscious facial reactions to emotional facial expressions.** *Psychol Sci* 2000, **11:**86–89.
17. Neta M, Norris CJ, Whalen PJ: **Corrugator muscle responses are associated with individual differences in positivity-negativity bias.** *Emotion* 2009, **9:**640–648.
18. Cacioppo JT, Petty RE, Losch ME, Kim HS: **Electromyographic activity over facial muscle regions can differentiate the valence and intensity of affective reactions.** *J Pers Soc Psychol* 1986, **50:**260–268.
19. Lang PJ, Greenwald MK, Bradley MM, Hamm AO: **Looking at pictures: affective, facial, visceral, and behavioral reactions.** *Psychophysiology* 1993, **30:**261–273.
20. Larsen JT, Norris CJ, Cacioppo JT: **Effects of positive and negative affect on electromyographic activity over zygomaticus major and corrugator supercilii.** *Psychophysiology* 2003, **40:**776–785.
21. Havas DA, Glenberg AM, Gutowski KA, Lucarelli MJ, Davidson RJ: **Cosmetic use of botulinum toxin-A affects processing of emotional language.** *Psychol Sci* 2010, **21:**895–900.
22. Finzi E, Wasserman E: **Treatment of depression with botulinum toxin A: a case series.** *Dermatol Surg* 2006, **32:**645–649. discussion 649-650.
23. Hexsel D, Brum C, Siega C, Schilling-Souza J, Dal'Forno T, Heckmann M, Rodrigues TC: **Evaluation of self-esteem and depression symptoms in depressed and nondepressed subjects treated with onabotulinumtoxinA for glabellar lines.** *Dermatol Surg* 2013, **39:**1088–1096.
24. Hennenlotter A, Dresel C, Castrop F, Ceballos-Baumann AO, Wohlschlager AM, Haslinger B: **The link between facial feedback and neural activity within central circuitries of emotion–new insights from botulinum toxin-induced denervation of frown muscles.** *Cereb Cortex* 2009, **19:**537–542.
25. Whalen PJ, Shin LM, McInerney SC, Fischer H, Wright CI, Rauch SL: **A functional MRI study of human amygdala responses to facial expressions of fear versus anger.** *Emotion* 2001, **1:**70–83.
26. American Society of Plastic Surgeons: **2013 Plastic Surgery Statistics Report.** [http://www.plasticsurgery.org/news/plastic-surgery-statistics/2013.html]
27. Becker-Wegerich P, Rauch L, Ruzicka T: **Botulinum toxin A in the therapy of mimic facial lines.** *Clin Exp Dermatol* 2001, **26:**619–630.
28. Tottenham N, Tanaka JW, Leon AC, McCarry T, Nurse M, Hare TA, Marcus DJ, Westerlund A, Casey BJ, Nelson C: **The NimStim set of facial expressions: judgments from untrained research participants.** *Psychiatry Res* 2009, **168:**242–249.
29. Friston KJ, Holmes AP, Price CJ, Buchel C, Worsley KJ: **Multisubject fMRI studies and conjunction analyses.** *Neuroimage* 1999, **10:**385–396.
30. Maldjian JA, Laurienti PJ, Kraft RA, Burdette JH: **An automated method for neuroanatomic and cytoarchitectonic atlas-based interrogation of fMRI data sets.** *Neuroimage* 2003, **19:**1233–1239.
31. Cox RW: **AFNI: software for analysis and visualization of functional magnetic resonance neuroimages.** *Comput Biomed Res* 1996, **29:**162–173.
32. Cousineau D: **Confidence intervals in within-subject designs: a simpler solution to Loftus and Masson's method.** *Tutorials Quant Meth Psych* 2005, **1:**42–45.
33. Gross JJ: **Antecedent- and response-focused emotion regulation: divergent consequences for experience, expression, and physiology.** *J Pers Soc Psychol* 1998, **74:**224–237.
34. Davis M, Whalen PJ: **The amygdala: vigilance and emotion.** *Mol Psychiatry* 2001, **6:**13–34.
35. Stein MB, Goldin PR, Sareen J, Zorrilla LT, Brown GG: **Increased amygdala activation to angry and contemptuous faces in generalized social phobia.** *Arch Gen Psychiatry* 2002, **59:**1027–1034.
36. Whalen PJ, Rauch SL, Etcoff NL, McInerney SC, Lee MB, Jenike MA: **Masked presentations of emotional facial expressions modulate amygdala activity without explicit knowledge.** *J Neurosci* 1998, **18:**411–418.
37. Williams MA, McGlone F, Abbott DF, Mattingley JB: **Differential amygdala responses to happy and fearful facial expressions depend on selective attention.** *Neuroimage* 2005, **24:**417–425.
38. Johnstone T, Somerville LH, Alexander AL, Oakes TR, Davidson RJ, Kalin NH, Whalen PJ: **Stability of amygdala BOLD response to fearful faces over multiple scan sessions.** *Neuroimage* 2005, **25:**1112–1123.
39. Manuck SB, Brown SM, Forbes EE, Hariri AR: **Temporal stability of individual differences in amygdala reactivity.** *Am J Psychiatry* 2007, **164:**1613–1614.

18

Influence of life stress, 5-HTTLPR genotype, and *SLC6A4* methylation on gene expression and stress response in healthy Caucasian males

Elif A Duman[1,5,6] and Turhan Canli[1,2,3,4*]

Abstract

Background: Previous research reported that individual differences in the stress response were moderated by an interaction between individuals' life stress experience and the serotonin transporter-linked polymorphic region (5-HTTLPR), a common polymorphism located in the promoter region of the serotonin transporter gene (*SLC6A4*). Furthermore, this work suggested that individual differences in *SLC6A4* DNA methylation could be one underlying mechanism by which stressful life events might regulate gene expression. The aim of this study was to understand the relation between early and recent life stress experiences, 5-HTTLPR genotype, and *SLC6A4* methylation. In addition, we aimed to address how these factors influence gene expression and cortisol response to an acute psychosocial stressor, operationalized as the Trier Social Stress Test (TSST). In a sample of 105 Caucasian males, we collected early and recent life stress measures and blood samples to determine 5-HTTLPR genotype and *SLC6A4* methylation. Furthermore, 71 of these participants provided blood and saliva samples before and after the TSST to measure changes in *SLC6A4* and *NR3C1* gene expression and cortisol response.

Results: Compared to S-group individuals, LL individuals responded with increased *SLC6A4* mRNA levels to the TSST ($t(66) = 3.71$, $P < .001$) and also showed increased global methylation as a function of ELS ($r\,(32) = .45$, $P = .008$) and chronic stress ($r\,(32) = .44$, $P = .010$). Compared to LL individuals, S-group individuals showed reduced *SLC6A4* mRNA levels ($r\,(41) = -.31$, $P = .042$) and increased F3 methylation ($r\,(67) = .30$, $P = .015$) as a function of ELS; as well as increased F1 methylation as a function of chronic stress and recent depressive symptoms ($r = .41$, $P < .01$), which correlated positively with *NR3C1* expression ($r\,(42) = .31$, $P = .040$).

Conclusions: Both early and recent life stress alter DNA methylation as a function of 5-HTTLPR genotype. Some of these changes are also reflected in gene expression and cortisol response, differentially affecting individuals' stress response in a manner that may confer susceptibility or resilience for psychopathology upon experiencing stressful life events.

Keywords: Early life stress, Serotonin transporter, Glucocorticoid receptor, Gene expression, DNA methylation, Hypothalamic-pituitary-adrenal axis, Depression

Background

Studies of gene-by-environment interactions (GxE) have begun to reveal important clues regarding the etiology of depression. Much of this research enterprise has been devoted to the serotonin transporter gene (*SLC6A4*) and its interaction with stressful life events (SLEs). Serotonin (5-hydroxytryptamine, 5-HT) is an important neurotransmitter regulating the hypothalamic-pituitary-adrenal axis (HPA) stress response [1,2] and has been implicated in various mood disorders such as depression. The serotonin transporter is responsible for the reuptake of excess serotonin in the synaptic cleft and is commonly targeted by a class of antidepressants known as selective serotonin reuptake inhibitors. A common variant (polymorphism) located in the promoter region of the gene (*SLC6A4*) encoding the transporter, the serotonin transporter-linked polymorphic region (5-HTTLPR), has been widely studied with regard to individual differences in trait neuroticism, anxiety, and depression. The

* Correspondence: turhan.canli@stonybrook.edu
[1]Integrative Neuroscience, Department of Psychology, Stony Brook University, Stony Brook, NY 11794-2500, USA
[2]Department of Radiology, Stony Brook University, Stony Brook, NY 11794, USA
Full list of author information is available at the end of the article

5-HTTLPR is characterized by a short (S) and a long (L) allele that differ in transcriptional efficiencies, with the S allele being less active than the L allele [3,4]. In addition to the 5-HTTLPR, an A/G single nucleotide polymorphism (SNP; rs25531) located within 5-HTTLPR is suggested to alter the transcriptional efficiency of the L allele, such that the L_G allele is considered functionally similar to the S allele [5].

A seminal longitudinal gene-by-environment (GxE) study by Caspi and colleagues reported that the S allele moderated increased risk for depression associated with childhood maltreatment [6]. Subsequent work has produced conflicting results [7-10], which may be due, in part, to variation across studies in the selection of the type and timing of stressful life events (SLEs), sample size, and assessment of depression [10-13]. With regard to SLEs, some studies have considered early life stress (ELS) such as childhood maltreatment, whereas others have focused on recent SLEs. Indeed, it now appears that the timing of SLEs is a critical variable in revealing an interaction with 5-HTTLPR genotype: the most recent, large-scale meta-analysis by Karg *et al.* [10] specifically investigated the effect of stressor type and discovered that 5-HTTLPR strongly moderated the relationship between depression and ELS, specifically childhood maltreatment.

Studies investigating the sequelae of ELS at the molecular level suggest that these effects may be stable and persist through adulthood, such as alterations in the expression of *SLC6A4* [14-17] but also see [18]. One of these studies reported an additive effect of ELS and 5-HTTLPR genotype, such that S carriers with ELS exhibited the lowest level of baseline *SLC6A4* expression [16]. Given known interactions between serotonergic and glucocorticoid systems [19], ELS-mediated regulation of *SLC6A4* and its effect on the glucocorticoid receptor (NR3C1) could be one mechanism by which ELS can affect the HPA response. Activity of HPA is regulated both by negative feedback of cortisol by binding to NR3C1 and also through the action of neurotransmitters, such as serotonin, in specific brain regions [20]. Indeed, one recent study in rats reported that ELS and a polymorphism in *SLC6A4* leads to altered hippocampal *NR3C1* expression and cortisol release [21], suggesting that 5-HTTLPR may alter HPA activity through its effects on *NR3C1* regulation.

Recent studies have begun to study GxE interactions using laboratory-based social stress tasks, such as the Trier Social Stress Test (TSST) [22]; or derivations of the TSST. For example, Alexander *et al.* [23] reported a significant interaction between SLEs and 5-HTTLPR genotype in healthy males such that S carriers with a high number of SLEs exhibited the highest cortisol response. Mueller *et al.* [24] reported the same interaction in young adults (but not in children or older adults) for SLEs during the first 5 years of life, which was associated with increased cortisol responses in S-allele carriers but decreased cortisol responses in homozygous L-allele carriers. These studies, along with other neuroimaging (such as [25]) and behavioral (such as [26]) studies suggest that 5-HTTLPR genotype moderates stress reactivity and vulnerability to psychopathology in interaction with environmental variables.

Other work has begun to address the underlying molecular mechanisms of these GxE interactions, with a particular focus on epigenetic changes [27]. The first epigenetic study investigating the impact of ELS was conducted in rats [28], focusing on DNA methylation, which involves the addition of a methyl group to a segment of DNA containing a CpG dinucleotide. DNA methylation can alter gene expression when it occurs across long sections of CpG-rich regions (so-called 'CpG islands') but also when it occurs at specific sites, such as binding sites for specific transcription factors (TF) [29]. Researchers showed that ELS, operationalized as poor maternal care with low levels of licking and grooming of pups, was associated with increased DNA methylation at a particular CpG site in the hippocampal *NR3C1*, which was associated with lower gene expression and with higher HPA activation in response to stress in adulthood [28]. Subsequent studies provided further evidence for a similar methylation pattern in the postmortem hippocampi of suicide victims exposed to childhood abuse [30], in the cord blood of infants with depressed mothers during pregnancy [31], and in the blood of adults exposed to childhood maltreatment [32]. The similarity of results across the range of species and tissues studied suggests that DNA methylation in *NR3C1* may be a highly conserved and ubiquitous mechanism by which life stress may alter gene expression.

Other studies examined DNA methylation in *SLC6A4*, focusing on a CpG island in the promoter region of this gene, spanning an untranslated exon [33]. Several studies in humans and in non-human primates reported associations between ELS and DNA methylation across the CpG island or at specific CpG sites [34-39]. In addition, some studies reported associations between methylation of the whole CpG island (or sections of it) and gene expression [16,37,40], whereas others reported reduced gene expression as a result of *in vitro* methylation of certain CpG sites [41,42]. 5-HTTLPR genotype appears to further differentiate *SLC6A4* methylation, as some studies reported increased methylation in S carriers [33,37] and suggested that methylation of the S allele may exacerbate the impact of ELS [34] (although some reported the reverse pattern in relation to unresolved trauma [43]).

One recent study examined the association between stressful life experiences, *SLC6A4* methylation, and individuals' cortisol response to during a modified form of the Trier Social Stress Test, TSST [38]. The study was based on 28 monozygotic twin pairs who were discordant for childhood bullying victimization [38] and reported that bullying victimization was associated with increased *SLC6A4* methylation and a blunted cortisol response to the TSST. The study did not address the putative moderating role of 5-HTTLPR genotype or the effect on *SLC6A4* mRNA gene expression. These questions were addressed across a set of two other studies. The first study was conducted in a population sample of 133 healthy young adults and reported an additive effect of early life stress (in the form of either prenatal stress or childhood maltreatment) and presence of the 5-HTTLPR S allele on reducing baseline *SLC6A4* mRNA gene expression [16]. These investigators also examined *SLC6A4* methylation and concluded that the observed differences in mRNA expression were unlikely to be mediated by methylation within this gene's CpG island. In a second, follow-up study with an enlarged sample of 200 healthy young adults, this group then used the TSST to show that *SLC6A4* methylation moderated the association between 5-HTTLPR genotype and cortisol response to the TSST such that S carriers with low *SLC6A4* methylation had higher cortisol responses than LL homozygotes [44]. There were no differences in cortisol response by 5-HTTLPR genotype in the high *SLC6A4* methylation group. However, authors did not report any associations between *SLC6A4* methylation and life stress.

In light of the fact that no single prior study combined all of the putative elements of a molecular GxE interaction, the aim of the current study was to first investigate the interaction between ELS and 5-HTTLPR on *SLC6A4* methylation and its association with *SLC6A4* and *NR3C1* expression and cortisol response following the TSST. In addition, we investigated whether chronic stress and recent depressive symptoms would be associated with *SLC6A4* methylation, gene expression, and cortisol response as a function of 5-HTTLPR genotype, given that several studies reported correlations between depressive symptoms, antidepressant response, and methylation of different CpG sites in the *SLC6A4* CpG island [36,40,45,46].

Methods

Participants

Participants were 105 Caucasian males aged 18 to 77 (M = 28.51, SD = 13.82) who were recruited from Stony Brook University and surrounding communities through flyers, newspaper, and online advertisements. Participants were screened by phone for eligibility. All participants reported no prior diagnosis of psychological disorders or use of any related medication. Details of other exclusion criteria are given in Additional file 1. Measures of early life and chronic stress, 5-HTTLPR genotype, and DNA methylation (see below) were available from all of these participants. A subset (N = 71) participated in the TSST (M_{age} = 29.79, SD_{age} = 15.24). Additional data on recent depressive symptoms, gene expression, and cortisol response to the TSST were available from these participants. The study was approved by the Stony Brook University Institutional Review Board, and participants provided written consents prior to participation in the experimental sessions. At the end of each session, participants were debriefed orally and in writing and compensated with $100 plus reimbursement for any public transportation costs.

Experimental sessions

To standardize biological measures under the influence of diurnal variation, all experimental sessions started between 12:00 and 14:00 h. Participants were instructed to refrain from eating, drinking (other than water), and exercise for at least 1 h before their arrival. The total procedure, which took about 4 h, included consenting, completion of questionnaires, the TSST, a life event interview, and debriefing. Participants also provided blood samples for genotyping and DNA methylation analyses, one at the beginning of the session (45 min before the TSST) and one at the end (105 min after the TSST). Cortisol levels were assessed using saliva samples collected at nine different time points throughout the session.

Assessment of early life stress

Early life stress was assessed with the Childhood Trauma Questionnaire (CTQ) [47], which is a commonly used measure of childhood maltreatment consisting of 28 items with subscales of physical, sexual, and emotional abuse and physical and emotional neglect. Each subscale consists of five items, plus three items that serve to control for denial of maltreatment. The items are rated on a 5-point Likert scale (1 to 5), with higher scores indicating higher levels of maltreatment. Scores are added up to calculate the CTQ total score, which can range from 25 to 125.

Assessment of chronic stress and recent depressive symptoms

Chronic stress for the last 3 months was assessed with the Trier Inventory of Chronic Stress (TICS) [48,49]. TICS is a 12-item self-report measure on the frequency of behaviors related to chronic stress, such as 'I worry that I will not be able to fulfill my tasks' and 'I experience having too much to do.' Each item is rated from 0 (never) to 4 (very often), and items are added up to calculate the total chronic stress score, which can range from 0 to 48.

Participants performing the TSST also completed the Beck Depression Inventory II BDI-II [50]; for assessing recent depressive symptoms. The BDI-II is a 21-item self-report measure of recent depressive symptoms (last 2 weeks) such as sadness, hopelessness, and self-blame. Each item is rated on a scale from 0 to 3, and scores can range from 0 to 63. Higher scores indicate higher depressive symptoms.

Assessment of cortisol levels and stress reactivity

For the assessment of cortisol levels in response to the TSST, participants' saliva samples were collected using salivettes (Sarstedt, Rommelsdorf, Germany). Forty-five minutes after the first blood draw and just prior to the beginning of the TSST, participants provided baseline saliva samples and were then taken to the TSST room. The TSST was performed as described in Kirschbaum *et al.* [22]. Briefly, the task consisted of a preparation phase (5 min), which was followed by a public speech (5 min) on why the participant would be the best candidate for his or her dream job and a backward-counting task (5 min). The task took place in front of a two-person committee that provided no verbal or non-verbal feedback. The active committee member, who gave instructions to the subject during the TSST, was always of the opposite sex (female); the inactive committee member, who did not communicate with the participant, was always of the same sex (male) as the participant. After the TSST, participants returned to the initial testing room and provided a second saliva sample right after the TSST and filled out an 8-item Visual Analog Scale (VAS) assessing the their experience of the TSST, such as finding it stressful, threatening, or challenging. Additional saliva samples were collected at 10, 20, 30, 45, 60, 90, and 105 min after the TSST. The saliva samples were stored at −20°C immediately after the session until being shipped to Brandeis University, Boston, for the analysis of cortisol concentration. Each sample was assayed in duplicates using a commercially available chemiluminescence immunoassay (RE62019) with a sensitivity of 0.16 ng/ml (IBL International, Toronto, ON, Canada). Inter- and intra-assay coefficients of variation were less than 7% and 4%, respectively. Cortisol peak increase was assessed as the difference between the peak cortisol level after the TSST and the baseline as used in prior studies [23,24]. For all participants, the highest response after the TSST was observed within 10 to 20 min after the TSST. We used peak response, rather than area under the curve, as a measure of cortisol reactivity, because the former is potentially more closely associated with changes in gene expression whereas the latter may be more closely associated with the overall hormonal output [51].

Processing blood samples

In order to start with a uniform group of cells, peripheral blood mononuclear cells (PBMCs) were isolated from blood immediately after the blood draw, using Leucosep® tubes (Greiner Bio-One Inc., Monroe, NC, USA) and Ficoll-Paque (GE Healthcare, Pittsburgh, PA, USA) separation medium according to manufacturer's protocol. The isolated PBMC pellets were stored at −80°C for subsequent DNA and RNA extraction procedures.

DNA and RNA extractions from PBMC pellets were carried out by the AllPrep DNA/RNA/Protein Mini kit (Qiagen, Valencia, CA, USA) according to manufacturer's instructions. Quantity and quality of the DNA and RNA were assessed through NanoDrop ND-1000 (Thermo Scientific, Wilmington, DE, USA), DNA samples were stored at −20°C, and RNA samples were stored at −80°C.

Genotyping of 5-HTTLPR and rs25531

5-HTTLPR genotype was determined through PCR amplification of 25 ng DNA at an annealing temperature of 67.5°C using primers employed in previous work [5]. A random subset of 24 samples was processed twice by a technician blind to the initial results to establish test-retest reliability, which was 100%. As a result of genotyping, individuals were genotyped as S/S, S/L, or L/L.

For genotyping the A/G SNP (rs25531), 6 μl of the 5-HTTLPR PCR products were digested with 5 Units of *Hpa*II restriction enzyme (New England Biolabs, Ipswich, MA, USA) for 3 h at 37°C. As a result, individuals were genotyped as S/S, S/L_A, S/L_G, L_A/L_A, L_A/L_G, and L_G/L_G. Given that expression of L_G allele was suggested to be similar to the S allele [52], the triallelic (S, L_A, L_G) classification scheme grouped S/L_G and L_G/L_G individuals as 'S/S' and L_A/L_G individuals as 'L/S'. Genotype distributions were in Hardy-Weinberg equilibrium according to both biallelic and triallelic classification schemes ($P > .05$).

DNA methylation analyses

For the analysis of DNA methylation, 500 ng DNA from each participant at baseline was bisulfite treated by using the Epitect Bisulfite kit (Qiagen, CA) according to manufacturer's instructions and stored at −20°C until used in methylation analyses. In addition, in all methylation analyses, 500 ng unmethylated (0%) and fully-methylated (100%) human DNA samples (Zymo Research, Irvine, CA, USA) were bisulfite treated along with participants' samples to be utilized as bisulfite conversion controls.

Global DNA methylation

The methylation of Long Interspersed Nuclear Element-1 (*LINE-1*) was used as a measure of global methylation both for investigation of associations with ELS (similar to [39]) and for controlling for global methylation when investigating gene-specific methylation (similar to [31]). *LINE-1* methylation was quantified in duplicates by using the PyroMark Q96 CpG LINE-1 kit (Qiagen, CA) in a PyroMark Q96 MD system at the Stony Brook University Genomics Core Facility according to manufacturer's protocol and with the commercial primers provided with the kit. Details of the procedure are given in Additional file 1.

SLC6A4 CpG island DNA methylation

Methylation of the CpG island upstream of *SLC6A4* was quantified by the Sequenom Epityper MassArray system (San Diego, CA, USA). Two sets of primers were designed to amplify the 79 CpG sites in the CpG island in two amplicons similar to Philibert *et al.* [40] by using the Epityper software (Sequenom, CA). With this technique, methylation of *CpG Units* is analyzed, which can consist of one or more adjacent CpG sites. A total of 37 CpG Units were covered by the two amplicons, consisting of 79 CpG sites. All samples were run in triplicates. After preprocessing, methylation data from 26 CpG Units in amplicons 1 and 2 were included in all analysis (Figure 1). Details of the procedure, primer sequences, and data analysis are given in Additional file 1.

Gene expression analyses

For each participant, two RNA samples were used for gene expression analyses, one 45 min before the TSST (baseline), and another 105 min after the TSST (response). Prior to quantification of gene expression, integrity of the RNA samples was assessed using the Agilent 2100 BioAnalyzer (Agilent Technologies, Santa Clara, CA, USA). RNA Integrity Numbers (RINs) of the samples were high (M = 7.94, SD = 1.32), and RINs of samples before and after the TSST did not differ significantly (P = .853). Afterwards, 1 μg of RNA from each time point was converted to cDNA using QuantiTect Reverse Transcription Kit according to the manufacturer's protocol (Qiagen, CA). The cDNA samples were then diluted five times, and 1 μl of the diluted cDNA was used for the gene expression analysis of the candidate genes by quantitative PCR (qPCR), using the Qiagen SYBR Green PCR + UNG kit (Qiagen, CA) and gene-specific primers designed from the Roche Universal Probe Library website (http://www.roche-applied-science.com/sis/rtpcr/upl/ezhome.html). The qPCR reactions were carried out in triplicates in the Roche 480 LightCycler system (Roche Applied Science, Indianapolis, IN, USA) at an annealing temperature of 60°C.

To identify the best reference genes in PBMCs, the expression of six candidate reference genes was analyzed from five individuals' RNA samples, obtained at baseline and response time points. This method identified *HPRT1* (hypoxanthine phosphoribosyltransferase 1) and *GAPDH* (glyceraldehyde 3-phosphate dehydrogenase) as the best reference genes in PBMCs. C_T values that were obtained by qPCR were then used to assess gene expression change between baseline and response samples, using the delta-delta-C_T method [53]. Changes in gene expression for each sample, normalized for reference genes, are shown as fold-change values, representing the fold change in *SLC6A4* and *NR3C1* after the TSST relative to baseline. Details of the qPCR analyses and primer sequences are given in Additional file 1.

Statistical analysis

All statistical analyses were performed using SPSS for Windows version 16.0 (Chicago, IL, USA), with significance level set at α = .05. In order to assess whether the TSST successfully evoked a cortisol response, we used a repeated measures ANOVA for the nine saliva samples collected throughout the experiment. Prior to all analyses, cortisol data were tested for normal distribution by the Kolmogorov-Smirnov test. Due to violation of normality for samples at multiple time points (P < .05), log transformation was applied to all cortisol data. Due to the violation of sphericity (P < .05), Greenhouse-Geisser correction was applied.

To examine correlations between variables of interest, Pearson's correlation coefficient (r) was used for the normally distributed variables, and Spearman's rho coefficient (rs) was used for the non-normally distributed variables. Partial correlations were used as necessary to

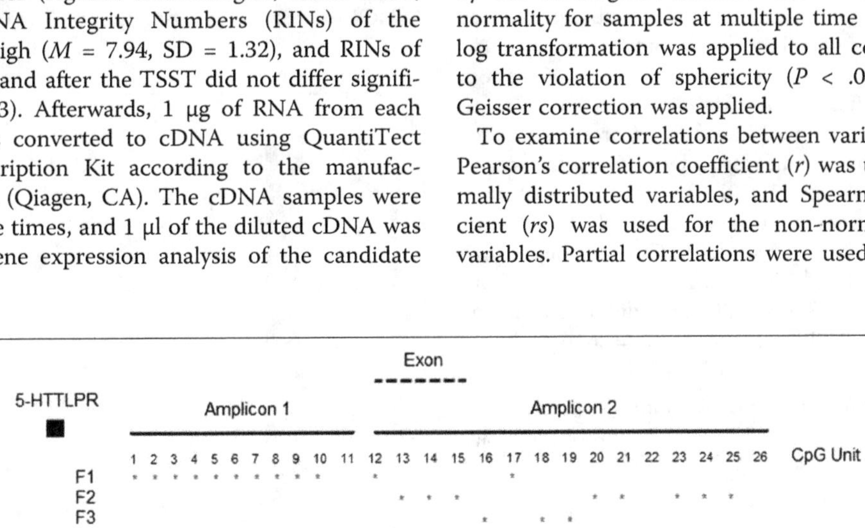

Figure 1 *SLC6A4* CpG island amplicons for DNA methylation analysis. Analyzed CpG Units are numbered from 1 to 26. The untranslated exon spans CpG Units 12 to 15 and 5-HTTLPR is located upstream of the CpG island. Asterisks show the CpG Units belonging to Factors 1, 2, and 3 (F1 to F3). F1 factor loadings ranged from .35 to .83, F2 factor loadings ranged from .37 to .76, and F3 factor loadings ranged from .73 to .87.

control for the effects of some variables such as age and *LINE-1* methylation.

In order to understand the methylation patterns across the CpG island and reduce the number of variables investigated, a factor analysis covering the 26 CpG Units across the island was conducted similar to Olsson *et al.* [41]. Kaiser-Meyer-Olkin measure of sampling adequacy (.834) and Bartlett's test of sphericity ($P < .001$) suggested that factor analysis is suitable for the data set. As a result of the analysis, five factors emerged explaining 75% of the variance. However, since fewer than three variables were loaded onto the last two factors, only the first three factors were considered: Factor 1 (F1), Factor 2 (F2), and Factor 3 (F3). Percentage of the variance explained by F1, F2, and F3 were 37, 15, and 12, respectively. Loadings on these factors were such that F1 primarily included CpG Units at the beginning of the CpG island up to the start of the exon, whereas F2 included those towards the end of the island and F3 included a shorter region towards the end of the island (Figure 1).

Results

Participant characteristics and response to the TSST

The study included 105 Caucasian males aged 18 to 77 ($M_{age} = 28.51$, $SD_{age} = 13.82$). The distribution of 5-HTTLPR genotype groups is shown in Table 1. Furthermore, age did not vary as a function of 5-HTTLPR genotype ($t(103) = 1.19$, $P = .238$; S group $M = 27.39$, SD = 13.12; LL group $M = 30.77$, SD = 15.07). ELS, as measured by CTQ total scores, ranged from 25 to 66 ($M = 34.83$, SD = 9.57). Only two participants reported past sexual abuse (scoring 7 within a range of 5 to 25). Apart from sexual abuse, all CTQ subscale scores were significantly correlated with each other ($r = .31$ to .63) and with the CTQ total score ($r = .67$ to .86; P values ≤.001; individual correlation coefficients are reported in Additional file 1: Table S1). Chronic stress for the last 3 months, as measured by TICS total scores, ranged from 0 to 42 ($M = 17.42$, SD = 9.70). None of these measures differed as a function of 5-HTTLPR genotype (S *vs.* LL; P values >.860). Current depressive symptoms (BDI-II) of TSST participants ranged from 0 to 30 ($M = 7.37$, SD = 7.20) and did not differ as a function of 5-HTTLPR genotype ($P = .646$).

Table 1 5-HTTLPR genotype distributions

	All	TSST participants only
SS	24	15
SL	46	30
LL	35	26
Total	105	71

Note. Genotypes are given according to the triallelic classification.

A repeated measures ANOVA showed a significant cortisol increase to the TSST as shown in Figure 2 ($F_{2.69,\ 70} = 61.41$, $P < .001$, partial $\eta^2 = .47$). 5-HTTLPR genotype was not associated with significant differences in the overall cortisol response ($P = .758$) or in baseline cortisol levels ($P = .900$).

SLC6A4 and *NR3C1* expression at baseline as a function of 5-HTTLPR genotype and early life stress

The first question we addressed was whether individuals differed in levels of serotonin transporter gene (*SLC6A4*) or glucocorticoid receptor gene (*NR3C1*) expression, as a function of either 5-HTTLPR genotype or early life stress, prior to any social stress exposure at baseline. We found no significant differences across any of our measures.

There were no significant differences in baseline *SLC6A4* expression as a function of 5-HTTLPR genotype ($t(66) = -.79$, $P = .430$; Additional file 2: Figure S1, panel A). There was also no significant correlation between baseline *SLC6A4* expression and ELS for the sample as a whole or as a function of 5-HTTLPR genotype (all r coefficients < .1, P values ≥ .539). The absence of any ELS effects was also noted when we converted measures of ELS from a continuous to a categorical variable: either by taking the median split of CTQ total scores ($F_{3,\ 63} = .86$, $P = .358$) or applying higher cut-off values used in prior studies to divide participants into 'no-ELS' or 'ELS' groups, $F_{3,\ 63} = .69$, $P = .410$ [similar to 16; detailed in Additional file 1]. There were also no effect of 5-HTTLPR and ELS interaction for both median split ELS scores ($F_{3,\ 63} = .08$, $P = .772$) or higher cut-off ELS scores ($F_{3,\ 63} = .01$, $P = .910$) on *SLC6A4* baseline expression.

There were no significant differences in baseline *NR3C1* expression as a function of 5-HTTLPR genotype

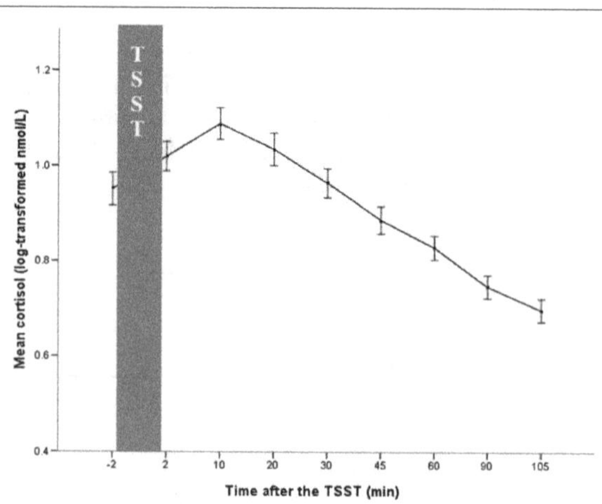

Figure 2 Cortisol response to the TSST. Cortisol levels (mean ± SE of mean) at different time points after the TSST.

($t(66) = .093$, $P = .926$; Additional file 2: Figure S1, panel C). There was also no significant correlation between baseline *NR3C1* expression and ELS for the sample as a whole or as a function of 5-HTTLPR genotype (all r coefficients < .1, P values ≥ .454). Similar results were obtained when utilizing categorical ELS values and investigating their interaction with 5-HTTLPR genotype (all P values ≥ .307).

SLC6A4 and *NR3C1* expression in response to the TSST as a function of 5-HTTLPR genotype and early life stress

The next question we addressed was whether individuals differed in levels of serotonin transporter gene (*SLC6A4*) or glucocorticoid receptor gene (*NR3C1*) expression, as a function of either 5-HTTLPR genotype or early life stress, in response to the TSST. We found differential effects for *SLC6A4* but not *NR3C1*.

In response to the TSST, we found that LL individuals responded with increased *SLC6A4* mRNA expression to the TSST whereas S-group individuals' expression values remained unchanged; LL individuals had significantly higher *SLC6A4* expression in response to the TSST than did S-group individuals ($t(66) = 3.71$, $P < .001$) (Additional file 2: Figure S1, panel B).

We also wanted to examine whether *SLC6A4* mRNA expression varied as a function of an interaction between 5-HTTLPR genotype and ELS. Although a formal interaction between 5-HTTLPR genotype and ELS was not significant ($F_{3,\ 63} = .91$, $P = .343$), we conducted exploratory analyses for each genotype separately, which showed that *SLC6A4* expression was inversely correlated with gene expression for S-group individuals (r (41) = −.31, $P = .042$) but not for LL individuals (r (23) = −.01, $P = .967$). Similar results were obtained when ELS was categorized as no-ELS *vs.* ELS ($F_{3,\ 63} = 5.83$, $P = .001$), such that LL individuals with ELS had the highest *SLC6A4* expression change, followed by LL with no-ELS, S carriers with no-ELS and S carriers with ELS. The results remained unchanged when a biallelic classification scheme was used.

NR3C1 expression in response to the TSST did not differ as a function of 5-HTTLPR genotype ($t(66) = -1.46$, $P = .149$; Additional file 2: Figure S1, panel D). *NR3C1* expression in response to the TSST also did not differ as a function of ELS for the entire sample, nor for any of the subsamples as a function of 5-HTTLPR genotype (all r coefficients < .2, P values ≥ .237).

Global DNA and *SLC6A4* methylation

Global methylation levels, as measured by *LINE-1* methylation, ranged from 71% to 80% ($M = 74.77$, SD = 2.38). There was a negative correlation between age and *LINE-1* methylation as expected [54]; $r(103) = -.25$, $P = .011$. There were no differences in *LINE-1* methylation as a function of 5-HTTLPR genotype ($P = .699$).

SLC6A4 CpG island average methylation ranged from 7% to 14% ($M = 8.85$, SD = 1.67), increasing from the 5′ to the 3′ end; intercorrelations between CpG Units were higher in the 5′ end than the 3′ end as previously reported [40].

Average *SLC6A4* methylation correlated positively with age ($r(103) = .33$, $P = .001$), consistent with the literature suggesting increases in promoter methylation by age [55]. Controlling for age, *SLC6A4* average methylation was also correlated with *LINE-1* methylation ($r(102) = .52$, $P < .001$).

Age was positively correlated with F2 (r_s (103) = .34, $P < .001$) and F3 (r_s (103) = .40, $P < .001$) but not with F1 methylation (r_s (103) = −.02, $P = .867$). Controlling for age, *LINE-1* methylation was positively correlated with F1 (r (102) = .60, $P < .001$) and F2 (r (102) = .33, $P = .001$) methylation but negatively with F3 methylation (r (102) = −.24, $P = .014$).

Early life stress: association with global DNA and *SLC6A4* methylation

In light of the previously discussed literature, we next addressed the question whether ELS is associated with either global DNA or *SLC6A4* methylation. There was no main effect and only a trend for a significant interaction between ELS and 5-HTTLPR ($F_{3,\ 67} = 3.74$, $p = .056$). An exploratory analysis for each genotype showed that ELS correlated positively with *LINE-1* methylation only in LL participants (r (32) = .45, $P = .008$), controlling for age. However, this correlation became non-significant once we controlled for chronic stress (r (31) = .27, $P = .136$).

There was no significant correlation between ELS and average *SLC6A4* methylation (r (103) = .09, $P = .380$), and results remained unchanged when controlling for age and *LINE-1* methylation. There was also no correlation between ELS and any of the three *SLC6A4* methylation factors, controlling for age and *LINE-1* methylation (r coefficients < .1, P values ≥ .090). However, when 5-HTTLPR genotype was taken into account (again controlling for age and *LINE-1* methylation), there was a significant interaction between 5-HTTLPR and ELS on F3 methylation ($F_{5,\ 99} = 7.98$, $P = .006$): ELS and F3 methylation correlated positively in S-group participants (r (67) = .30, $P = .015$) but not for LL participants (r (31) = −.28, $P = .118$). There were no significant correlations between ELS and F1 or F2 methylation by 5-HTTLPR genotype (Additional file 1: Table S3).

SLC6A4 methylation: association with *SLC6A4* and *NR3C1* expression and with cortisol release

Given that DNA methylation can regulate gene expression, we next addressed the question whether *SLC6A4* methylation was associated with differential gene expression of

Table 2 Correlations between *SLC6A4* methylation and *NR3C1* expression

NR3C1 expression	F1 methylation		F2 methylation		F3 methylation		Average methylation	
	S	LL	S	LL	S	LL	S	LL
Baseline	.21	.35	.14	.34	−.05	−.12	.09	.16
Response	*.31**	.20	−.03	.06	.14	−.37	*.34**	−.02

Note. $^{*}P < .05$. Significant correlations are shown in italics.

either *SLC6A4* or *NR3C1*. There was no significant correlation between *SLC6A4* methylation and *SLC6A4* expression overall, for any of the three factors, or as a function of 5-HTTLPR genotype (r coefficients < .2, P values ≥ .203).

There was also no significant correlation between *SLC6A4* methylation and *NR3C1* expression overall (r (68) = .21, P = .082), nor a significant interaction (F3, 66 = 2.21, P = .142). Exploratory analyses showed a significant correlation between overall *SLC6A4* methylation and *NR3C1* expression for S-group participants only (r (42) = .34, P = .023). In particular, there was also a correlation between F1 methylation and *NR3C1* expression in S-group participants only, (r (42) = .31, P = .040). Neither F2 nor F3 methylation were correlated with *NR3C1* expression for any of the genotype groups (Table 2).

To further assess the functional significance of these observations, we conducted additional correlational analyses with participants' cortisol responses. There was no significant correlation between *NR3C1* expression and cortisol response in any of the genotype groups; nor was there a significant correlation between *SLC6A4* F1 methylation and cortisol response in any of the genotype groups. Only when *SLC6A4* F1 methylation results were further subdivided into tertiles did some differential effects emerge genotype (Additional file 3: Figure S2).

We also addressed the functional significance of *SLC6A4* methylation in regard to cortisol release in response to the TSST. There were no significant correlations between cortisol release and *SLC6A4* methylation (overall or for F1 to F3) for the sample overall or as a function of 5-HTTLPR genotype (all r coefficients < .2, P > .110).

Chronic stress, recent depressive symptoms: association with global DNA and *SLC6A4* methylation

As discussed in the introduction, a meta-analysis of GxE interactions differentiated between early life stress and other stressors. Having examined ELS in the previous sections, we now turned to the association of chronic stress and recent depressive symptoms with global DNA and *SLC6A4* methylation.

Chronic stress (controlling for age) correlated significantly with global DNA methylation, as measured by *LINE-1* methylation, for the overall sample (r (102) = .23, P = .019). This correlation was driven by LL participants (r (32) = .44, P = .010) but not by S-group carriers (r (67) = .15, P = .219). This effect remained unchanged when controlling for ELS, as well. Recent depressive symptoms did not correlate significantly with *LINE-1* methylation for the overall sample (r (68) = .19, P = .111), nor as a function of 5-HTTLPR genotype (S carriers: r (42) = .19, P = .209; LL: r (23) = .22, P = .284).

Chronic stress (controlling for age and *LINE-1* methylation) did not correlate significantly with overall *SLC6A4* methylation for the overall sample, nor as a function of 5-HTTLPR genotype (Table 3). Recent depressive symptoms correlated only marginally with overall *SLC6A4* methylation (r(67) = .22, P = .064; Table 3). When we investigated the association of chronic stress and recent depressive symptoms for each *SLC6A4* methylation factor separately, there was a significant interaction between 5-HTTLPR and chronic stress ($F_{5,\ 99}$ = 4.01, P = .048) but not for recent depressive symptoms ($F_{5,\ 66}$ = 1.17, P = .283) on F1 methylation. A follow-up analysis by genotype found that the correlations were driven by the S group (r = .41, P < .01) but not LL participants (r = -.16, P > .519; Table 3). The results remained unchanged when controlling for ELS as well.

A summary of the current study findings is given in Table 4.

Discussion

This study aimed to address mechanisms of GxE interactions shaping individual differences in social stress

Table 3 Partial correlations between SLC6A4 methylation, chronic stress, and recent depressive symptoms

	SLC6A4 methylation			
	Average	F1	F2	F3
All				
Recent depressive symptoms	.22	*.30**	.08	−.17
Chronic stress	.05	*.20**	−.04	−.16
S group				
Recent depressive symptoms	.28	*.41***	.08	−.16
Chronic stress	.20	*.41***	.01	−.25
LL				
Recent depressive symptoms	−.02	.14	−.11	−.23
Chronic stress	−.16	−.11	.04	−.10

Note. Partial correlations controlling for age and *LINE-1* methylation. $^{*}P < .05$; $^{**}P < .01$. Significant correlations are shown in italics.

Table 4 Summary of the major study findings

	DNA methylation	Gene expression change in response to the TSST
		SLC6A4 expression: LL > S-group
Early life stress ↑	LINE-1 methylation: S-group ↔ LL ↑	*SLC6A4* expression: S-group ↓ LL ↔
	F3 methylation: S-group ↑ LL ↔	
Chronic stress ↑	LINE-1 methylation: S-group ↔ LL ↑	F1 methylation correl w/ *NR3C1* expression: S-group ↑ LL ↔
	F1 methylation: S-group ↑ LL ↔	

Note. Arrows pointing up or down indicate significantly increased or decreased methylation/expression, respectively. Sideway arrows indicate no significant change.

reactivity. Using the TSST as a well-validated social stress paradigm, we investigated the relationship between SLEs and genetic and epigenetic variations, as well as their downstream effects on gene expression and HPA activity. We focused in particular on *SLC6A4*, which has been shown to moderate the effects of stressful life events and HPA reactivity.

We began our analyses with an *in vivo* blood-based assessment of serotonin transporter (*SLC6A4*) or glucocorticoid receptor (*NR3C1*) mRNA expression at baseline, as a function of either 5-HTTLPR genotype or ELS. We found no significant differential gene expression at baseline as a function of genotype or life stress, nor an interaction between these two variables. One other group, focusing on *SLC6A4*, conducted a similar study and did report lower levels of *SLC6A4 mRNA* expression as a function of 5-HTTLPR genotype and ELS, as well as an additive effect of these two variables [16]. Our sample was about 20% smaller, and it is therefore possible that we lacked statistical power to detect a difference.

When we turned our attention to the dynamic regulation of *SLC6A4* expression following exposure to the TSST, we found evidence for a regulatory role of 5-HTTLPR genotype: LL homozygotes showed a 1.5-fold increase in gene expression following the stressor, whereas S-group individuals' expression levels remained unchanged. This finding is consistent with Mueller *et al.*'s study showing increased responsiveness to the TSST in LL homozygotes (when collapsed across SLEs), as measured by cortisol activation [24]. This finding is also consistent with Glatz *et al.*'s study [56] that reported less expression of the S allele following glucocorticoid stimulation. One reason for the difference in dynamic gene expression as a function of 5-HTTLPR genotype may be related to structural features in the promoter region of *SLC6A4* (as determined by the PROMO software; [57]), which contains several transcription factor binding sites (for example, AP-2, GR-α, Sp1) that are important in the glucocorticoid system [3,56]. Another reason may be differential affinity for methylation-related proteins as a function of 5-HTTLPR genotype [58]. To our knowledge, previous human studies did not consider the effect of 5-HTTLPR genotype on stress-related dynamic changes in PBMC *SLC6A4* expression. Thus, replication of this result in larger samples would be important.

Although change in *SLC6A4* expression was not affected as a function of ELS *per se*, it was affected as a function of the interaction between ELS and 5-HTTLPR genotype: ELS further exacerbated the reduced rate of change in *SLC6A4* expression to the TSST in S carriers but not in LL homozygotes. This result is similar to a set of rhesus macaque studies, which reported that ELS was associated with decreased *SLC6A4* expression in response to a stressor [14,59]. However, these studies did not report a differential effect of 5-httlpr genotype, which may reflect lacking statistical power due to the low number of subjects, particularly of SS genotype. The life stress effects we observed were specific to ELS, because we did not find a correlation between recent stress events and *SLC6A4* expression, consistent with another recent study [16]. Thus, our data suggest a model by which ELS appears to differentially amplify the genotype effects on dynamic *SLC6A4* expression in S carriers, which may render them vulnerable for psychopathology following stress exposure.

ELS may alter gene expression through modifications in DNA methylation [33]. To address this question, we considered both global *LINE-1* and gene-specific *SLC6A4* methylation. Indeed, ELS (as well as chronic stress) correlated positively with *LINE-1* methylation but only in LL participants. These results are consistent with a recent study in LL macaques that also reported an association between animals' stress response and global and *SLC6A4* methylation in individuals who had experienced ELS [39]. ELS and chronic stress may affect *LINE-1* methylation through a common pathway, because when we controlled for chronic stress, the correlation between ELS and *LINE-1* methylation became nonsignificant. Future work conducted with larger samples should replicate this finding and examine possible molecular mechanisms by which chronic stress and ELS may alter *LINE-1* methylation.

ELS did not correlate significantly with average *SLC6A4* methylation, nor with methylation of any of the three *SLC6A4* methylation factors (F1 to F3). However, ELS may be associated with site-specific *SLC6A4* methylation as a function of 5-HTTLPR genotype: ELS correlated positively with F3 (but not with F1 or F2) methylation but only in S-Group participants. This finding suggests that not all CpG regions within *SLC6A4* may be equally sensitive to ELS as a function of 5-HTTLPR genotype. Given our small sample, this conclusion remains speculative until replicated in a larger sample.

One way to assess whether methylation of a particular CpG region is functionally significant is to consider it in the context of gene expression. Here, we found no evidence that F3 methylation, as a function of ELS and 5-HTTLPR genotype, correlated significantly with *SLC6A4* mRNA expression. Indeed, there was no evidence for any relation between *SLC6A4* methylation and *SLC6A4* mRNA expression overall, for any of the three factors, or as a function of 5-HTTLPR genotype. This observation is consistent with another study that concluded that methylation of *SLC6A4* was unlikely to moderate its expression [16].

It is possible, however, that *SLC6A4* methylation may exert an effect through indirect pathways, by regulating *NR3C1* expression [21]. Indeed, we discovered that there was a significant correlation between overall *SLC6A4* (as well as F1) methylation and *NR3C1* expression but only for S-group participants. This association did not, however, produce a corresponding differential cortisol response as one might expect [21], casting some doubt on the functional significance of this association.

In addition to ELS, we also examined the association of chronic stress and current depressive symptoms with global and with *SLC6A4* methylation (albeit, the exclusion of participants with a history of, or current, depression restricted the range of observed depressive symptoms). We found that both chronic stress and recent depressive symptoms were positively correlated with F1 methylation (a region in the 5′ end of the *SLC6A4* CpG island) in S group but not LL participants. Importantly, these results remained significant when we controlled for age, *LINE-1* methylation, and ELS. Given that short allele carriers exposed to life stress are more likely to show depressive symptoms [6], these findings are in line with previous studies that associated higher *SLC6A4* methylation with depression [36,40,45]. Our F1 region overlaps with a region examined in a study of MZ twins that reported a positive association between BDI scores and methylation [45]. This F1 region also overlaps with one examined in a study of job burnout in nurses [60]: when adjusted for working environment (high *vs.* low stress), methylation of this region was positively associated with increased burnout. The study found no influence of 5-HTTLPR genotype, which may reflect limited statistical power due to sample size. Taken together, our results and these other studies suggest that the region overlapping with F1 of the *SLC6A4* CpG island may be particularly plastic and sensitive to the effects of chronic or recent (as opposed to early) stressors.

SLC6A4 F1 methylation may exert its effects by regulating gene expression. Although there was no association between *SLC6A4* F1 methylation and *SLC6A4* expression, there was a link with *NR3C1* expression. This link may reflect underlying structural features of the F1 region, which contains multiple binding sites for glucocorticoid receptors as determined by the PROMO software [57]. The link between *SLC6A4* F1 methylation and *NR3C1* expression was genotype specific: F1 methylation was positively correlated with *NR3C1* expression in S group but not LL individuals. The functional significance of this observation remains tentative because there was no significant correlation between either *SLC6A4* F1 methylation or *NR3C1* expression, on the one hand, and cortisol response to the TSST, on the other. Exploratory data suggest that level of F1 methylation may be a moderating factor, but our sample was too small to make any conclusive statements (Additional file 3: Figure S2).

Strengths and limitations

One of the strengths of this study is that our sample was homogeneous. We limited enrollment to Caucasians to minimize ethnic stratification. We enrolled only males to minimize the confounding effects of steroid hormones on HPA reactivity. We excluded individuals with a previous diagnosis of psychopathology and related medication use. These criteria are important considering their confounding effects on DNA methylation [46,61], brain activity, and physiology [62].

The homogeneity of our sample comes at the cost of limited generalizability, since our data cannot be extrapolated to non-Caucasians, women, or individuals with psychopathology. Furthermore, the exclusion of individuals with diagnosed psychopathology may have limited the number of study participants with high levels of ELS ($N = 18$). Thus, the results of our analyses involving ELS should be considered preliminary, particularly when this cohort is further divided by 5-HTTLPR genotype. We also did not correct for multiple testing due to the exploratory nature of the study. Therefore, we suggest that future studies recruit broader and larger samples of the population (women, minorities) and also recruit specifically for individuals with high levels of early life stress history and statistically control for diagnosis of psychopathology.

The exclusion of patients with psychopathology also limited the number of participants with large numbers of ELS events or with specific types of ELS, such as sexual abuse. On the other hand, even gazing through this narrow window of ELS, we observed important changes in DNA methylation, gene expression, and cortisol response. Use of different measures for ELS, chronic stress, and depressive symptoms allowed us to investigate their contributions as well as control for their effects on each other.

The study design was cross-sectional and based in large part on retrospective self-report, so that some variables of interest, such as ELS, are difficult to verify objectively. Furthermore, as is common in human studies of this kind, our observations are by necessity correlational. Thus, future longitudinal studies in humans, as well as studies based on animal models and *in vitro* processes, will be crucial to complement these results and to further develop mechanistic models of GxE interactions observed here.

A strength of this study is that it classified 5-HTTLPR genotype according to both biallelic and triallelic coding schemes [4,5,52]. However, due to sample size, we lacked the power to analyze each genotype group separately. Future studies with higher sample sizes should investigate these groups separately together with their interactions with early and recent stress measures.

A particularly strong feature of our study was the focus on dynamic changes in gene expression in response to the TSST in a within-subject study design. However, because blood samples were only analyzed for changes between baseline and 105 min after the TSST, it is possible that we did not capture the peak in gene expression. On the other hand, for a subset of the participants, we had gene expression data 45 min after the TSST (*unpublished results*), which suggested a gradual increase in the expression of *SLC6A4* and *NR3C1* from baseline to 105 min after the TSST. In addition, a study by Nater *et al.* [63] reported changes in gene expression in stress- and immune-related pathways as early as 60 min following the TSST, although another study reported continued gene expression changes up to 24 h following stress exposure [64]. Taken together, future studies should measure the expression of candidate genes at multiple time points after the stressor.

Finally, this study had two strong features with regard to its epigenetic analyses: it controlled for global methylation effects [31], and it included the majority of the CpG Units in the *SLC6A4* CpG island. The latter feature is important, because considering only a part of CpG sites maybe misleading, as different CpG sites may vary substantially in terms of their TF binding sites and infrastructure to attract methylation-related proteins [61,65].

One important limitation of this study is that our epigenetic analyses are based on peripheral biomarkers, that is, PBMCs, rather than brain tissue from regions involved in stress processing. Yet, there is growing evidence that DNA methylation patterns may be similar across tissues and species [66-68]. This may also apply to stress-related changes in methylation. For example, in relation to *NR3C1* methylation, the same region associated with ELS was found to be highly methylated in rat [28] and human postmortem hippocampus [30], human leukocytes [32], and cord blood [31]. In addition, there is also recent evidence suggesting effects of peripheral DNA methylation of candidate genes such as *SLC6A4* and catechol-o-methyl transferase on brain activity [42,69]. A multi-pronged approach combining a variety of species *in vivo*, *in vitro*, and postmortem will be required to further elucidate the underlying mechanisms of stress affecting gene expression.

Future research

In light of the limitations discussed above, future research should be extended to ethnically diverse populations, to women, and to patient populations in order to examine the differential impact of stress and 5-HTTLPR genotype on gene expression, DNA methylation, and HPA response [24,33,70-72].

Future TSST study designs could be further strengthened by including an active control condition. For example, Het and colleagues [73] introduced a placebo version of the TSST, which retained the free speech and arithmetic aspects of the task but removed its stressful features of uncontrollability and social evaluation. Inclusion of an active control condition could further define social stress-related aspects of gene expression and serve as a control condition against possibly spurious correlations. This would also be beneficial to dissociate gene expression changes due to diurnal variation and those induced by stressors like the TSST.

Future work also needs to address causal mechanisms. For example, studies investigating the impact of ELS on *NR3C1* expression across different species and in different tissues (hippocampus to blood) have provided important insights. This multi-pronged approach would also allow us to better understand the neuroanatomical bases of these interactions similar to [74]. In addition, *in vitro* studies investigating the effects of TF binding and methylation at target sites on expression and glucocorticoid response would complement these studies.

Indeed, future studies should focus on mechanistic explanations for differential gene expression, by focusing on the putative role of TF expression and binding *in vitro*. In addition, it would be important to investigate the effect of *SLC6A4* in concert with other genes, such as brain-derived neurotrophic factor (*BDNF*). Previous GxE studies suggested combined effects of 5-HTTLPR, a polymorphism in *BDNF*, and life stress on HPA activity and depression such as [75-77], and a recent review suggested complementary effects of these polymorphisms on the development and chronicity of depression [78]. The association of ELS and *BDNF* methylation is also under investigation [79], making it an ideal gene to investigate its genetic and epigenetic interactions with *SLC6A4*.

Conclusions

We conclude that individuals respond differently to stress as a function of 5-HTTLPR genotype, both at the level of *SLC6A4* and *NR3C1* gene expression and at the level of gene methylation. Compared to S-group individuals, LL individuals responded with increased *SLC6A4* mRNA levels to the TSST and also show increased global methylation as a function of ELS and chronic stress. Compared to LL individuals, S-group individuals showed reduced *SLC6A4* mRNA levels and increased F3 methylation as a function of ELS; as well as increased F1 methylation as a function of chronic stress and recent depressive symptoms, which correlated positively with *NR3C1* expression. These findings highlight the complex interplay by which an individual's genotype and type of life stressor may affect DNA methylation and gene expression with relevance to HPA activity, to contribute to individual differences in disease susceptibility or resilience.

Additional files

Additional file 1: Supplementary information. This file contains more detailed information on exclusion criteria, ELS categorization details, DNA methylation, and qPCR protocols.

Additional file 2: Figure S1. *SLC6A4* (A-B) and *NR3C1* (C-D) gene expression at baseline and in response to the TSST as a function of 5-HTTLPR genotype. There were no significant differences in gene expression by 5-HTTLPR genotype, except for *SLC6A4* expression in response to the TSST. LL individuals increased *SLC6A4* mRNA expression to the TSST whereas S-group individuals remained unchanged; LL individuals had significantly higher *SLC6A4* expression in response to the TSST than did S-group individuals (***$P < .001$).

Additional file 3: Figure S2. *NR3C1* expression and cortisol peak response as a function of 5-HTTLPR genotype in the top tertile of *SLC6A4* F1 methylation. For individuals in the lower two tertiles of F1 methylation, there was no correlation between *NR3C1* expression and cortisol response for any of the genotype groups (all P values >.05). For individuals in the top tertile, *NR3C1* expression correlated positively with cortisol peak response for S-group participants (r (18) = .60, P = .006), but not LL participants (r (9) = −.22, P = .523).

Abbreviations

5-HT: 5-hydroxytryptamine; 5-HTT: 5-hydroxytryptamine transporter; 5-HTTLPR: 5-hydroxytryptamine transporter-linked polymorphic region; BDI: Beck Depression Inventory; CTQ: Childhood Trauma Questionnaire; ELS: early life stress; GAPDH: glyceraldehyde 3-phosphate dehydrogenase; GxE: gene-environment interaction; GR: glucocorticoid receptor; HPA: hypothalamic-pituitary-adrenal axis; HPRT1: hypoxanthine phosphoribosyltransferase; LINE-1: Long Interspersed Nuclear Element-1; NGFI-A: nerve growth factor-inducible protein A; NR3C1: nuclear receptor subfamily 3 group C member 1; PBMC: peripheral blood mononuclear cell; SLC6A4: solute carrier family 6 member 4; SLE: stressful life event; SNP: single nucleotide polymorphism; TICS: Trier Inventory of Chronic Stress; TF: transcription factor; TSST: Trier Social Stress Test; UNG: uracil-N-glycosylase.

Competing interests

The authors declare that they have no competing interests.

Authors' contributions

EAD contributed to the design of the study as part of her dissertation, conducted the behavioral, genetic, and epigenetic procedures and data analysis, and writing of the first draft of the manuscript. TC supervised the design and execution of the study and wrote and edited the manuscript. All authors read and approved the final manuscript.

Acknowledgements

This work was funded by NSF BCS-0843346 awarded to TC. We thank Anett Mueller-Alcazar and Yael Isler for TSST training, Anatoly Mikhailik and Indra Jayatilaka for technical assistance in the collection and processing of blood samples, and the entire Canli Lab for their help running the experimental sessions and data entry.

Author details

[1]Integrative Neuroscience, Department of Psychology, Stony Brook University, Stony Brook, NY 11794-2500, USA. [2]Department of Radiology, Stony Brook University, Stony Brook, NY 11794, USA. [3]Program in Neuroscience, Stony Brook University, Stony Brook, NY 11794, USA. [4]Program in Genetics, Stony Brook University, Stony Brook, NY 11794, USA. [5]Department of Psychology, Bogazici University, Bebek, 34342 Istanbul, Turkey. [6]Center for Life Sciences and Technologies, Bogazici University, Bebek, 34342 Istanbul, Turkey.

References

1. Herman J, Prewitt C, Cullinan W. Neuronal circuit regulation of the hypothalamo-pituitary-adrenocortical stress axis. Crit Rev Neurobiol. 1996;10:371–94.
2. Jørgensen H, Knigge U, Kjær A, Møller M, Warberg J. Serotonergic stimulation of corticotropin-releasing hormone and pro-opiomelanocortin gene expression. J Neuroendocrinol. 2002;14:788–95.
3. Heils A, Teufel A, Petri S, Stöber G, Riederer P, Bengel D, et al. Allelic variation of human serotonin transporter gene expression. J Neurochem. 1996;66:2621–4.
4. Lesch K, Bengel D, Heils A, Sabol S, Greenberg B, Petri S, et al. Association of anxiety-related traits with a polymorphism in the serotonin transporter gene regulatory region. Science. 1996;274:1527–31.
5. Wendland J, Martin B, Kruse M, Lesch K, Murphy D. Simultaneous genotyping of four functional loci of human SLC6A4, with a reappraisal of 5-HTTLPR and rs25531. Mol Psychiatry. 2006;11:224–6.
6. Caspi A, Sugden K, Moffitt T, Taylor A, Craig I, Harrington H, et al. Influence of life stress on depression: moderation by a polymorphism in the 5-HTT gene. Science. 2003;301:386–9.
7. Munafò MR, Durrant C, Lewis G, Flint J. Gene × environment interactions at the serotonin transporter locus. Biol Psychiatry. 2009;65:211–9.
8. Caspi A, Hariri AR, Holmes A, Uher R, Moffitt TE. Genetic sensitivity to the environment: the case of the serotonin transporter gene and its implications for studying complex diseases and traits. Am J Psychiatry. 2010;167:509–27.
9. Risch N, Herrell R, Lehner T, Liang KY, Eaves L, Hoh J, et al. Interaction between the serotonin transporter gene (5-HTTLPR), stressful life events, and risk of depression. JAMA. 2009;301:2462–71.
10. Karg K, Burmeister M, Shedden K, Sen S. The serotonin transporter promoter variant (5-HTTLPR), stress, and depression meta-analysis revisited: evidence of genetic moderation. Arch Gen Psychiatry. 2011;68:444–54.
11. Uher R, McGuffin P. The moderation by the serotonin transporter gene of environmental adversity in the etiology of depression: 2009 update. Mol Psychiatry. 2010;15:18–22.
12. Uher R, McGuffin P. The moderation by the serotonin transporter gene of environmental adversity in the aetiology of mental illness: review and methodological analysis. Mol Psychiatry. 2008;13:131–46.
13. Duncan LE, Keller MC. A critical review of the first 10 years of candidate gene-by-environment interaction research in psychiatry. Am J Psychiatr. 2011;168:1041–9.
14. Kinnally E, Tarara E, Mason W, Mendoza S, Abel K, Lyons L, et al. Serotonin transporter expression is predicted by early life stress and is associated with

disinhibited behavior in infant rhesus macaques. Genes Brain Behav. 2010;9:45–52.

15. Lee J-H, Kim HJ, Kim JG, Ryu V, Kim B-T, Kang D-W, et al. Depressive behaviors and decreased expression of serotonin reuptake transporter in rats that experienced neonatal maternal separation. Neurosci Res. 2007;58:32–9.
16. Wankerl M, Miller R, Kirschbaum C, Hennig J, Stalder T, Alexander N. Effects of genetic and early environmental risk factors for depression on serotonin transporter expression and methylation profiles. Transl Psychiatry. 2014;4:e402.
17. Own LS, Iqbal R, Patel PD. Maternal separation alters serotonergic and HPA axis gene expression independent of separation duration in c57bl/6 mice. Brain Res. 2013;1515:29–38.
18. Gardner KL, Hale MW, Lightman SL, Plotsky PM, Lowry CA. Adverse early life experience and social stress during adulthood interact to increase serotonin transporter mRNA expression. Brain Res. 2009;1305:47–63.
19. Hellstrom IC, Dhir SK, Diorio JC, Meaney MJ. Maternal licking regulates hippocampal glucocorticoid receptor transcription through a thyroid hormone–serotonin–NGFI-A signalling cascade. Philos Trans R Soc B. 2012;367:2495–510.
20. Ulrich-Lai YM, Herman JP. Neural regulation of endocrine and autonomic stress responses. Nat Rev Neurosci. 2009;10:397–409.
21. Belay H, Burton CL, Lovic V, Meaney MJ, Sokolowski M, Fleming AS. Early adversity and serotonin transporter genotype interact with hippocampal glucocorticoid receptor mRNA expression, corticosterone, and behavior in adult male rats. Behav Neurosci. 2011;125:150–60.
22. Kirschbaum C, Pirke K, Hellhammer D. The 'Trier Social Stress Test' - a tool for investigating psychobiological stress responses in a laboratory setting. Neuropsychobiology. 1993;28:76–81.
23. Alexander N, Kuepper Y, Schmitz A, Osinsky R, Kozyra E, Hennig J. Gene-environment interactions predict cortisol responses after acute stress: implications for the etiology of depression. Psychoneuroendocrinology. 2009;34:1294–303.
24. Mueller A, Armbruster D, Moser DA, Canli T, Lesch K-P, Brocke B, et al. Interaction of serotonin transporter gene-linked polymorphic region and stressful life events predicts cortisol stress response. Neuropsychopharmacology. 2011;36:1332–9.
25. Canli T, Qiu M, Omura K, Congdon E, Haas BW, Amin Z, et al. Neural correlates of epigenesis. Proc Natl Acad Sci U S A. 2006;103:16033–8.
26. Taylor SE, Way BM, Welch WT, Hilmert CJ, Lehman BJ, Eisenberger NI. Early family environment, current adversity, the serotonin transporter promoter polymorphism, and depressive symptomatology. Biol Psychiatry. 2006;60:671–6.
27. Bagot R, Meaney M. Epigenetics and the biological basis of gene x environment interactions. J Am Acad Child Adolesc Psychiatry. 2010;49:752–71.
28. Weaver I, Cervoni N, Champagne F, D'Alessio A, Sharma S, Seckl J, et al. Epigenetic programming by maternal behavior. Nat Neurosci. 2004;7:847–54.
29. Szyf M, Weaver I, Meaney M. Maternal care, the epigenome and phenotypic differences in behavior. Reprod Toxicol. 2007;24:9–19.
30. McGowan P, Sasaki A, D'Alessio A, Dymov S, Labonté B, Szyf M, et al. Epigenetic regulation of the glucocorticoid receptor in human brain associates with childhood abuse. Nat Neurosci. 2009;12:342–8.
31. Oberlander TF, Weinberg J, Papsdorf M, Grunau R, Misri S, Devlin AM. Prenatal exposure to maternal depression, neonatal methylation of human glucocorticoid receptor gene (NR3C1) and infant cortisol stress responses. Epigenetics. 2008;3:97–106.
32. Tyrka AR, Price LH, Marsit C, Walters OC, Carpenter LL. Childhood adversity and epigenetic modulation of the leukocyte glucocorticoid receptor: preliminary findings in healthy adults. PLoS One. 2012;7:e30148.
33. Philibert R, Madan A, Andersen A, Cadoret R, Packer H, Sandhu H. Serotonin transporter mRNA levels are associated with the methylation of an upstream CpG island. Am J Med Genet B Neuropsychiatr Genet. 2007;144:101–5.
34. Beach SRH, Brody GH, Todorov AA, Gunter TD, Philibert RA. Methylation at 5HTT mediates the impact of child sex abuse on women's antisocial behavior: an examination of the Iowa adoptee sample. Psychosom Med. 2011;73:83–7.
35. Devlin AM, Brain U, Austin J, Oberlander TF, Feil R. Prenatal exposure to maternal depressed mood and the MTHFR C677T variant affect SLC6A4 methylation in infants at birth. PLoS One. 2010;5:12201.
36. Kang H-J, Kim J-M, Stewart R, Kim S-Y, Bae K-Y, Kim S-W, et al. Association of SLC6A4 methylation with early adversity, characteristics and outcomes in depression. Prog Neuro-Psychopharmacol Biol Psychiatry. 2013;44:23–8.
37. Kinnally EL, Capitanio JP, Leibel R, Deng L, LeDuc C, Haghighi F, et al. Epigenetic regulation of serotonin transporter expression and behavior in infant rhesus macaques. Genes Brain Behav. 2010;9:575–82.
38. Ouellet-Morin I, Wong C, Danese A, Pariante C, Papadopoulos A, Mill J, et al. Increased serotonin transporter gene (SERT) DNA methylation is associated with bullying victimization and blunted cortisol response to stress in childhood: a longitudinal study of discordant monozygotic twins. Psychol Med. 2012;43(9):1–11.
39. Kinnally EL, Feinberg C, Kim D, Ferguson K, Leibel R, Coplan JD, et al. DNA methylation as a risk factor in the effects of early life stress. Brain Behav Immun. 2011;25:1548–53.
40. Philibert RA, Sandhu H, Hollenbeck N, Gunter T, Adams W, Madan A. The relationship of 5HTT (SLC6A4) methylation and genotype on mRNA expression and liability to major depression and alcohol dependence in subjects from the Iowa Adoption Studies. Am J Med Genet B Neuropsychiatr Genet. 2008;147:543–9.
41. Olsson C, Foley D, Parkinson-Bates M, Byrnes G, McKenzie M, Patton G, et al. Prospects for epigenetic research within cohort studies of psychological disorder: a pilot investigation of a peripheral cell marker of epigenetic risk for depression. Biol Psychol. 2010;83:159–65.
42. Wang D, Szyf M, Benkelfat C, Provençal N, Turecki G, Caramaschi D, et al. Peripheral SLC6A4 DNA methylation is associated with in vivo measures of human brain serotonin synthesis and childhood physical aggression. PLoS One. 2012;7:e39501.
43. van IJzendoorn MH, Caspers K, Bakermans-Kranenburg MJ, Beach SR, Philibert R. Methylation matters: interaction between methylation density and serotonin transporter genotype predicts unresolved loss or trauma. Biol Psychiatry. 2010;68:405–7.
44. Alexander N, Wankerl M, Hennig J, Miller R, Zänkert S, Steudte-Schmiedgen S, et al. DNA methylation profiles within the serotonin transporter gene moderate the association of 5-HTTLPR and cortisol stress reactivity. Translational Psychiatry. 2014;4:e443.
45. Zhao J, Goldberg J, Bremner JD, Vaccarino V. Association between promoter methylation of serotonin transporter gene and depressive symptoms: a monozygotic twin study. Psychosom Med. 2013;75:523–9.
46. Domschke K, Tidow N, Schwarte K, Deckert J, Lesch K-P, Arolt V, et al. Serotonin transporter gene hypomethylation predicts impaired antidepressant treatment response. Int J Neuropsychopharmacol. 2014;17(8):1167–76.
47. Bernstein DP, Fink L, Handelsman L, Foote J, Lovejoy M, Wenzel K, et al. Initial reliability and validity of a new retrospective measure of child abuse and neglect. Am J Psychiatr. 1994;151:1132–6.
48. Schulz P, Schlotz W. The Trier Inventory for the Assessment of Chronic Stress (TICS): scale construction, statistical testing, and validation of the scale work overload. Diagnostica. 1999;45:8–19.
49. Schulz P, Schlotz W, Becker P. Trierer Inventar zum Chronischen Stress (TICS) [Trier Inventory for Chronic Stress (TICS)]. Gottingen: Hogrefe; 2004.
50. Beck AT, Steer RA, Brown GK. Beck Depression Inventory BDI-II Manual. 2nd ed. Orlando, FL: Psychological Corporation; 1996.
51. Pruessner JC, Kirschbaum C, Meinlschmid G, Hellhammer DH. Two formulas for computation of the area under the curve represent measures of total hormone concentration versus time-dependent change. Psychoneuroendocrinology. 2003;28:916–31.
52. Hu X, Oroszi G, Chun J, Smith TL, Goldman D, Schuckit MA. An expanded evaluation of the relationship of four alleles to the level of response to alcohol and the alcoholism risk. Alcohol Clin Exp Res. 2005;29:8–16.
53. Livak KJ, Schmittgen TD. Analysis of relative gene expression data using real-time quantitative PCR and the 2-[Delta][Delta] CT method. Methods. 2001;25:402–8.
54. Kim J, Kim JY, Issa JPJ. Aging and DNA methylation. Curr Chem Biol. 2009;3:1–9.
55. Richardson B. Impact of aging on DNA methylation. Ageing Res Rev. 2003;2:245–61.
56. Glatz K, Mössner R, Heils A, Lesch K. Glucocorticoid regulated human serotonin transporter (5 HTT) expression is modulated by the 5 HTT gene promotor linked polymorphic region. J Neurochem. 2003;86:1072–8.
57. Messeguer X, Escudero R, Farré D, Núñez O, Martínez J, Albà MM. PROMO: detection of known transcription regulatory elements using species-tailored searches. Bioinformatics. 2002;18:333–4.

58. Vasiliou SA, Ali FR, Haddley K, Cardoso MC, Bubb VJ, Quinn JP. The SLC6A4 VNTR genotype determines transcription factor binding and epigenetic variation of this gene in response to cocaine in vitro. Addict Biol. 2012;17:156–70.
59. Kinnally E, Lyons L, Abel K, Mendoza S, Capitanio J. Effects of early experience and genotype on serotonin transporter regulation in infant rhesus macaques. Genes Brain Behav. 2008;7:481–6.
60. Alasaari JS, Lagus M, Ollila HM, Toivola A, Kivimäki M, Vahtera J, et al. Environmental stress affects DNA methylation of a CpG rich promoter region of serotonin transporter gene in a nurse cohort. PLoS One. 2012;7:e45813.
61. Sugawara H, Bundo M, Ishigooka J, Iwamoto K, Kato T. Epigenetic regulation of serotonin transporter in psychiatric disorders. J Genet Genomics. 2013;40:325–9.
62. Nestler EJ, Barrot M, DiLeone RJ, Eisch AJ, Gold SJ, Monteggia LM. Neurobiology of depression. Neuron. 2002;34:13–25.
63. Nater U, Whistler T, Lonergan W, Mletzko T, Vernon S, Heim C. Impact of acute psychosocial stress on peripheral blood gene expression pathways in healthy men. Biol Psychol. 2009;82:125–32.
64. Morita K, Saito T, Ohta M, Ohmori T, Kawai K, Teshima-Kondo S, et al. Expression analysis of psychological stress-associated genes in peripheral blood leukocytes. Neurosci Lett. 2005;381:57–62.
65. Meaney MJ. Epigenetics and the biological definition of gene × environment interactions. Child Dev. 2010;81:41–79.
66. Byun H-M, Siegmund KD, Pan F, Weisenberger DJ, Kanel G, Laird PW, et al. Epigenetic profiling of somatic tissues from human autopsy specimens identifies tissue-and individual-specific DNA methylation patterns. Hum Mol Genet. 2009;18:4808–17.
67. Davies MN, Volta M, Pidsley R, Lunnon K, Dixit A, Lovestone S, et al. Functional annotation of the human brain methylome identifies tissue-specific epigenetic variation across brain and blood. Genome Biol. 2012;13:R43.
68. Provençal N, Suderman MJ, Guillemin C, Massart R, Ruggiero A, Wang D, et al. The signature of maternal rearing in the methylome in rhesus macaque prefrontal cortex and T cells. J Neurosci. 2012;32:15626–42.
69. Ursini G, Bollati V, Fazio L, Porcelli A, Iacovelli L, Catalani A, et al. Stress-related methylation of the catechol-O-methyltransferase Val 158 allele predicts human prefrontal cognition and activity. J Neurosci. 2011;31:6692–8.
70. Kudielka B, Buske-Kirschbaum A, Hellhammer D, Kirschbaum C. HPA axis responses to laboratory psychosocial stress in healthy elderly adults, younger adults, and children: impact of age and gender. Psychoneuroendocrinology. 2004;29:83–98.
71. Carpenter LL, Tyrka AR, Ross NS, Khoury L, Anderson GM, Price LH. Effect of childhood emotional abuse and age on cortisol responsivity in adulthood. Biol Psychiatry. 2009;66:69–75.
72. DeSantis SM, Baker NL, Back SE, Spratt E, Ciolino JD, Maria MS, et al. Gender differences in the effect of early life trauma on hypothalamic-pituitary-adrenal axis functioning. Depress Anxiety. 2011;28:383–92.
73. Het S, Rohleder N, Schoofs D, Kirschbaum C, Wolf O. Neuroendocrine and psychometric evaluation of a placebo version of the 'Trier Social Stress Test'. Psychoneuroendocrinology. 2009;34:1075–86.
74. Jasinska AJ, Lowry CA, Burmeister M. Serotonin transporter gene, stress and raphe-raphe interactions: a molecular mechanism of depression. Trends Neurosci. 2012;35:395–402.
75. Kaufman J, Yang B, Douglas-Palumberi H, Grasso D, Lipschitz D, Houshyar S, et al. Brain-derived neurotrophic factor-5-HTTLPR gene interactions and environmental modifiers of depression in children. Biol Psychiatry. 2006;59:673–80.
76. Comasco E, Åslund C, Oreland L, Nilsson KW. Three-way interaction effect of 5-HTTLPR, BDNF Val66Met, and childhood adversity on depression: a replication study. Eur Neuropsychopharmacol. 2013;23:1300–6.
77. Dougherty L, Klein D, Congdon E, Canli T, Hayden E. Interaction between 5-HTTLPR and BDNF Val66Met polymorphisms on HPA axis reactivity in preschoolers. Biol Psychol. 2010;83:93–100.
78. Uher R. Gene-environment interactions in common mental disorders: an update and strategy for a genome-wide search. Soc Psychiatry Psychiatr Epidemiol. 2014;49:3–14.
79. Roth TL, Lubin FD, Funk AJ, Sweatt JD. Lasting epigenetic influence of early-life adversity on the BDNF gene. Biol Psychiatry. 2009;65:760–9.

Permissions

All chapters in this book were first published in BMAD, by BioMed Central; hereby published with permission under the Creative Commons Attribution License or equivalent. Every chapter published in this book has been scrutinized by our experts. Their significance has been extensively debated. The topics covered herein carry significant findings which will fuel the growth of the discipline. They may even be implemented as practical applications or may be referred to as a beginning point for another development.

The contributors of this book come from diverse backgrounds, making this book a truly international effort. This book will bring forth new frontiers with its revolutionizing research information and detailed analysis of the nascent developments around the world.

We would like to thank all the contributing authors for lending their expertise to make the book truly unique. They have played a crucial role in the development of this book. Without their invaluable contributions this book wouldn't have been possible. They have made vital efforts to compile up to date information on the varied aspects of this subject to make this book a valuable addition to the collection of many professionals and students.

This book was conceptualized with the vision of imparting up-to-date information and advanced data in this field. To ensure the same, a matchless editorial board was set up. Every individual on the board went through rigorous rounds of assessment to prove their worth. After which they invested a large part of their time researching and compiling the most relevant data for our readers.

The editorial board has been involved in producing this book since its inception. They have spent rigorous hours researching and exploring the diverse topics which have resulted in the successful publishing of this book. They have passed on their knowledge of decades through this book. To expedite this challenging task, the publisher supported the team at every step. A small team of assistant editors was also appointed to further simplify the editing procedure and attain best results for the readers.

Apart from the editorial board, the designing team has also invested a significant amount of their time in understanding the subject and creating the most relevant covers. They scrutinized every image to scout for the most suitable representation of the subject and create an appropriate cover for the book.

The publishing team has been an ardent support to the editorial, designing and production team. Their endless efforts to recruit the best for this project, has resulted in the accomplishment of this book. They are a veteran in the field of academics and their pool of knowledge is as vast as their experience in printing. Their expertise and guidance has proved useful at every step. Their uncompromising quality standards have made this book an exceptional effort. Their encouragement from time to time has been an inspiration for everyone.

The publisher and the editorial board hope that this book will prove to be a valuable piece of knowledge for researchers, students, practitioners and scholars across the globe.

List of Contributors

Patti Waters and Cheryl M McCormick
Department of Psychology and Centre for Neuroscience, Brock University, St Catharines, Ontario, Canada

Sophie A George, Stephanie A Stout and Melissa Tan
Department of Psychiatry, University of Michigan, 4250 Plymouth Road, Ann Arbor, MI 48109, USA

Dayan Knox
Department of Psychiatry, University of Michigan, 4250 Plymouth Road, AnnArbor, MI 48109, USA
Present address: Department of Psychology, University of Delaware, 108 Wolf Hall, Newark, DE 19716, USA

Israel Liberzon
Department of Psychiatry, University of Michigan, 4250 Plymouth Road, Ann Arbor, MI 48109, USA
Ann Arbor Veterans Affairs Hospital, 2215 Fuller Road, Ann Arbor, MI 49105, USA

Scott P Orr, Natasha B Lasko and Michael L Macklin
Department of Psychiatry, Massachusetts General Hospital and Harvard Medical School, Charlestown, MA, USA
Department of Veterans Affairs Medical Center, Manchester, NH, USA

Suzanne L Pineles
National Center for PTSD, Women's Health Sciences Division, VA Boston Healthcare System, Boston, MA, USA
Department of Psychiatry, Boston University School of Medicine, Boston, MA, USA

Yuchiao Chang
General Medicine Division, Massachusetts General Hospital and Harvard Medical School, Boston, MA, USA

Roger K Pitman
Department of Psychiatry, Massachusetts General Hospital and Harvard Medical School, Charlestown, MA, USA

Cristina Cusin and Darin D Dougherty
Division of Neurotherapeutics, Department of Psychiatry, Massachusetts General Hospital, 149 13th Street, Rm 2612, Charlestown, MA 02129, USA

Michal Ziv, Philippe R Goldin, Hooria Jazaieri, Kevin S Hahn and James J Gross
Department of Psychology, Stanford University, Jordan Hall, Bldg. 420, Stanford, CA, USA

Catherine Belzung
U930, UFR Sciences et Techniques, Parc Grandmont, Rue Monge, Tours, 37200, France

Maël Lemoine
Université François-Rabelais, UFR Médecine, 10 Bd Tonnellé, Tours Cedex, 37032, France

Orna Issler, Adi Neufeld-Cohen, Yael Kuperman and Alon Chen
Department of Neurobiology, Weizmann Institute of Science, Rehovot 76100, Israel

Roderick N Carter, Jonathan R Seckl, and Pauline M Jamieson
Centre for Cardiovascular Science, Queens Medical Research Institute, 47 Little France Crescent, Edinburgh EH16 4TJ, UK

Evan D Paul and Christopher A Lowry
Department of Integrative Physiology and Center for Neuroscience, University of Colorado Boulder, Boulder, CO 80309, USA

Paul AT Kelly and Henry J Olverman
Centre for Cognitive and Neural Systems, University of Edinburgh, 1 George Square, Edinburgh EH8 9JZ, UK

Timothy Hall
Discipline of Psychiatry, School of Medicine, University of Adelaide, Adelaide, Australia

Cherrie Galletly
Discipline of Psychiatry, School of Medicine, University of Adelaide, Adelaide, Australia
Ramsay Health Care (SA) Mental Health Services, Adelaide, South Australia
Northern Mental Health, Adelaide Metro Mental Health Directorate, Adelaide, South Australia

C Richard Clark
Cognitive Neuroscience Laboratory and School of Psychology, Flinders University of South Australia, Adelaide, Australia

Melinda Veltmeyer
Veterans Affairs Medical Centre Research Service, Manchester, New Hampshire, England
Harvard Medical School, Boston, USA

Mark W Gilbertson
Veterans Affairs Medical Centre Research Service, Manchester, New Hampshire, England

Scott P Orr and Roger K Pitman
Massachusetts General Hospital and Harvard Medical School, Boston, USA

lexander McFarlane
The Centre of Military and Veterans' Health, Adelaide, Australia

Christopher C Conway
Department of Psychology, University of California, Los Angeles, Box 951563, Los Angeles, CA 90095-1563, USA

George M Slavich
Department of Psychology, Cousins Center for Psychoneuroimmunology, University of California, Los Angeles CA, USA
Department of Psychiatry and Biobehavioral Sciences, University of Los Angeles, CA, USA

Constance Hammen
Department of Psychology, University of California, Los Angeles, Box 951563, Los Angeles, CA 90095-1563, USA
Department of Psychiatry and Biobehavioral Sciences, University of California Los Angeles, CA, USA

Jennifer Y F Lau and Kevin Hilbert
Department of Experimental Psychology, University of Oxford, South Parks Road, Oxford OX1 3UD, UK

Robert Goodman And Thalia C Eley
Institute of Psychiatry, King's College London, London, UK

Alice M Gregory
Psychology Department, Goldsmiths, London, UK

Daniel S Pine
Mood and Anxiety Program, National Institute of Mental Health, Bethesda, USA

Essi M Viding
Department of Psychology, University College London, London, UK

Alan N Simmons, Dewleen G Baker, Heather K Donovan and Martin P Paulus
Veterans Affairs San Diego Healthcare System, 3350 La Jolla Village Drive, San Diego, CA 92161, USA
University of California San Diego, 9500 Gilman Drive, La Jolla, CA 92093, USA
Center of Excellence in Stress and Mental Health, VASDHS, 3350 La Jolla Village Drive, San Diego, CA 92161, USA

Scott C Matthews and Arame Motezadi
Veterans Affairs San Diego Healthcare System, 3350 La Jolla Village Drive, San Diego, CA 92161, USA University of California San Diego, 9500 Gilman Drive, La Jolla, CA 92093, USA
Center of Excellence in Stress and Mental Health, VASDHS, 3350 La Jolla Village Drive, San Diego, CA 92161, USA

Research Service & VA Mental Illness Research, Education and Clinical Center, VASDHS, 3350 La Jolla Village Drive, San Diego, CA 92161, USA

Irina A Strigo
University of California San Diego, 9500 Gilman Drive, La Jolla, CA 92093, USA
Center of Excellence in Stress and Mental Health, VASDHS, 3350 La Jolla Village Drive, San Diego, CA 92161, USA

Murray B Stein
Veterans Affairs San Diego Healthcare System, 3350 La Jolla Village Drive, San Diego, CA 92161, USA
University of California San Diego, 9500 Gilman Drive, La Jolla, CA 92093, USA

Matthew D Sacchet and Ian H Gotlib
Neurosciences Program, Stanford University, Stanford, CA, USA
Department of Psychology, Stanford University, Jordan Hall, Building 01-420, 450 Serra Mall, Stanford, CA 94305, USA

Gautam Prasad
Department of Psychology, Stanford University, Jordan Hall, Building 01-420, 450 Serra Mall, Stanford, CA 94305, USA
Imaging Genetics Center, Institute for Neuroimaging and Informatics, Keck School of Medicine of USC, Los Angeles, CA, USA

Lara C Foland-Ross
Department of Psychology, Stanford University, Jordan Hall, Building 01-420, 450 Serra Mall, Stanford, CA 94305, USA

Shantanu H Joshi
Ahmanson-Lovelace Brain Mapping Center, Department of Neurology, UCLA, Los Angeles, CA, USA

J Paul Hamilton
Laureate Institute for Brain Research, Tulsa, OK, USA

Paul M Thompson
Imaging Genetics Center, Institute for Neuroimaging and Informatics, Keck School of Medicine of USC, Los Angeles, CA, USA

Shani Ofrat and Robert F Krueger
University of Minnesota, 75 East River Road, Minneapolis, MN, USA

Daniella J Furman, J Paul Hamilton and Ian H Gotlib
Department of Psychology, Stanford University, 450 Serra Mall, Stanford, CA 94305-2004, USA

Kathryn MacPherson, Marguerite Camp, Ozge Gunduz-Cinar and Andrew Holmes
Laboratory of Behavioral and Genomic Neuroscience, National Institute on Alcohol Abuse and Alcoholism, NIH, Bethesda, MD, USA

Nigel Whittle and Nicolas Singewald
Department of Pharmacology & Toxicology, Institute of Pharmacy and CMBI, University of Innsbruck, Innsbruck, Austria

Sharmin Ghaznavi and Thilo Deckersbach
Massachusetts General Hospital, Boston, MA, USA

M Justin Kim, Todd F Heatherton and Paul J Whalen
Department of Psychological and Brain Sciences, Dartmouth College, 6207 Moore Hall, Hanover, NH 03755, USA

Maital Neta
Department of Psychology, B84 East Stadium, University of Nebraska-Lincoln, Lincoln, NE 68588-0156, USA

F Caroline Davis
US Army Natick Soldier Research Development and Engineering Center, Cognitive Science Research Team, 10 Kansas St., Natick, MA 01760, USA
Department of Psychology, Tufts University, 490 Boston Avenue, Medford, MA 02155, USA

Erika J Ruberry
Department of Psychology, University of Washington, 119A Guthrie Hall, Seattle, WA 98195, USA

Diana Dinescu
Department of Psychology, University of Virginia, 102 Gilmer Hall, Charlottesville, VA 22904, USA

Mitchell A Stotland
Department of Surgery (Plastic) and Pediatrics, Geisel School of Medicine at Dartmouth, Dartmouth-Hitchcock Medical Center, Lebanon, NH 03756, USA
Department of Surgery (Plastic and Craniofacial), Sidra Research and Medical Center, Doha, Qatar

Elif A Duman
Integrative Neuroscience, Department of Psychology, Stony Brook University, Stony Brook, NY 11794-2500, USA
Department of Psychology, Bogazici University, Bebek, 34342 Istanbul, Turkey
Center for Life Sciences and Technologies, Bogazici University, Bebek, 34342 Istanbul, Turkey

Turhan Canli
Integrative Neuroscience, Department of Psychology, Stony Brook University, Stony Brook, NY 11794 2500, USA
Department of Radiology, Stony Brook University, Stony Brook, NY 11794, USA
Program in Neuroscience, Stony Brook University, Stony Brook, NY 11794, USA
Program in Genetics, Stony Brook University, Stony Brook, NY 11794, USA

Index

www.ingramcontent.com/pod-product-compliance
Lightning Source LLC
LaVergne TN
LVHW080604210926
848485LV00003B/102

* 9 7 8 1 6 3 2 4 1 4 5 8 8 *